Acupuncture Techniques

Tianjun Wang · Weixiang Wang
Editors

Acupuncture Techniques

A Practical Manual

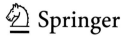
Springer

Editors
Tianjun Wang
London Academy of Chinese Acupuncture
London, UK

Weixiang Wang
Dutch Acupuncture Academy
Amsterdam, The Netherlands

ISBN 978-3-031-59271-3   ISBN 978-3-031-59272-0 (eBook)
https://doi.org/10.1007/978-3-031-59272-0

© The Editor(s) (if applicable) and The Author(s), under exclusive license to Springer Nature Switzerland AG 2024

This work is subject to copyright. All rights are solely and exclusively licensed by the Publisher, whether the whole or part of the material is concerned, specifically the rights of translation, reprinting, reuse of illustrations, recitation, broadcasting, reproduction on microfilms or in any other physical way, and transmission or information storage and retrieval, electronic adaptation, computer software, or by similar or dissimilar methodology now known or hereafter developed.
The use of general descriptive names, registered names, trademarks, service marks, etc. in this publication does not imply, even in the absence of a specific statement, that such names are exempt from the relevant protective laws and regulations and therefore free for general use.
The publisher, the authors and the editors are safe to assume that the advice and information in this book are believed to be true and accurate at the date of publication. Neither the publisher nor the authors or the editors give a warranty, expressed or implied, with respect to the material contained herein or for any errors or omissions that may have been made. The publisher remains neutral with regard to jurisdictional claims in published maps and institutional affiliations.

This Springer imprint is published by the registered company Springer Nature Switzerland AG
The registered company address is: Gewerbestrasse 11, 6330 Cham, Switzerland

If disposing of this product, please recycle the paper.

Foreword by Prof. Dr. Shuhuai He

Acupuncture, encompassing needling and moxibustion as its key elements, is a vital component of traditional Chinese medicine. These techniques represent the various methods of acupuncture practices, crucial for clinical application and understanding their principles of action. Mastering these skills, principles, and their clinical applications is essential for an acupuncturist, significantly enhancing the efficacy of acupuncture treatments.

The history of acupuncture is rich, with needling originating from Bian stone acupuncture and moxibustion from fire cauterization. During the Jin, Yuan, and Ming dynasties, acupuncture flourished, and notable contributions include Dou Hanqing's "Fourteen-Character Technique," as well as the "Eight Methods of Treating Diseases" and "Four Methods of Moving Qi" from the Ming Dynasty's "Jin Zhen Fu." Yang Jizhou's "Zhen Jiu Da Cheng" systematically summarized previous methods, combined with personal experiences, introducing techniques like the "Twelve-Character Sequential Method" and "Eight Methods of Manipulation," innovating various acupuncture skills. Subsequent generations continued to refine these techniques based on clinical experiences, forming a comprehensive system of acupuncture and moxibustion.

Acupuncture treatments are characterized by "pattern differentiation," where pattern differentiation involves determining the cause, location, and nature of the disease. Treatment principles include selecting appropriate meridians, acupoints, and specific needling and moxibustion techniques.

The principle of acupuncture is to regulate Yin and Yang, nourish the deficient, and reduce the excess, as stated in "Ling Shu·Gen Jie": "The essence of using needles is to balance Yin and Yang." By stimulating meridians and acupoints with various techniques, acupuncture adjusts the body's functional states, shape, Qi, and spirit, as expressed in "Ling Shu·Jiu Zhen Shi Er Yuan": "Effective results are like the wind blowing the clouds, as clear as seeing the sky, thus concluding the way of needling." From "Su Wen·Bao Ming Quan Xing Lun": "The essence of needling is first to treat the spirit." "Ling Shu·Guan Zhen": "In using needles, remember their spirit." Mastery of these techniques is crucial for achieving the therapeutic effects of balancing Yin and Yang, nourishing the deficient, and reducing excess.

Skill in acupuncture is critical to its effectiveness. Different tools, needle insertion depths, techniques, stimulation intensities, directions of needling, and sensations during needling produce varying effects and outcomes. Familiarity with the indications for various tools and mastery of techniques are vital. Only through skilled practice can acupuncture effectively regulate Yin and Yang, nourish the deficient, and reduce excess.

The diversity of acupuncture tools and techniques, along with varied perspectives and schools of thought, has led to some confusion and impacted its widespread application. Therefore, a systematic introduction of these techniques and indications is essential for clinicians to select and master appropriate acupuncture methods, enhancing treatment efficacy. In light of this, Prof. Dr. Tianjun Wang and Prof. Dr. Weixiang Wang invited 17 renowned experts from China and the West to comprehensively introduce ancient and modern needling and moxibustion techniques, their scope, and precautions in the book *Acupuncture Techniques*. The publication of this book is set to improve the effectiveness of acupuncture further and promote its development and proliferation.

Former Dean of the Acupuncture and Tuina School of Beijing University of Chinese Medicine, Former Director of the Acupoint Research Society of the China Acupuncture Association, Former Dean of the Villa Jiada College of Chinese Medicine in Italy, Honorary Chairman of the World Floating Needle Acupuncture Society, and Honorary Dean of the Qi Huang College of Traditional Chinese Medicine in Italy.

Rome, Italy　　　　　　　　　　　　　　　　　　　　　　　Prof. Dr. Shuhuai He
October 2023

针灸技法大全

序

针灸是中医学的重要组成部分，针法和灸法是针灸学的重要内容.针法和灸法是指各种针灸技术的操作方法，是临床应用及作用原理的重要内容.熟练地掌握其操作技能、操作原理、临床应用对一个针灸师是非常重要的，是提高针灸治疗效果的重要手段.

针灸学历史悠久，针法始于砭刺，灸法始于火灼，书载始见于《内经》、《难经》，并奠定了刺灸手法的基础，在金元明时期得到昌盛发展，有金元窦汉卿的十四字手法、明代《金针赋》的"治病八法"和"飞经走气"四法、杨继洲的《针灸大成》，系统地总结了前人的刺灸方法，并结合自家的经验，提出了"十二字分次第手法"和"下手八法"，创造了多种刺灸的方法和技能.之后历代医家结合自己的临床经验对刺灸的技能不断补充完善，形成了一套较完善的刺灸法体系.

针灸治疗的特点是"辨证论治"，辩证是确定疾病的病因、病位和病证的性质.论治是指治疗时确定治疗的原则、治疗的经络、治疗的腧穴、刺法和灸法的具体操作.

针灸治疗的原则是调节阴阳，补虚泻实，《灵枢·根结》篇曰："用针之要，在于调阴与阳."针灸治病时采用各种刺灸方法刺激经络腧穴，发挥其调整机体的功能状态，调形、调气、调神.正如《灵枢·九针十二原》所说："气至而有效，效至信，若风之吹云，明乎若见苍天，刺之道毕矣."《素问·宝命全形论》："凡刺之真，必先治神."《灵枢·官针》篇："用针之要，勿忘其神."只有如此才能达到调节阴阳、补虚泻实的治疗作用，所以刺灸手法的技能是针灸治病的重要手段.

刺灸的技能是发挥针灸作用的关键内容，针灸时采用针具不同、针刺的深浅不同、针刺的手法不同、刺激的强度不同、针刺的方向不同，针刺时的针感不同，所产生的作用不同，效果不同，所以熟悉掌握各种针具的适应症，各种手法的操作技能是非常重要的.只有熟练地掌握刺灸的技能，才能较好地实现针灸调阴阳、补虚泻实的功能.

针刺的针具很多，手法操作各异，医家见解不一，流派众多，致使学者莫衷一是，影响了针灸的推广应用.因此非常需要系统地介绍各种手法的操作技能、适应症，以便使临床工作者选择适合自己适用的针灸法，准确掌握其技能，提高治疗效果. 鉴于此, 王维祥、王天俊二位教授邀请国内外和西方17位刺灸法大家, 结合科研成果和自己的经验全面介绍古今针刺和灸法的操作技能、适应范围, 注意事项, 汇集成书, 名为《针灸技法大全》. 本书的出版定能进一步提高针灸疗效, 促进针灸的推广和发展.

何树槐

何树槐
原北京中医药大学针灸推拿学院院长
原中国针灸学会腧穴研究会主任
原意大利Villa jiada中医学院院长
世界针灸浮刺学会荣誉主席
意大利岐黄中医学院荣誉院长
2023年10月于意大利罗马

Foreword by Dr. Yair Maimon

In the realm of acupuncture, where ancient wisdom meets modern science, Prof. Weixiang Wang and Tianjun Wang have crafted a well-written book that delves into the rich tapestry of both time-honored and contemporary acupuncture techniques. This book explores different techniques that are part of the vast landscape of acupuncture practices.

In our rapidly advancing world, the fusion of ancient healing arts with modern science is providing new insights into acupuncture techniques. Acupuncture, deeply rooted in profound logic that has withstood the test of centuries, now encounters the investigation of modern scientific exploration. As we navigate these junctures of tradition and progress, we find ourselves uniquely positioned to appreciate the depth of ancient medicine through the lens of a modern approach.

The synthesis presented in this book serves as a bridge connecting three crucial pillars of Chinese medicine: first, ancient knowledge, a repository of wisdom passed down through generations; second, invaluable clinical experience shared through the mentorship of seasoned practitioners, at conferences, and in personal teachings; and third, rigorous research that provides the objective evidence necessary for assessing the effectiveness of various techniques. This book integrates these pillars, offering clinicians a coherent and thoughtful exploration that expands their clinical perspectives.

The inclusion of a wealth of clinical examples, well-referenced, ranges from micro-acupuncture systems, which draw parallels between the human microcosm and the macrocosm of the universe, to a nuanced understanding of how each area of the body reflects the entirety of our being. The clarity with which these systems are presented opens new avenues for clinicians, enhancing their repertoire of treatment options for a myriad of conditions. It is noteworthy to encounter a book that clearly summarizes a variety of approaches, seamlessly weaving together both ancient and modern techniques.

Congratulations to Prof. Weixiang Wang and Prof. Tianjun Wang for their commendable effort. My sincere wish is that readers, through the pages of this book, expand their knowledge and embrace novel healing techniques which were not known to them before. May this newfound wisdom translate into enhanced health and healing for their patients.

With the utmost respect and best wishes to the readers, I express my gratitude to Prof. Weixiang Wang and Prof. Tianjun Wang for their valuable contribution to the field.

Dr. Yair Maimon
President of the ETCMA
The European TCM Association

Acknowledgments

The realization of this book has been made possible through the unwavering support of our families, colleagues, friends, students, and patients.

Bringing together eighteen authors from diverse countries, each with distinct educational backgrounds, practice styles, native languages, and residing in different time zones, to collaborate closely on such an extensive team and project initially appeared to be a daunting challenge. Nevertheless, we transformed the seemingly impossible into reality, and we extend our sincere gratitude to our dedicated team for their creative and exceptional contributions.

Our heartfelt appreciation goes to Prof. Shuhuai He, former Dean of the Acupuncture and Tuina School at Beijing University of Chinese Medicine, and Dr. Yair Maimon, President of the European TCM Association, for their generous and highly commendatory forewords. Their insightful words not only add depth and breadth to the book but also serve as a source of great encouragement for acupuncturists worldwide.

We would also like to express our gratitude to the lecturers and students from the London Academy of Chinese Acupuncture (LACA), Dutch Acupuncture Academy (DAA), and the Second Teaching Hospital of Nanjing University of Chinese Medicine for their steadfast support and empowerment throughout this journey.

Finally, our deepest thanks go to Prof. Dr. Benlin You, one of the most esteemed alumni of Nanjing University of Chinese Medicine, a distinguished Chinese calligrapher, and a practitioner of Chinese Medicine, who graciously contributed his art for the book's Chinese title all the way from Australia.

Contents

Introduction

Introduction to Acupuncture Techniques 3
Tianjun Wang

Techniques of Filiform Needling

Prior to Needling 19
Weixiang Wang

Basic Needling 35
Weixiang Wang

Prevention and Management of Possible Accidents in Acupuncture Practice 59
Lin Chen

Classical Needling: Huang Di Nei Jing and Nanjing 69
Linjun Xia and Yun Ding

Jinzhenfu Needling Methods and Needling Technique on Reinforcement and Reduction 85
Linjun Xia and Yun Ding

The Simple Burn-Penetrate Method in Acupuncture 99
Ying Wang

Dao-Qi Needling Technique 111
Zunli Guo

Moxibustion and Cupping

Moxibustion 125
Phoebus Tian

xiii

Cupping Therapy 143
Lin Chen

Micro Acupuncture Systems

Scalp Acupuncture 167
Tianjun Wang and Katherine Dandridge

Auricular Acupuncture 185
Jun She

Cheek Acupuncture 205
Yongzhou Wang and Yongzheng Wu

Wrist-Ankle Acupuncture 219
Yu Sun and Katherine Dandridge

Acupuncture Techniques with Special Needles

Yuan Li Needling 239
Songyan Chen

Fire Needling 255
Defeng Wang and Shunchang Wang

Three-Edged Needle, Plum-Blossom Needle and Gua Sha 273
Bo Sheng

Electric Acupuncture and Laser Acupuncture

Electroacupuncture 291
Zunli Guo

Laser Acupuncture 305
Rongxian Zhang

Summary

Summary and Combination 323
Weixiang Wang and Tianjun Wang

Editors and Contributors

About the Editors

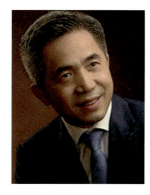

Prof. Dr. Tianjun Wang (王天俊) (*Chief Editor*) graduated from Nanjing University of Chinese Medicine (NUCM) in 1989. He completed his Ph.D. of Acupuncture at NUCM. Tianjun moved to the UK and joined the University of East London UK as Senior Lecturer and Director of Acupuncture Clinic 2007–2014. He is Guest Professor of NUCM.

Currently Prof. Wang is Principal of the London Academy of Chinese Acupuncture (LACA). He is also Vice President of the Scalp Acupuncture Committee of World Federation of Chinese Medicine Societies (WFCMS) and President of the Academy of Scalp Acupuncture UK (ASA). He owns TJ Acupuncture Clinic and Brain Care Centre in London.

Prof. Wang has authored and co-authored more than 50 academic papers as well as been Peer-Reviewer to many international journals. His authored book *Acupuncture for Brain: Treatment for Neurological and Psychologic Disorders* was published by Springer 2021.

Author of

Chapter One: Introduction to Acupuncture Techniques

Chapter Eleven: Scalp Acupuncture

Chapter Twenty: Summary and Combination

xv

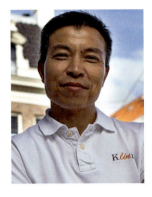

Prof. Dr. Weixiang Wang (王维祥) (*Chief Editor*), a Ph.D. graduate of Nanjing University of Chinese Medicine (NUCM), has played a pivotal role in advancing TCM in the Netherlands. Formerly serving at the Second Clinical College of NUCM until 2003, he co-founded the European Academy of Traditional Medical Science and currently acts as Academic Dean of the Dutch Acupuncture Academy (DAA). With a rich background, Dr. Wang has led the Dutch Association of TCM (NVTCG Zhong) as Chairman for six years, contributing an additional three years as Board Member. Additionally, he serves as Executive Member of the European Association of TCM (ETCMA). Driven by a commitment to elevate educational standards and integrate TCM into healthcare systems, his lectures on the integrative practice of TCM are highly sought-after in academic institutions and TCM congresses. As Accomplished Author, Dr. Wang has written and co-authored 11 TCM books in China since the commencement of his TCM career in 1989. Currently practicing at Klinic in Amsterdam, he holds the prestigious position of President for one of the most influential TCM events, the International Dutch TCM Congress (DTCMC).

Author of
Chapter Two: Prior to Needling
Chapter Three: Basic Needling
Chapter Twenty: Summary and Combination

Contributors

Lin Chen Klinic, Amsterdam, The Netherlands

Songyan Chen London Academy of Chinese Acupuncture, London, UK

Katherine Dandridge Muthill, Perthshire, Scotland

Yun Ding Mosonmagyaróvár, Hungary

Zunli Guo London Academy of Chinese Acupuncture, London, UK

Jun She London Confucius Institute for Traditional Chinese Medicine, London, UK

Bo Sheng Confucius Institute for Traditonal Chinese Medicine, London, UK

Yu Sun Sunny International (UK) Ltd., Brighton, UK

Phoebus Tian London Academy of Chinese Acupuncture, London, UK

Defeng Wang France Académie Wang de MTC, Toulouse, France

Shunchang Wang France Académie Wang de MTC, Toulouse, France

Tianjun Wang London Academy of Chinese Acupuncture, London, UK

Weixiang Wang Dutch Acupuncture Academy, Amsterdam, The Netherlands; Dutch Acupuncture Academy, Amsterdam, The Netherlands

Ying Wang Dr Ying Chinese Medical Centre, Lowestoft, UK

Yongzhou Wang International Cheeks Acupuncture Therapy Institute, Paris, France

Yongzheng Wu CNRS UMR3691, Cellular Biology and Microbial Infection Unit, Institut Pasteur, Université Paris Cité, Paris, France

Linjun Xia Mosonmagyaróvár, Hungary

Rongxian Zhang The Second Affiliated Hospital of Nanjing University of Chinese Medicine, Nanjing City, Jiangsu Province, China

Introduction

Introduction to Acupuncture Techniques

Tianjun Wang

Learning Objectives
- To understand the history and development of acupuncture and moxibustion.
- To emphasise the role of acupuncture techniques.
- To develop practitioner knowledge about the role of acupuncture techniques.
- To understand the limitations of acupuncture technique training in the West.

1 History of Acupuncture Techniques

Acupuncture techniques were gradually developed and progressed with the evolving needs of medical practice and disease development, the creation of needles and the improvement of material technology. The history of acupuncture needling and moxibustion is explained in detail.

1.1 History of acupuncture needling

The need for medical treatment has prompted people to create needles. Needles have grown from thick to thin, and their materials have developed from stone, bamboo, and bone to iron, copper, gold, silver, and stainless steel, gradually becoming more delicate and finer. The acupuncture techniques and methods changed from simple to complex and then from broad to complex, reflecting the progress and academic development of acupuncture.

T. Wang (✉)
London Academy of Chinese Acupuncture, 70 Springfield Dive, London IG2 6QS, UK
e-mail: info@tjacupuncture.co.uk

© The Author(s), under exclusive license to Springer Nature Switzerland AG 2024
T. Wang and W. Wang (eds.), *Acupuncture Techniques*,
https://doi.org/10.1007/978-3-031-59272-0_1

The origin of acupuncture needling

The origin of piercing can be traced back to the Stone Age. The most primitive acupuncture and cutting tool in ancient times was called "Bian stone". Bian stones are the most primitive medical tools, which are small cone-shaped or wedge-shaped stone tools that have been ground and are used to tap a certain part of the skin of the body, sometimes with light puncture and bleeding as well as cutting methods and draining pus. Bian stone needling is the predecessor of acupuncture.

In ancient times, it was not possible to cast iron, so stones were used as needles. Later, needles were developed on this basis.

In addition to Bian Stone, ancient acupuncture tools also include bone needles and bamboo needles. The bone needles unearthed thus far have a history of six or seven thousand years.

They come in a variety of forms, some with a point at one end and no hole at the other, and some with both ends pointed. Such bone needles are often used as medical tools. In addition, judging from the shape of the ancient "Zhen" Chinese language character, there were needles made from bamboo.

The formation of acupuncture needling

From the advancement of Bian Stone through to the development of Jiu Zhen (Nine Needles) is an important change in the history of acupuncture progress, and it is also a symbol of the formation of needling methods.

In the Huang Di Nei Jing (The Yellow Emperor's Classic of Internal Medicine), the 'bible of TCM', particularly the second section the Ling Shu (Spiritual Axis), which mainly discusses the 'nine needles'. Thus, the Ling Shu is also called Zhen Jing (the Classic of Needling).

'Nine needles' are formed on the basis of the original 'Bian stone' or 'needle stone' and developing 'Bianshi' or 'needle methods' after a long historical period, continuous improvement and gradual perfection. The hardness of the nine needles is equivalent to that of Bian Stone, their elasticity, toughness, and sharpness are better than those of Bian Stone, and they are skilfully manufactured.

Because it has nine different shapes, it not only retains the function of cutting swelling and discharging pus but also greatly expands the scope of application and has a variety of therapeutic functions. Various acupuncture methods have gradually been formed and improved. (Details of techniques for the nine needles will be discussed in Chap. 5: Classical Needling).

The development of acupuncture needling

Acupuncture needling has been continuously enriched with the establishment of TCM theory. The Huangdi Neijing has summarised a relatively complete needling system, which includes the principle of holding the needle, the type of needling, the operation of reinforcing and reducing needling (RRN) techniques, the strength of needling, etc. The majority recorded in this text was filiform needling, that is a process of needling with a solid needle of material which was capable of acupressure and acupuncture itself. There were several different filiform needling rotation procedures, including by quantity of five, nine and twelve rotations. In terms of the reinforcing and reducing methods of needling that were described in the text, there were Xuji (slow and fast) RRN, breathing RRN, twirling RRN, Yingsui (against and following) RRN, and opening and closing RRN. These kinds of needling techniques laid the foundation for the acupuncture techniques of later generations. Later another classic text, the Nanjing, which was developed from the Neijing, proposed another needling method; Ying-Wei RRN which emphasised the importance of the use of both hands during acupuncture needling, which had a great influence on later generations of acupuncture practice and methodology.

After which, generations of acupuncturists, based on the Neijing, combined with their respective experiences at the various times and locations, created and used a variety of acupuncture methods. During the Song and Jin Dynasties, the Ziwuliuzhu technique was created. Then during the Yuan Dynasty, Hanqing Dou developed "Fourteen Methods of Acupuncture" in the text 'Guide to Acupuncture Classics'. In the 'Shen Ying Jing' written by Hui Chen in the early Ming Dynasty, he put forward the "Qi invigorating Method". Several other books were published in the Ming Dynasty as well. For example, 'Jing Zhen Fu (Golden Needle Ode)' recorded a compendium of reinforcing and reducing methods and systematically discussed methods of "Shao Shan Huo (Burning Mountain Fire)" and 'Tao Tian Liang (Penetrating the Sky)'. Jizhou Yang's 'Zhen Jiu Da Cheng (The Great Compendium of Acupuncture)' collected the great achievements of acupuncture techniques before the Ming Dynasty and proposed many concepts including 'needling does have a dosage', 'a large reinforcing method, a large reducing method', 'even reinforcing and reducing methods', 'twelve methods of acupuncture', and 'eight methods of manipulation'. After the middle of the Qing Dynasty, acupuncture medicine gradually declined, and acupuncture techniques developed slowly.

After the 1950s, acupuncture techniques were again greatly developed and research on techniques and manipulation also entered a new era.

After the 1950s acupuncture technology developed significantly and research on manipulation entered a new and exciting period: from clinical studies and experimental research to mechanistic exploration. Acupuncture techniques then received increasing attention because the directly relate to the enhanced therapeutic effects of acupuncture treatments. In addition, with the integration of traditional acupuncture with modern technology, many new techniques have been established. Some of them focus on specific parts of the body, such as scalp acupuncture, ear acupuncture, wrist-ankle acupuncture and some are combined with modern technology, such as electro-acupuncture and laser acupuncture. These developments not only expand the scope of acupuncture treatment but also promote the development of acupuncture medicine. All these techniques will be described in relevant chapters.

1.2 History of Moxibustion

Moxibustion is a warming therapy inherited from ancient times. Moxibustion, like acupuncture, is a main component of the variety of acupuncture techniques available.

The origin of moxibustion

When the ancient predecessors warmed up by the fire or cooked food, they were occasionally burned by fire somewhere on the body and this at times relieved various kinds of pain. They were informed by this experience that burning can help heal and benefit physical ailments. In addition, moxibustion is based on the needs of ancient people to treat and soothe the issue of diseases caused by internal and external cold.

At the beginning of the development of moxibustion practice, branches and firewood may have been used to make a fire for smoking, ironing, burning, and scalding the body to relieve pain and other ailments. Later, with the deepening of a structured medical practice, 'moxa' was gradually selected as the main material of moxibustion, this is the herb 'artemesia vulgaris'.

The formation of moxibustion

Moxibustion has been widely used among the people of the Qin period. The Huangdi Neijing was written before the Qin and Han dynasties and contains a large number of records about moxibustion. The principle of moxibustion treatment, operating procedures, scope of application, reinforcing and reducing methods and precautions are all detailed within.

Moxibustion became more popular in the Wei and Jin Dynasties. The first monograph on moxibustion was 'Cao's Moxibustion', written by Xi Cao during the Three Kingdoms period. A suppurative moxibustion method was first recorded in 'The ABC of Acupuncture' written by Fumi Huang in the Jin Dynasty.

Hong Ge, a famous doctor, recorded 109 acupuncture prescriptions in his text 'Elbow Reserve Emergency Prescriptions', 94 of which were moxibustion prescriptions. He proposed using moxibustion for emergencies, and that moxibustion could nourish Yang, a concept which further developed moxibustion. At the same time, various moxibustion materials were used and a method of partition moxibustion was first used, which is the method of using a material between the moxa and the skin. As an additional contribution to this famous book, Professor Youyou Tu was inspired by it and invented her famous methods to treat malaria and was awarded the Nobel Prize in 2015.

Simiao Sun, the 'king' of herbal medicine in the Tang Dynasty, once vigorously advocated moxibustion to treat diseases. In his book 'Thousands of Golden Prescriptions', there are garlic-partitioned moxibustion, salt-partitioned moxibustion, etc. In addition, in the Tang Dynasty, there were doctors who specialised in moxibustion, called 'moxibustion masters. It can be seen that moxibustion developed into an independent discipline in the Tang Dynasty.

In the Song Dynasty, there were several texts on moxibustion, such as 'Children Mingtang Moxibustion Classic', 'Xifangzi Mingtang Moxibustion Classic' and

'Gonghuangshu Point Moxibustion', which formed a unique school in theory and practice and enriched the content of moxibustion science. In addition, there are many records about 'Heavenly Moxibustion' and 'Self-Moxibustion in many acupuncture books. This includes the therapeutic administration of certain irritating herbs such buttercup leaves, white mustard seeds and eclipse grass to relevant acupoints and causing blisters for healing various disorders.

After the Yuan and Ming Dynasties, moxibustion began to improve toward painless warming practices and the more primitive moxibustion tended to decline. At the same time, the Ming and Qing dynasties there was more attention towards the use of moxibustion equipment which laid the foundation for the development of moxibustion equipment in later generations.

The development of moxibustion

Moxibustion has a long history in the treatment of disease. At first it was a simple method, mostly using direct moxibustion (applying repetitive moxa cones directly on the skin and often lifting before the burning and scarring of the skin ensued) and the moxa cones were relatively large and strong. To alleviate pain and burning scars, from the Ming and Qing dynasties to the present, modern moxibustion methods mostly use smaller moxa sticks and the cones tend to be applied for fewer times. In addition, a variety of moxibustion methods have been derived since, such as traditional moxa sticks, various herbal stick moxa, warming moxa devices, warming needle moxibustion, and heavenly moxibustion. According to different conditions, indirect moxibustion is now commonly used which either is the procedure of holding a moxa implement over the acupoint or applying moxa cones separated from the skin with ginger slices, garlic slices, salt, tempeh cake, aconite cake, etc.

Since the 1950s, moxibustion has been valued clinically for the unique therapeutic effects, particularly in China. Great progress has been made in the scope, methods and equipment of moxibustion. With the combination of moxibustion with modern technology, new moxibustion technologies, such as laser moxa, electric moxa and electrothermal moxa have been developed, and various moxibustion instruments have also been developed (Details will be discussed in Chap. 10: Moxibustion).

2 Types of Acupuncture and Moxibustion Techniques

The range of acupuncture techniques include five categories: filiform needling, special needle acupuncture, special area acupuncture, moxibustion and special acupoint therapy.

Filiform needling refers to the method of stimulating acupoints by the manipulation of filiform needles. The basic operation techniques include the various methods of holding the needle, of inserting the needle, moving the needle, reorienting the needle and the methods of withdrawing the needle. This group forms the basis of a variety of acupuncture techniques, which configure the basic methods and operation skills that the acupuncturist must grasp.

Special needle acupuncture refers to the method of using special acupuncture tools other than filiform needles to act on meridians, acupoints or special parts of the human body to prevent and treat diseases. It includes three-edged needling, skin needling, intradermal needling, the long needle method, fire needling, 'di' needling (spoon needling or thick needling), Yuan-li needling, etc. Special needle needling techniques are generally used to treat special diseases and have the characteristics of strong results and curative effects for specific disorders.

Special area acupuncture refers to various methods of diagnosing and treating systemic diseases but uses needling and other methods to act on relatively independent specific parts of the human body. It is named because the stimulating parts are different from traditional meridian points. Special area acupuncture, such as scalp acupuncture, ear acupuncture, eye acupuncture, tongue acupuncture, face acupuncture, check acupuncture, nose acupuncture, has the characteristics of concentrated acupoints, easy operation, and unique curative effects.

Moxibustion refers to the method of using moxa or other flammable materials to burn, smoke and iron certain parts or acupoints of the human body to prevent and treat diseases. According to different moxibustion materials, moxibustion can be divided into moxibustion with wormwood and moxibustion without wormwood. Moxibustion methods include moxa cone moxibustion, moxa roll moxibustion, warming needle moxibustion and warming moxa device moxibustion. Moxibustion without wormwood methods include sky moxibustion, lamplight moxibustion, yellow wax moxibustion, herbal ingot moxibustion, herbal twist moxibustion, herbal pen moxibustion and herbal thread moxibustion.

Special acupoint therapy refers to the application of various natural and artificial physical factors (electricity, sound, light, heat, magnetism, etc.) and chemical factors (Chinese and Western medicines) that act on meridians and acupoints and achieve the purpose of preventing and treating diseases through the adjustment of the body. These include acupoint sticking therapy, acupoint electrotherapy, acupoint magnetic therapy, acupoint laser irradiation therapy, acupoint microwave radiation therapy, acupoint infrared radiation therapy, acupoint drug iontophoresis, etc.

The above acupuncture and moxibustion methods have their own characteristics and they can be used alone in clinical applications or can be used according to actual clinical needs to cooperate with each other to achieve the best clinical effect. All these techniques will be described in relevant chapters.

3 The Role of Acupuncture Techniques

3.1 The Elements to Achieve Better Acupuncture Results

Acupuncture treatment stimulates the body's natural healing processes. To achieve better results, there are several elements that should be considered:

Proper diagnosis: Before starting acupuncture treatment, proper assessments and diagnoses should be made. This involves understanding the patient's chief complaints, current symptoms, related symptoms, medical diagnosis and treatment history, family history, lifestyle factors that may contribute to their condition, pulse presentation, tongue reading, relevant physical assessments, etc. Sometime should be combined with western medicine diagnosis as well.

Individualised treatment plan: Acupuncture treatment should be tailored to the individual's needs by selecting the appropriate points and the proper acupuncture techniques to target based on the patient's diagnosis and symptoms.

Lifestyle advice: In addition to acupuncture treatment, lifestyle changes may be recommended to support the body's natural healing process. This can include changes in diet, exercise, and stress management techniques. Based on TCM principles, Taiji/Tai Chi, Qigong, dietary adjustments, etc., may be advised to relevant patients.

Acupuncture technique selection: Unlike herbal medicine treatment, after proper diagnosis and treatment plans and acu-points are made, acupuncture treatment needs to select suitable techniques based on the diagnosis and treatment plan. These could be basic filiform needling, moxibustion or other special techniques. This selection might be based on the knowledge of the practitioner training. As an example, the acupuncturists who have learned scalp acupuncture may select it to treat stroke patients alongside filiform needles. This selection may improve the results for the treatment of stroke. The Dao-qi technique on DU-26 Renzhong could successfully awaken the brain to restore consciousness from coma. For chronic pelvic floor disorders, Baliao point plus electro-acupuncture may be added to general needling treatment.

Acupuncture technique performance: Acupuncture treatment is not only based on acupuncture theory and technique selection but also depends on the techniques being skilfully applied. Skilled training of basic needling may achieve pain-free insertion or minimal discomfort. Scalp acupuncture with fast needling of 200 movements per minute could generate healthy electric waves in the brain to achieve better results for brain conditions.

There are several ways to help practitioners improve technique selection and performance, including continuing education, clinical practice and experience, patient communication, patient comfort analysis and adjustments, practitioner self-care, clinical mentor system, etc.

By selection and performance, acupuncture techniques bridge the basic theories, such as between TCM foundation and diagnosis, acupuncture channels and points, to the actual clinical practice and efficacy of patient treatment.

3.2 The Dosage of Acupuncture Techniques

The dosage of acupuncture techniques can vary depending on the specific condition being treated, the individual patient and the practitioner's treatment plan. The dosage of acupuncture treatment involves the consideration of several elements.

In one session of treatment, the dosage of acupuncture may involve the number of needles, the type of needles, the area of acupoints, the direction and depth of needling, the intensity of needling manipulation, the duration of needle retention, etc. For example, fewer needles may be used with a gentle insertion technique for more sensitive, frail or ailing patients, while a larger number of needles may be used for a more intensive treatment or for the more robust patient. In a course of acupuncture treatment, the dosage may relate to the quantity or multiple sessions, the frequency of sessions, and the dosage of each session with regards to needling, strength of treatment and duration.

Generally speaking, the elements to strengthen the dose of acupuncture treatment are to increase the number of needles, use of larger needles, some special needles such as fire needling, Yuanli needling, or needling methods such as scalp acupuncture, Dao-qi needling and then also the use of strong manipulation, longer duration of needle retention, more frequency and more sessions of treatment.

3.3 Outline of Research on Acupuncture Techniques

Research of acupuncture techniques has grown significantly in recent years, with many studies examining its effectiveness and safety for various conditions. Below is a basic outline of the research on acupuncture techniques:

Clinical trials: Randomised controlled trials are considered the gold standard for evaluating the efficacy of acupuncture. Many clinical trials have been conducted on acupuncture, often comparing it to sham acupuncture or standard care. These trials have examined a range of conditions, including pain, nausea, depression, and fertility issues. For example, the treatment for women with stress urinary incontinence by electroacupuncture involving the lumbosacral region, compared with sham electroacupuncture, resulted in less urine leakage after 6 weeks [7].

Mechanism of action: Researchers are also interested in understanding how acupuncture works from a biological perspective. Studies have shown that acupuncture can modulate the activity of the nervous system, increase blood flow and release endorphins, among other effects. A recent study indicated that the efficacy of scalp acupuncturein treating brain diseases, especially ischemic strokes, is mostly achieved by stimulating the scalp nerves, especially the trigeminal nerve, to improve cerebral blood flow (CBF) [6].

Safety: Acupuncture is generally considered safe when administered by a qualified and licenced practitioner who uses sterile needles. However, there have been reports of adverse effects, such as bruising, bleeding, and infection. Research has examined the safety of acupuncture and identified risk factors that can increase the likelihood of adverse effects. Recently, Baumler and colleagues [1] reported on BMJ Open that acupuncture-related adverse effects were 1.01 per 10,000 patients and 7.98 per million treatments. Mild adverse effects, such as bleeding, pain or flares at the needle site, occurred in less than 10% of the treatments (9.4/100).

Neuroimaging studies: Brain imaging studies have been used to examine the neural mechanisms underlying acupuncture. These studies have shown that acupuncture can activate specific regions of the brain, which may be responsible for its therapeutic effects. Maeda et al. [9] reported that their clinical study used fMRI brain scans to investigate selected patients with carpal tunnel syndrome (CTS) and showed that when particular fingers were manipulated to increase the pressure on the meridian nerve, the brain scans showed areas of the brain as blurry. The real electroacupuncture (EA) groups were superior to the sham group in producing improvements in neurophysiological outcomes, both local to the wrist and in the brain. Moreover, greater improvement in second/third interdigital cortical separation distance following real acupuncture predicted sustained improvements in symptom severity at the 3-month follow-up, while sham patients did not. Acupuncture at local versus distal sites may improve median nerve function at the wrist by somatopicapic arrangement and distinct neuroplasticity in the primary somatosensory cortex following therapy. The same part of the brain was rescanned following the acupuncture treatment and showed that the area remapping immediately following therapy was linked with better long-term symptom reduction. The study further suggests that improvements in primary somatosensory cortex somatotopy can predict long-term clinical outcomes for CTS.

Patient-reported outcomes: Patient-reported outcomes, such as pain scores, quality of life, satisfaction with treatment, and MYMOP (Measure Your Medical Outcome Profile), have also been used widely to evaluate the effectiveness of acupuncture. In an exploratory single-arm observational clinical study [2], participants received seven individualised treatments (S1) and six optional additional treatments (S2). The MYMOP, SF-36 and PANAS were administered at baseline, during each series, and at follow-up 4 and 12 weeks after the end of treatment. The primary outcome was the change in the MYMOP score at the end of each series. This small study suggests that acupuncture plus moxibustion is an acceptable and useful adjunct to usual care for cancer survivors with lymphoedema.

4 The Development of Acupuncture Techniques

Acupuncture has been used for thousands of years in traditional Chinese medicine, and it has continued to evolve and develop over time. In modern times, acupuncture techniques have undergone significant changes and advancements to become more effective, efficient, and safe. Here are some of the ways that acupuncture techniques have been modernized:

Improved Needle Materials

Modern acupuncture needles are made mainly from stainless steel, which makes them more hygienic and durable than traditional needles made of bone or stone.

Thinner needle size

Compared to the materials developed from bone, stone, copper, silver and gold, the modern stainless steel needles are much thinner. Generally, the thinner the needle is, the less pain there is during needling insertion.

Single-Use Needles

Acupuncture needles are now designed for single-use only to prevent cross-contamination and reduce the risk of infection rather than using an autoclave for sterilisation. This modern approach to acupuncture has made it a safer and more reliable treatment option.

Developing modern acupuncture techniques

Combined or integrated with modern medicine knowledge and technology, many new acupuncture techniques have been developed. Here are some examples of this development.

- Electroacupuncture is the combination of needling combined with electricity.
- Integrating traditional acupuncture theory and techniques with modern neurological knowledge meant that scalp acupuncture was created.
- Merging acupuncture needling and the holographic theory, ear acupuncture was developed.

Most of these developing modern acupuncture techniques will be explained in detail in the book, including scalp acupuncture (SA), ear acupuncture (EA), wrist-ankle acupuncture (WAA), cheek acupuncture (CA), fire needling (FN), yuan li needling (YLN), plum blossom needling and three-edged needles, electric acupuncture (ELA), and laser acupuncture (LA).

5 Limitations of Acupuncture Technique in Western Medicine

Acupuncture has been introduced to countries in the West gradually over hundreds of years, which spread from China or through other Asian countries. Many of the aspects of Chinese acupuncture have been well communicated, including the TCM foundations and diagnosis methods, acupuncture channel and points, the application of acupuncture for clinical treatments, etc. Unfortunately, acupuncture techniques have not been well presented and initiated and therefore have not been sufficiently practiced in most Western countries.

5.1 Lack of Technique Training for Acupuncture Education in Western Medicine

Acupuncture education in Western countries has no national curriculum. Different institutions may have their own program structure. Based on our teaching experiences or as external examiners with backgrounds in a variety of Western acupuncture institutions, a peculiar phenomenon has been noticed for many years; a lack of training in acupuncture techniques.

Many colleges provide acupuncture education, including TCM foundation and diagnosis, acupuncture meridian and points, TCM pattern identification, treatment of common disorders, clinical skills and practice, personal development, acupuncture research, etc. Basic needling and moxibustion are also covered. Unfortunately, further needling techniques and the development of modern techniques are not well understood or communicated.

5.2 Weaknesses of Techniques in Acupuncture Practice

Due to a lack of acupuncture technique training in colleges and later in continuing professional development (CPD), many Western acupuncturists and lecturers have little technique knowledge or skill. The results therefore of general acupuncture practice in the West are often not as effective as those in China, or there are at least fewer quick positive therapeutic responses. Many acupuncturists only insert needles at points with a shortage of suitable depth, direction, angle, and insufficient needling sensation. As an example, scalp acupuncture has been part of the national curriculum in China since the 1980s. In Western countries, even in 2020, few acupuncture colleges still teach scalp acupuncture as part of their routine curriculum.

5.3 Confusion of Techniques Among Acupuncture Studies

In the last two to three decades, acupuncture research in Western countries has been rapidly developing. There are many successful studies. Unfortunately, one of the strange phenomena among acupuncture studies in the west is that many results are inconclusive, or sometimes the conclusion that acupuncture is no more than a placebo. One of the reasons for this anomaly is that the methodology of acupuncture research in western countries is limited to a basic technical level. Many of them do not explain techniques or just mention the basic 'de qi' sensation. For example, acupuncture treatment in China is used frequently and for patients who suffer a stroke, supported with many successful clinical studies, including many well-designed high-quality trials. Several systematic reviews and meta-analyses have proven the effectiveness of acupuncture for stroke. Looking back at the use of acupuncture in the West, there are very few acupuncture studies on stroke or other neurological disorders. A few of them resulted in negative results or results with efficacy defined as less than a placebo level. One of the reasons may be attributed to the lack of specific acupuncture techniques used, such as scalp acupuncture and/or the Du-mai Dao-qi technique, and the use of only general body acupuncture.

5.4 Concern About Using Acupuncture Techniques for Western Patients

Some acupuncturists believe that Western patients are more sensitive to needling. Thus, the needles used by many Western acupuncturists are thinner and shorter. Many acupuncturists only put the needles in with tube guiding needles but do not operate any needling technique. In addition, further traditional techniques, such as reinforcing and reducing, or modern acupuncture techniques, such as electro-acupuncture and scalp acupuncture, are not commonly used. Well-trained acupuncturists with skill and training in techniques can practice acupuncture needling that is pain-free or with very little sensation on needle insertion. Furthermore, most chronic or treatment-resistant conditions require a sufficient dosage of acupuncture. Bearable, slightly strong needling may generate much quicker and more efficient results. Of course, it is important to provide a full explanation and agreement with the patients. Based on clinical experience, most patients are happy to receive a suitable and more beneficial acupuncture technique for their disorder if it means increased efficacy.

6 The Need for a Comprehensive Book on Acupuncture Techniques

There are a great number of acupuncture books in Western countries. Most Western acupuncture books are focused on acupuncture meridians and points, such as A Manual of Acupuncture [3], and some are focused on the treatment of diseases, such as The Practice of Chinese Medicine [8]. In terms of the acupuncture technique books, some only introduce very basic needling and some only focus on one technique, such as ear acupuncture [12], Chinese scalp acupuncture [4], and electro-acupuncture [10]; some covered several techniques, such as in the text by Hecker et al only introduced microsystems acupuncture [5].

There are few books that cover most used acupuncture techniques, not only traditional techniques but also modern techniques. There is a need to have a book to cover comprehensive acupuncture techniques.

The uniqueness of this book, Acupuncture Techniques—A Practical Manual, covers basic needling techniques, further techniques, moxibustion, cupping and most commonly used modern developed acupuncture techniques, such as scalp acupuncture, ear acupuncture, cheek acupuncture, electroacupuncture and laser acupuncture.

7 Summary

The array of acupuncture techniques, including acupuncture needling and moxibustion, have a long history in China and have spread via various channels and doctors to Western countries for hundreds of years. Acupuncture technique plays an important role in acupuncture education and practice. Unfortunately, compared to the other elements of acupuncture education, which is in part a basis of Chinese medicine, many acupuncture techniques have not been well introduced and developed and resulted in a lack of technique training for training of acupuncture professionals in the West. These weaknesses of technique in acupuncture practice, confusion of technique in acupuncture studies, worry about the stronger stimulation techniques for Western patients and therefore, the need for a comprehensive book on acupuncture techniques to share with Western training providers and acupuncture schools.

Comprehension/Review Questions
- Describe the concept of applying acupuncture techniques?
- Describe the different types of acupuncture needling and moxibustion techniques?
- How should an acupuncture technique be selected?

References

1. Bäumler P, Zhang W, Stübinger T, et al. Acupuncture-related adverse events: systematic review and meta-analyses of prospective clinical studies. BMJ Open. 2021;11:e045961. https://doi.org/10.1136/bmjopen-2020-045961.
2. De Valoisa BA, Young TE, Melsome E. Assessing the feasibility of using acupuncture and moxibustion to improve quality of life for cancer survivors with upper body lymphoedema. Eur J Oncol Nurs. 2012;16:301–9.
3. Deadman P, Al-Khafaji M, Baker KA. Manual of acupuncture. Fifth Imprint. East Sussex: JCM publications; 2003.
4. Hao JJ, Hao LL. Chinese scalp acupuncture. Blue poppy press. Boulder, USA; 2011.
5. Hecker H-U, Steveling A, Peuker E-T. Microsystems acupuncture-the complete guide: ear-scalp-mouth-hand. Stuttgart, New York: Thieme; 2006.
6. Jin G-Y, Jin LL, Jin BX, et al. Neural control of cerebral blood flow: scientific basis of scalp acupuncture in treating brain diseases. Front Neurosci. 2023;17:1210537. https://doi.org/10.3389/fnins.2023.1210537.
7. Liu ZS, Liu Y, Xu HF, et al. Effect of electroacupuncture on urinary leakage among women with stress urinary incontinence a randomized clinical trial. JAMA. 2017;317(24):2493–501. https://doi.org/10.1001/jama.2017.7220.
8. Maciocia G. The practice of chinese medicine 2nd edition. The treatment of diseases with acupuncture and chinese herbs. Edinburgh: Churchill Livingstone; 2007.
9. Maeda Y, Kim H, Ketter N, et al. Rewiring the primary somatosensory cortex in carpal tunnel syndrome with acupuncture. Brain. 2017;140(4):914–27.
10. Mayor D. Electroacupuncture: a practical manual and resource. London: Churchill Livingstone. Elsevier; 2001.
11. O' Connor J, Bensky D (trans). Acupuncture: a comprehensive text. Seattle: Eastland Press; 1981.
12. Oleson T. Auriculotherapy manual Chinese and western systems of ear acupuncture, 4e. London: Elsevier Health Sciences; 2013.

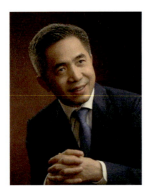

Prof. Dr. Tianjun Wang (王天俊) graduated from Nanjing University of Chinese Medicine (NUCM) in 1989. He completed his PhD of Acupuncture at NUCM. Tianjun moved to the UK and joined the University of East London UK as a Senior Lecturer and the Director of Acupuncture Clinic 2007–2014. He is a Guest Professor of NUCM.

Current Prof. Wang is the Principal of the London Academy of Chinese Acupuncture (LACA). He is also the Vice President of the Scalp Acupuncture Committee of World Federation of Chinese Medicine Societies (WFCMS) and the president of the Academy of Scalp Acupuncture UK (ASA). He owns TJ Acupuncture Clinic and Brain Care Centre in London.

Prof. Wang has authored and co-authored more than 50 academic papers as well as peer reviewers to many international journals. His authored book "Acupuncture for Brain: Treatment for Neurological and Psychologic Disorders" published by Springer 2021.

Techniques of Filiform Needling

Prior to Needling

Weixiang Wang

Learning Objectives

1. Explore the details of needle structure, materials, and the strategic selection of needle size, length, and gauge.
2. Examine the advantages of disposable needles and the shift towards modern sterilization practices.
3. Gain practical insights into needle storage, examination, and the importance of the practitioner's finger strength.
4. Comprehend the preparatory steps before needling, including patient body postures for optimal treatment outcomes.

1 About Filiform Needles

In the field of acupuncture, needles are fundamental tools for practitioners, comparable to the implements used by a carpenter. Among the various needles used in clinical settings, the filiform needle is particularly noteworthy and essential, commonly known simply as a 'needle.' This seemingly straightforward yet influential instrument is a core element in acupuncture practice, enabling the precise stimulation of acupuncture points as part of the therapeutic process.

Filiform needles, also known as Hao Zhen 毫针 in China (literally meaning mini needles), are slender, metallic instruments that play a pivotal role in acupuncture therapy. Unlike the hypodermic needles used for injections, filiform needles are designed to be incredibly fine and flexible. This design ensures minimal discomfort during insertion and allows for precise placement on acupuncture points. The term "filiform" aptly describes their thinness, emphasising their non-invasive nature.

W. Wang (✉)
Dutch Acupuncture Academy, Amsterdam, The Netherlands
e-mail: tcmdao@gmail.com

The primary function of filiform needles is to stimulate specific acupuncture points on the body, promoting the flow of qi and facilitating the body's natural healing processes. Acupuncture theory posits that the body's energy circulates through meridians or channels, and disruptions in this flow can lead to pain, illness, or imbalance. Filiform needles regulate the flow of qi and restore the body and mind harmonization.

Filiform needles possess several key attributes that make them suitable for acupuncture practice. Their slender composition ensures that the insertion process is relatively painless and minimally disruptive to the surrounding tissues. They are available in various lengths to accommodate different treatment depths and body areas. In modern practice, filiform needles are typically sterile and disposable, adhering to stringent hygiene standards. The fine nature of these needles reduces the risk of tissue damage or bleeding, making them suitable for sensitive areas and patients with a low pain threshold. Additionally, their design allows for precise targeting of acupuncture points, ensuring accurate stimulation and therapeutic outcomes.

Despite their unassuming appearance, filiform needles have the power to influence the body profoundly. Their insertion triggers a series of responses, including the release of endorphins (natural painkillers), modulation of the nervous system, and enhancement of blood circulation. These combined effects contribute to pain relief, relaxation, and the restoration of balance within the body's systems.

2 Needle Structure (See Fig. 2.1)

Acupuncture needles, seemingly straightforward tools, harbour a complex design aimed at ensuring precision, comfort and therapeutic efficacy.

Needle Handle

The handle of an acupuncture needle acts as the bridge between the practitioner's hand and the patient's body. Handles come in diverse designs, catering to various techniques and practitioner preferences. Textured or ergonomically shaped handles enhance grip, facilitating nuanced manipulations. The handle's length affects tactile perception and control during insertion [1].

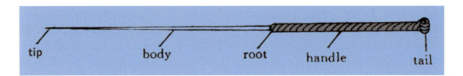

Fig. 2.1 Needle structure

Needle Tail

Extending from the handle to the body, the needle tail, often overlooked, plays a pivotal role in manipulation. Its length influences flexibility, allowing subtle adjustments during treatment. A longer tail provides a greater range, facilitating precise positioning and stimulating acupuncture points [1].

Needle Tip

The needle tip, which is finely honed, makes contact with the skin and acupuncture points. Its design minimizes discomfort during insertion, often described as a mild pinprick. Tapering ensures smooth penetration while reducing tissue impact. A well-crafted tip allows practitioners to access points accurately [1].

Needle Body

Needle body has different lengths accommodate insertion depths, from 15 to 100 mm. Body diameter affects strength and flexibility, influencing needle responsiveness and acupuncture stimulating dosage [1].

Needle Root

Positioned where the needle meets the handle, the root bolsters stability during manipulation. A secure connection prevents separation, ensuring seamless treatment. Root design impacts balance and control during insertion and movement, and prevent from any needling incidence [1].

3 Needle Materials Across Different Countries

China

Chinese acupuncture needles embrace diversity and innovation. They may employ materials such as stainless steel, copper, or silver. Needles may have longer tails, more suited for warm-needling techniques where moxa is applied on top for enhanced therapeutic effects.

Japan

Japanese acupuncture needles, known to be extremely thin, prioritise patient comfort. In ancient time materials such as gold or silver had been used to reduce skin resistance during insertion. Longer tails and slender bodies align with Japan's gentle needling approach.

South Korea

South Korean acupuncture needles blend Chinese and Japanese characteristics. Materials such as surgical stainless steel offer durability. The design balances manipulation control with patient comfort, reflecting effective yet comfortable treatments.

4 Needle Size: Length and Gauge

One of the foundational considerations in acupuncture practice is the selection of needle length, a nuanced aspect that significantly influences treatment precision, patient comfort, and therapeutic efficacy.

4.1 Anatomy Dictates Needle Length

Antomic structure is one the first considerations to choose the needle length. Points may be distributed across different regions of the body, necessitating varying depths of insertion for optimal therapeutic outcomes. This underscores the essential connection between anatomical difference and needle length selection.

Short Acupuncture Needles (3–7 mm)

In instances where treatment involves superficial areas, such as the face, hands, ears, or scalp, the use of short acupuncture needles proves invaluable. Ranging from 3 to 7 mm, these needles are adept at accessing points that lie closer to the skin's surface. Their shortened length minimises the risk of inadvertent overpenetration and ensures a gentler needling experience in delicate regions. These needles are often chosen for Jing-Well, Ying-Spring points.

Medium Length Acupuncture Needles (13–40 mm)

The category of medium-length needles, spanning from 13 to 40 mm, constitute the versatile workhorses of acupuncture practice. These needles can be applied on the face, hands, feet, arms, lower legs, abdomen, shoulders, and back. Their adaptability allows practitioners to effectively address a wide range of conditions and therapeutic needs.

Long Acupuncture Needles (50 mm and Above)

Long acupuncture needles, surpassing 50 mm in length, are employed when targeting areas characterised by greater muscular or adipose tissue depth, such as the legs or the gluteal region. These extended needles are also chosen for points that require deep stimulation, such as those situated in the lower back and hip areas, like GB-30 Huan Tiao.

Patient-specific attributes play a pivotal role in determining the appropriate needle length. The patient's build, sensitivity and anatomical variations influence the choice, ensuring both safety and efficacy.

4.2 Selection of the Right Needle Length

Selecting the correct needle length is essential not only for patient safety but also for the efficacy of the treatment. Too short a needle may not reach the intended depth, while needles that are excessively long might inadvertently cause discomfort or damage.

The selection of needle length is far from arbitrary; it involves a fine and calculated approach. A balanced choice between safety and effectiveness, needle length is the key to stimulate the acupoints while precision, efficacy, and personalised care are three main goals.

A Prerequisite for Needle Length Selection

A. **Facial and Head Points**

The needle length chosen for facial points is guided by their superficial nature. Short acupuncture needles, within the range of 0.03–7 mm, are employed.

B. **Extremities—Hands and Limbs**

When needling points on the hands or limbs, practitioners often turn to medium-length acupuncture needles (13–40 mm). Their moderate length allows practitioners to effectively access points that range from more superficial to moderately deep locations.

C. **Back and Abdominal Points**

The back and abdomen house acupuncture points of varying depths. Medium-length needles are frequently selected (13–40 mm) due to the dynamic nature of abdominal points. The choice balances accessibility, depth, and patient comfort, facilitating effective stimulation for diverse conditions. The selection of needle length should consider the patient's build and the needling direction. Avoid to harm any internal Zang Fu organs should always be the first consideration.

D. **Patient's Build**

When choosing the needle length, the patient's body size and composition need to be considered as well. Smaller individuals may benefit from shorter needles, while larger patients might require longer needles to reach target points effectively.

E. **Patient Sensitivity**

Patients with heightened sensitivity may prefer shorter and thinner needles to ensure minimal discomfort during insertion.

F. **Muscular Athletes**

Individuals with robust musculature might necessitate longer needles to penetrate deeper layers of tissue effectively. These needles are useful for sports-related injuries or muscle tension.

G. **Safety and Effectiveness**

When selecting the appropriate needle length, prioritizing safety in practice takes precedence over treatment effectiveness. In cases of uncertainty, it is advisable to opt for a shorter needle length.

4.3 Needle Gauge in Acupuncture

Choosing the right thickness of the needle is crucial in everyday acupuncture. The thickness, or gauge, of the needle has a big impact on how it feels during acupuncture and how well it works. As practitioners balance patient comfort, treatment results, and the specifics of the body, understanding the importance of needle thickness is really important.

The essence of needle gauge resides in its numerical representation—in the Chinese needle system a gauge of 30 (0.32 mm) indicates a thicker needle compared to a gauge of 32 (0.28 mm). The standard array of acupuncture needles spans from 26 (0.45 mm) to 33 (0.26 mm) gauges. For Japanese and Korean needles the gauge 0, 1, 2, 3… 8 are often used to stand for the size from 0.14 to 0.30 mm. it is advisable to check the individual supplier and brand of needle to ascertain which gauge is finer or sturdier [2].

4.4 Balancing Needle Length and Gauge in Acupuncture Practice

In acupuncture, the balance between needle length and gauge is not merely a technical consideration; it is an assessment and concentration by a trained practitioner that is fundamental to effective needling. This synchronisation between practitioner skills and knowledge of needle length and gauge and the relationship to the patient presentation that ensures that each acupuncture session best outcome.

5 Choice of Needles

5.1 Needle Material

The choice of needle material accentuates the precision in application that characterises effective acupuncture practice. Each needle material possesses distinct qualities, lending a unique touch to the needling experience.

Stainless Steel Needles: Stainless steel needles are the cornerstone of modern acupuncture. Revered for their precision and sterility, these needles embody reliability and ease of use. Their nonreactive nature ensures minimal discomfort during insertion and enhances patient safety. The practitioners' choice for most clinical applications, stainless steel needles epitomize the fusion of tradition and contemporary standards.

Gold and Silver Needles: Gold and silver needles have been used in the history of acupuncture. Due to their high costs and less flexibility and resilience, they are kept in the acupuncture museum nowadays.

Disposable Needles: Disposable needles have become increasingly popular due to their single-use design, minimizing the risk of cross-contamination. Crafted from stainless steel or other materials, disposable needles underscore the paramount importance of hygiene in modern healthcare practices. Their convenience and safety make them a go-to choice for practitioners and patients alike.

Specialized Needles: The practice of acupuncture extends to specialized needles designed for specific applications. Intradermal needles, for example, are ultrafine needles inserted into the skin's surface for cosmetic or pain management purposes. In the past decades more and more needles have been renovated in the needs of acupuncture practice such as Fu Zhen (superficial needling), Jin Zhen (sinew needling) etc.

5.2 The Strategic Selection of Needle Size

Acupuncture offers a spectrum of needle sizes, allowing practitioners to finely tailor treatments to individual patients and specific points. Smaller needles, often ranging from 0.16 to 0.25 mm in diameter, cater to sensitive areas or those requiring more delicate manipulation. Medium-sized needles, spanning 0.25–0.30 mm, prove versatile, finding application across various anatomical regions. Thicker needles, typically 0.30–0.40 mm, are selected for points demanding stronger stimulation or deeper penetration.

5.3 Inspection of Needle Packages

In acupuncture practice, patient safety is paramount, so the act of procuring needles entails a pivotal step: inspecting the needle packages.

First and foremost, the packaging must be intact, unopened, and devoid of any signs of tampering. Any breaches in the packaging's integrity could compromise the sterility of the needles and potentially pose risks to patients.

Furthermore, confirming the product's authenticity is essential. Verifying the manufacturer's seal, lot number, and expiration date imprint confidence in the quality of the needles.

5.4 Examination of the Needle Structure

Examining the needle structure is pivotal in ensuring that the instrument is not only safe but also primed for optimal therapeutic efficacy.

The needle's tip and body are focal points of inspection. A needle's tip should be free of irregularities, deformities, or blemishes that could hinder smooth insertion or cause discomfort to the patient. Similarly, the body should be straight and uniform, devoid of any bends or defects that might impede needling precision.

The needle handle, often equipped with a guide tube, must be intact and seamlessly integrated. The guide tube, if present, ensures controlled insertion, safeguarding against potential needle contamination.

5.5 Needle Sterilization

In the contemporary practice of acupuncture, a transformational shift has taken root in the realm of needle sterilization. This shift is characterized by the widespread adoption of disposable needles among Western acupuncture practitioners, and in China more and more doctors are using the disposable needles as well in demand of patients. This transition, resonating with principles of patient safety, hygiene, and efficiency, embodies a profound evolution in the practice of acupuncture, aligning it with the demands of modern healthcare standards [2, 3].

5.6 Key Advantages of Disposable Needles

Enhanced Patient Safety: The adoption of disposable needles is inherently aligned with contemporary healthcare practices that prioritize patient safety. By eliminating the risk of cross-contamination and infections associated with reusability.

Hygiene and Consistency: Disposable needles are packaged under controlled conditions, ensuring a sterile and pristine environment. The standardized packaging guarantees uniform hygiene across treatment sessions, bolstering both patient confidence and practitioner credibility.

Patient-Centric Approach: The utilization of disposable needles attests to the practitioner's commitment to patient-centric care.

5.7 Needle Storage

Maintaining impeccable hygiene and safety standards is paramount in an acupuncture clinic, both during the treatment process and when handling used needles. Proper storage of used needles is a crucial element same as the storing unused needles. Here is a detailed guide on the best practices for storing used and unused acupuncture needles.

Storing Used Needles: The Special Yellow Box Approach

In alignment with healthcare protocols, consider using a designated sharps container for storing used acupuncture needles. These containers are often marked with a distinct yellow color and are designed to prevent accidental needlestick injuries and contamination. The special yellow box serves as a secure repository for used needles, safeguarding both practitioners and clinic staff.

> **Selecting a sharps container:** Choose a sharps container that is sturdy, leak-proof, and puncture-resistant. Ensure that it is appropriately sized to accommodate the volume of used needles generated in the clinic.
> **Proper Placement:** Position the sharps container in a conspicuous and easily accessible location within the treatment room. This encourages immediate disposal of used needles after treatments, minimizing the risk of needlestick injuries.
> **Secure Sealing:** Once the container is approximately three-quarters full, seal it securely to prevent any spillage. Follow local regulations for disposing of full sharps containers.

5.8 Storing Unused Needles

Unused acupuncture needles are valuable instruments that need proper storage to maintain their efficacy and sterility. How to ensure the integrity of unused needles:

> **Clean and Dry Environment:** Designate a dry, clean, and well-ventilated area for storing unused needles. This prevents moisture and dust accumulation that could compromise needle sterility.

Shaded Area: Store the unused needles away from direct sunlight or harsh lighting. Ultraviolet rays and excessive heat can affect the integrity of the needle materials and packaging.

Organized Arrangement: Arrange unused needles systematically to facilitate easy access during treatments. Store them in their original packaging to maintain sterility until they are ready for use.

Adhering to Expiry Dates: Keep a close watch on the expiration dates of the needles. Discard any needles that have surpassed their expiration to ensure patient safety and treatment efficacy.

6 Needle Practice

6.1 Practice of Finger Strength

In acupuncture, the practice of finger strength emerges as a foundational skill that practitioners diligently cultivate. Aspiring acupuncturists embark gradual conditioning and targeted exercises, preparing the fingers for the intricate task of needling. In China the education of acupuncture is at university level, lots of emphasis and finger power practice are in the core curriculum while in most of the western acupuncture education institutes, it is often been omitted.

Here is a more detailed insight into mastering the practice of finger strength:
Targeted Exercises: Practitioners engage in exercises that enhance finger dexterity and strength. Activities such as squeezing stress balls, using finger grippers, or practicing finger push-ups against resistance contribute to building finger strength.

Gradual Progression: practitioners gradually increase the resistance and intensity of their finger exercises. This incremental progression ensures that finger strength develops in a controlled and sustainable manner.

Point Location: In the practice of acupuncture, accurate point location requires not only precision but also finger strength. Practitioners practice palpating and locating acupuncture points on their colleagues, enhancing their touch sensitivity and finger coordination.

6.2 Practice of Needling Manipulation

A. **Practice on a Soft Tissue Paper Bag (See Fig. 2.2)**

Prepare a small bag by folding soft tissue paper into a compact shape—approximately 8 cm in length, 5 cm in width, and 2–3 cm in thickness. Wrap this bag with gauze and secure it by tying with thread to form a structure "#." To practice needle

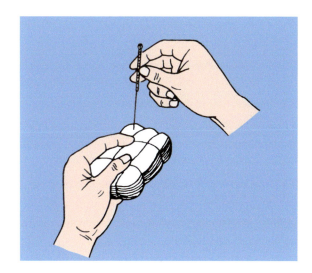

Fig. 2.2 Practice needle on a paper bag

manipulation techniques, hold the bag in your left hand while gripping the acupuncture needle handle about an inch along your right hand's thumb, index, and middle fingers, akin to holding a pen or brush [4].

Position the needle's tip on the package and, using your right thumb, index, and middle fingers, rotate the handle in both clockwise and counterclockwise directions, gradually applying pressure. Repeat this exercise multiple times in various positions. This practice is particularly beneficial for enhancing finger strength and refining the delicate skills necessary for precise manipulation and rotation during acupuncture.

B. **Practice on Yourself**

Needling one's own acupuncture points offers profound insights into the patient's experience and a deep connection with acupuncture.

Needling oneself enhances empathy as practitioners experience first-hand sensations, pain thresholds, and subtle energetic shifts that patients encounter. This personal encounter deepens their understanding of the therapeutic process. Practitioners may started from selecting points that resonate with their personal needs or needling the upper legs where no main meridian routes pass by.

C. **Practice on Your Fellows**

Practitioners learn from each other, exchange insights. Practitioners take turns needling each other's points, offering real-time feedback on sensations, techniques, and therapeutic responses. This dynamic learning process enriches their understanding of different needling approaches.

Variety of Experiences: Practitioners encounter various pain thresholds, anatomical variations, and how soon or late to get the arrival of Qi while needling their colleagues. This exposure contributes to a well-rounded understanding of acupuncture's impact.

6.3 Preparation Before Needling [4, 5] (Please delete 13.4)

The steps taken before needling are about not only technique but also creating an environment that fosters trust and optimal healing outcomes.

(1) Sterilization of the Needle

As mentioned before, the landscape of acupuncture has shifted toward the use of disposable needles which is a commitment to patient safety, minimizing the risk of infection transmission and cross-contamination.

(2) Sterilization of Hands of the Practitioner

The practitioner's hands are the pivots through acupuncture flows. Ensuring their sterility is a fundamental aspect that maintains the sanctity of the therapeutic encounter. Here is a step-by-step guide to the practitioner's hand sterilization:

Step 1: Washing Hands: The process begins with washing hands using soap and water for at least 20 s. Thorough hand washing includes cleaning under the nails and between the fingers, addressing potential hiding places for microorganisms.

Step 2: Application of the hand sanitizer: Following thorough washing, an alcohol-based hand sanitizer is applied. When dispensing an appropriate amount, practitioners rub their hands together, ensuring that they cover all surfaces, until the sanitizer has dried.

Step 3: Rubbing Hands Together: The vigorous rubbing of hands continues until the hand sanitizer is completely dry.

Attention: in some countries acupuncture practitioners are requested to put on disposable gloves to prevent the transfer of microorganisms between your hands and the patient's skin.

(3) Sterilization of the Body Surface of the patient

The patient's body surface, where acupuncture points will be needled, is prepared with meticulous care to ensure optimal hygiene. Patients are often advised to take certain steps to contribute to this process:

Preparation Before the Appointment: Patients are encouraged to take a shower before their acupuncture appointment, especially if they have been engaged in intense physical activities or have sweated profusely. Clean skin provides an ideal canvas for acupuncture needling and minimizes the chances of bacterial presence.

Practitioners may also advise patients to inform them of any skin conditions, irritations, or allergies that might affect the needling process. This communication ensures a tailored approach to sterilization and needling, accommodating individual patient needs.

Prior to Needling

On the area for acupuncture needles: Select an antiseptic solution, such as rubbing alcohol (isopropyl alcohol) or an iodine-based solution. Ensure the solution is suitable for skin disinfection. Dip cotton balls or swabs into the chosen antiseptic solution. Squeeze out excess liquid to avoid dripping. Gently wipe the area where the acupuncture needles will be inserted with the soaked cotton balls or swabs. Use a back-and-forth motion to cover the entire area. Let the antiseptic solution air dry on the skin and then insert the needles.

7 Choice of Patient's Body Postures (See Fig. 2.3)

7.1 Supine Position

It is necessary to choose the right body posture which contributes to both the patient's comfort and the practitioner's ability to access acupuncture points with precision. The patient reclines on their back in the supine position, arms resting gently at their sides. This posture is often chosen for addressing digestive issues, such as bloating

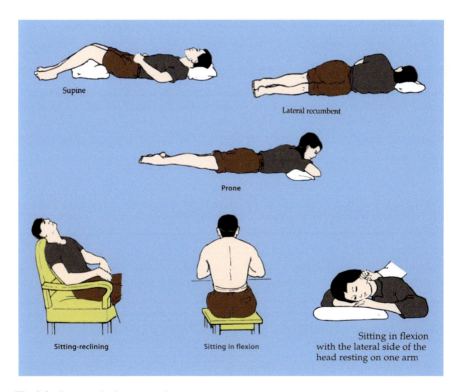

Fig. 2.3 Common body postures in acupuncture

or discomfort. Acupoints on the abdomen, chest, head, face and upper limbs become easily accessible, offering an open canvas for treatment. The supine position not only encourages relaxation but also enables the practitioner to foster a sense of ease, making it an ideal choice for patients seeking a soothing and calming acupuncture experience [4].

7.2 Prone Position

The patient take a face down in the prone position, their face resting in a comfortable face cradle. This posture is well suited for treating lower back pain or sciatica. The practitioner can focus on accessing points along the back, spine, and lower limbs with precision. By addressing these areas, the practitioner aims to alleviate discomfort and promote musculoskeletal balance. The prone position facilitates a targeted approach to addressing specific pain points on the posterior side of the body from the Du Mai, bladder meridian and gallbladder meridians [3].

7.3 Lateral Recumbent Position: Balancing Yin and Yang

The patient lie down on their side, knees slightly bent, in the lateral recumbent position. This posture is often selected for treating conditions that involve both sides of the body, such as hormonal imbalances. The practitioner can easily access points on both the front and back of the body, promoting a balanced flow of Qi. The lateral recumbent position embodies the principles of yin and yang, offering a holistic approach to treatment, often combining acupoints of Front-Mu points and Back-Shu points [4, 5].

7.4 Sitting in Flexion: Active Engagement

The Patient seated comfortably, knees bent and feet flat on the floor, in a flexed posture. This position is suitable for conditions that require active movement during treatment, such as frozen shoulder. By involving the patient in gentle movements while needling, the practitioner aims to restore joint mobility and alleviate stiffness. The sitting-in-flexion posture encourages patient engagement, fostering a collaborative treatment process.

7.5 Sitting-Reclining Position: Comfort and Accessibility

The patient takes in a slightly inclined position, supported by cushions, in the sitting-reclining posture. This choice is ideal for addressing respiratory issues, such as asthma or allergies. Points on the upper body, including the chest and neck, become easily accessible. The comfortable recline supports relaxation while allowing the practitioner to target specific areas related to the respiratory system [3].

7.6 Sitting in Flexion with Lateral Head Resting: Targeting the Neck and Upper Extremities

The patient sits on a treatment table, knees drawn close to their chest, and their lateral head resting on one arm. This posture is often utilized for treating tension headaches. The flexion and lateral head resting positions provide optimal access to points on the neck, shoulders, and upper extremities [4].

Review Questions

1. What is the primary function of filiform needles in acupuncture therapy?
2. Discuss the key attributes that make filiform needles suitable for acupuncture practice.
3. How does needle length selection correlate with anatomical differences and patient-specific attributes?
4. What are the advantages of using disposable needles in acupuncture, and how do they contribute to patient safety?
5. Explain the importance of finger strength in acupuncture practice and the targeted exercises involved.
6. What are the key considerations in selecting the right needle gauge in acupuncture?
7. Describe the steps involved in the sterilization of hands for practitioners before needling.
8. Explore the various patient body postures and their significance in acupuncture treatment.

References

1. Liu Y. Diagrams of acupuncture. 1st ed. Shanghai: Shanghai Scien&tech Pulishing House; 2003.
2. Qiu ML. Chinese acupuncture and moxibustion. 1st ed. London: Churchill Liverstone; 1993.
3. Yang JS. Zhen Jiu Xue. 1st ed. Beijing: People's Publishing House; 1989.
4. Liang FR, Wang H. Zhen Jiu Xue. 4th ed. Beijing: China TCM Publishing House; 2018.
5. Wang H, Du YH. Zhen Jiu Xue. 3rd ed. Beijing: China TCM Publishing House; 2012.

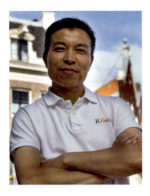

Prof. Dr. Weixiang Wang (王维祥) A PhD graduate of Nanjing University of Chinese Medicine (NUCM) (NJUCM), has played a pivotal role in advancing TCM in the Netherlands. Formerly serving at the Second Clinical College of NUCM until 2003, he co-founded the European Academy of Traditional Medical Science and currently act as the academic dean of the Dutch Acupuncture Academy (DAA). With a rich background, Dr. Wang has led the Dutch Association of TCM (NVTCG Zhong) as chairman for six years, contributing an additional three years as a board member. Additionally, he serves as an executive member of the European Association of TCM (ETCMA). Driven by a commitment to elevate educational standards and integrate TCM into healthcare systems, his lectures on the integrative practice of TCM are highly sought-after in academic institutions and TCM congresses. An accomplished author, Dr. Wang has written and co-authored 11 TCM books in China since the commencement of his TCM career in 1989. Currently practicing at Klinic in Amsterdam, he holds the prestigious position of president for one of the most influential TCM events, the International Dutch TCM Congress (DTCMC).

Basic Needling

Weixiang Wang

Learning Objectives

1. Understanding Techniques: Grasp the nuances of Puncturing hand and Pressing hand techniques, along with single and double-handed needle insertion methodologies.
2. Factors in Insertion: Comprehend the considerations in depth, angle, and direction of needle insertion based on various patient and anatomical factors.
3. Needling Manipulations: Explore the significance of primary and auxiliary needling manipulations and their impact on therapeutic outcomes.
4. De Qi and Therapeutic Efficacy: Understand the concept of De Qi and its pivotal role in therapeutic effectiveness.
5. Tonifying and Reducing Techniques: Learn how tonifying and reducing techniques contribute to restoring meridian balance.
6. Retaining and Withdrawing the Needle: Understand the importance of these phases in stimulating healing responses and harmonizing Qi flow.

1 Needle Insertion: Puncturing Hand and Pressing Hand (See Fig. 3.1)

For acupuncturists, needle insertion is more than just a physical act—it is a blend of technique, intention, and precision. Two of the distinct methods that practitioners employ are "Puncturing hand" and "Pressing hand," each representing a unique approach to needle insertion.

W. Wang (✉)
Dutch Acupuncture Academy, Amsterdam, The Netherlands
e-mail: tcmdao@gmail.com

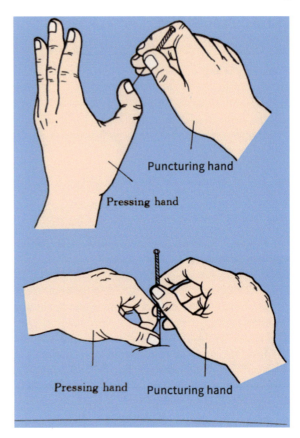

Fig. 3.1 Puncturing hand and pressing hand

Puncturing Hand: Puncturing Hand—Guiding the Needle with Finesse

The "Puncturing hand" technique, often referred to as the "puncturing hand," exemplifies the practitioner's finesse in guiding the needle's trajectory. This method involves the delicate and precise use of the practitioner's hand to control the needle's entry into the skin. By holding the needle between the thumb and the middle finger, with the index finger poised to guide, the practitioner ensures that the needle's insertion is accurate and controlled.

The primary function of "Puncturing hand" is to facilitate the needle's entry into the acupuncture point with minimal resistance or discomfort. This technique is particularly valuable when targeting points that are located beneath thin layers of tissue or points that require precise alignment with the body's meridian pathways. The practitioner's hand, guided by a deep understanding of anatomy and the flow of Qi, gently navigates through the layers, creating a pathway for the needle's therapeutic achievement [1–3].

Pressing Hand: Pressing Hand—Anchoring the Point with Purpose

On the other hand, the "Pressing hand" technique, or the "pressing hand," serves as an anchor for needle insertion. This technique involves applying slight pressure to the skin surrounding the acupuncture point before inserting the needle. The practitioner's thumb or fingers gently press against the skin, stabilizing the area and creating a supportive foundation for needle placement.

The primary function of "Pressing hand" is to ensure accuracy and stability during needle insertion. By stabilizing the tissues surrounding the acupuncture point, the practitioner minimizes the risk of unintended movement, discomfort, or pain during needling. This technique is particularly valuable when dealing with points located in areas with varying tissue densities or when targeting points that are sensitive or prone to movement.

Incorporating the "Puncturing hand" and "Pressing hand" techniques into acupuncture practice showcases the practitioner's ability to harmonize the physical act of needle insertion with the intention to restore the balance of body and mind.

Insertion Technique: Inserting the Needle with One Hand (See Fig. 3.2)

The method of single-handed needle insertion, as the name suggests, involves inserting the acupuncture needle using a single hand. While seemingly straightforward, the technique lies in the practitioner's ability to merge technique, intention, and anatomical awareness to create a harmonious and effective needling experience.

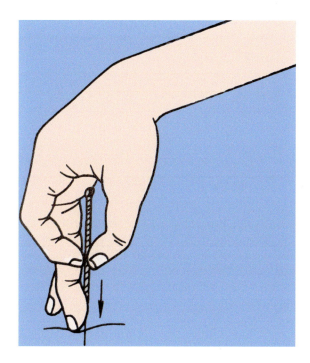

Fig. 3.2 Inserting the needle with one hand

Technique: Single-handed needle insertion demands a choreography that melds skill and mindfulness (it is called "shou shen" in Chinese). The practitioner holds the acupuncture needle between their thumb, index, and middle fingers of one hand. With gentle yet purposeful control, they guide the needle's entry into the designated acupuncture point. The supporting hand stabilizes the surrounding tissue, ensuring that the insertion is smooth and controlled [2].

The significance of single-handed needle insertion extends beyond its apparent simplicity. This technique allows for a heightened sensory connection between the practitioner and the patient's body. As the practitioner's hand guides the needle's path, their fingertips become attuned to the body's subtle responses, aiding in precise needle placement.

Advantages of Single-Handed Needle Insertion

Precision Single-handed insertion facilitates precise targeting of acupuncture points, which is crucial for optimizing therapeutic outcomes. The practitioner's tactile awareness aids in navigating meridians and tissues accurately.
Comfort: Patients often experience greater comfort during single-handed needle insertion due to the controlled and focused approach. The steady yet gentle touch of the practitioner's hand minimizes discomfort or sudden movements.
Efficiency: The seamless integration of technique and intention streamlines the needling process. This can be especially advantageous when treating multiple points during a session.

2 Insertion Technique: Inserting the Needle with Both Hands

In the practice of acupuncture, the technique of inserting the needle with both hands, the puncturing and pressing hands, represents a coordinated precision.

2.1 *Zhi Qie Fa: Inserting the Needle Aided by Pressure from the Pressing Hand*

The Zhi Qie Fa technique is a practice of harmony between the puncturing hand and the pressing hand. As the needle is gently guided into the acupuncture point by the puncturing hand, the finger of the pressing hand exerts subtle pressure on the skin around the insertion site. This method ensures precise needle placement and minimizes tissue resistance, allowing for smooth entry and a comfortable experience for the patient.

Basic Needling

2.2 Jia Chi Fa: Inserting the Needle by Coordinating the Puncturing and Pressing Hands

Jia Chi Fa embodies a synchronized approach to needle insertion. Both hands, working in tandem, seamlessly execute the technique. The puncturing hand gently guides the needle's entry, while the pressing hand provides delicate support to stabilize the surrounding tissue.

2.3 Ti Nie Fa: Inserting the Needle by Pinching Up the Skin (See Fig. 3.3)

Ti Nie Fa, characterized by its distinctive pinching motion, adds a unique dimension to needle insertion. The puncturing hand pinches up a small fold of skin around the acupuncture point before inserting the needle. This pinch creates a slight elevation, enhancing needle entry accuracy and reducing discomfort. This technique is particularly valuable when targeting points located in areas with varying tissue densities.

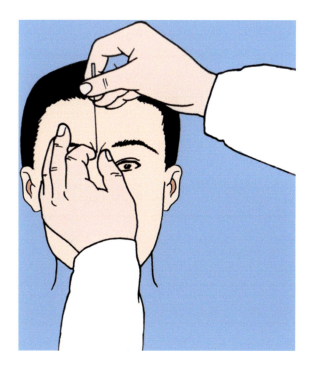

Fig. 3.3 Inserting the needle by pinching up the skin

2.4 Shu Zhang Fa: Inserting the Needle by Stretching the Skin (See Fig. 3.4)

Shu Zhang Fa encompasses a technique of stretching the skin before needle insertion. The puncturing hand gently stretches the skin taut around the intended acupuncture point. This tension allows for enhanced visibility and accessibility to the point, ensuring precise needle placement. Shu Zhang Fa is often favored when needling points are situated in regions where skin laxity might otherwise pose a challenge [3].

3 Angle and Depth of Needle Insertion (See Fig. 3.5)

The three primary insertion angles —Perpendicular, Oblique, and Horizontal —each carry a distinct purpose, facilitating optimal needle placement for different points and conditions [4].

Perpendicular Insertion

Perpendicular insertion is characterized by a direct and vertical approach (90°), with the needle inserted perpendicular to the skin's surface. This angle is commonly chosen when needling points are located on the limbs or trunk and require deep penetration to access the underlying meridians. The perpendicular angle is particularly effective for points where the depth to the target is relatively consistent.

Example: Nei Guan (PC-6)

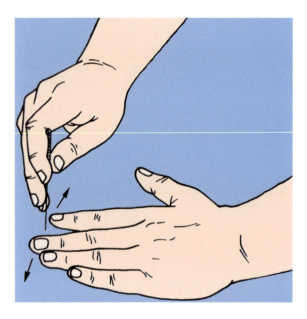

Fig. 3.4 Inserting the needle by stretching the skin

Fig. 3.5 Angles of needle insertion

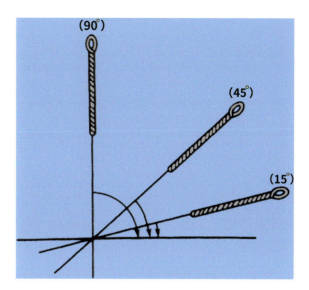

Nei Guan, PC-6, is a point frequently used for nausea and vomiting. To access this point, a perpendicular insertion angle is employed. The needle is inserted directly through the skin, penetrating to the desired depth along the pericardium meridian. The perpendicular approach ensures that the needle reaches the intended target area, allowing for optimal therapeutic effect.

Oblique Insertion

Oblique insertion involves inserting the needle at an angle, usually approximately 45°, to the skin's surface. This angle is often selected for points located along the meridian pathways, allowing the practitioner to follow or against the energetic flow. Oblique insertion can be advantageous when points are located near tendons, ligaments, or bone, as it offers a pathway that minimizes interference with these structures.

Example: Yang Ling Quan (GB-34)

Yang Ling Quan, GB- 34, is an important point for treating musculoskeletal and tendon issues such as knee pain. When needling GB34, an oblique angle is chosen to follow the gallbladder meridian's trajectory. This angle ensures that the needle glides smoothly along the meridian, addressing the energy imbalance in the affected area.

Horizontal Insertion

Horizontal insertion involves inserting the needle parallel to the skin's surface, typically at a shallow depth. This angle is often employed for points located on the head, face, and neck, where the skin is thinner and points are relatively superficial. Horizontal insertion is also favored for points that require a broader therapeutic impact over a larger area.

Example: Shuai Gu (GB-8)

Shuai Gu (GB-8) is situated on top of the ears. For needling Shuai Gu (GB-8), a horizontal insertion angle is utilized due to the point's location on the head and the thinner skin in this area. The shallow insertion aims to stimulate the local energy flow and address conditions such as headache and eye discomfort.

4 Direction of Needle Insertion

The direction of needle insertion determine the course of Qi flow along the body's meridians. The orientation of the needle—whether along the meridian, against the meridian's flow, or directed toward specific points—is a vital consideration that integrates anatomical understanding, meridian pathways, and treatment objectives [3].

Along or Against the Meridian

Inserting the needle along the meridian involves aligning the needle parallel to the meridian's trajectory. This approach is often employed to stimulate the flow of Qi along a specific meridian, addressing imbalances related to that meridian's functions. For instance, needling along the gallbladder meridian's path can aid in resolving issues related to gallbladder and liver functions (tonifying function).

On the other hand, inserting the needle against the meridian's flow involves needling in a direction opposite to the natural flow of Qi. This technique is often employed to redirect stagnant or blocked energy and to promote a rebalancing effect (reducing function). When targeting points along the stomach meridian for digestive concerns, inserting against the meridian's flow can aid in promoting smoother digestion.

Pointing the Needle for Safety

In certain cases, the direction of needle insertion is chosen for safety reasons. Points that are located near vulnerable structures, such as eyes, internal organs, blood vessels or nerves, may require specific orientations to minimize the risk of injury. For instance, when needling the Feng Chi (GB-20) point, which is situated at the base of the skull, the needle tip should point but no higher than the tip of the nose. This orientation ensures that the needle is safely inserted without risking contact with sensitive areas.

Inserting the Needle Based on Treatment Requirements

The third direction of needle insertion involves pointing the needle based on the treatment requirements. When addressing specific health issues, practitioners may choose to direct the needle toward the location of the ailment or discomfort. For example, when BL40 (Weizhong) is chosen to treat lower back pain or sciatica, the direction of needle insertion is toward the location of the lower back or sciatica, which is called the Zhen (needle) zhi (reach) bing (disease) suo (location) in Acupuncture.

Basic Needling

Depth of Needle Insertion in Acupuncture
The depth of needle insertion requires a delicate balance between precision and intuition. The depth at which a needle is inserted can greatly influence the therapeutic outcome, and several factors come into play when determining the optimal depth.

Constitution
The constitution of a patient plays a pivotal role in determining the appropriate depth of needle insertion. Patients with a robust constitution may require slightly deeper insertions to access deeper Qi layers, while those with a delicate constitution may respond better to shallower insertions. Tailoring the depth to the patient's constitution ensures a harmonious balance between the needle's influence and the body's response.

Patient Age
Patient age is another critical factor in depth determination. Children and the elderly tend to have more delicate tissues, necessitating shallower insertions. The energetic vitality of young people may allow for slightly deeper insertions, while aging tissues may require gentler approaches. Adapting the depth based on age ensures patient comfort and safety while optimizing therapeutic outcomes.

Anatomic Location to Needle
The body is a landscape of diverse tissue densities and structures. The depth of needle insertion must account for these variations. Points located near bones, tendons, or sensitive structures may require shallower insertions to prevent injury, while points situated within muscular areas may permit slightly deeper penetration.

Depth of meridians
The depth of the meridians beneath the skin's surface varies across the body. Deeper meridians may require deeper insertions to effectively access the energy flow, while more superficial meridians may respond well to shallower insertions. The acupuncturist's knowledge of meridian depths guides them in choosing the depth that ensures optimal interaction with the energetic pathways.

Nature of the Disease
The nature of the disease being treated also influences the depth of needle insertion. Conditions with deeper-seated imbalances or chronic issues may call for deeper insertions to access underlying energy blockages. Acute conditions or superficial-level disturbances may benefit from shallower insertions that stimulate immediate responses. Adapting the depth to the disease's nature supports a targeted and effective approach.

Seasonal considerations
Traditional Chinese Medicine holds a profound connection between the seasons and the body's energy dynamics. During spring and summer, when energy is abundant and active, shallower insertions are favored. In contrast, during autumn and winter, when energy tends to be more internal and subdued, deeper insertions are preferred. This approach harmonizes the treatment with the natural cycles of the body and the environment.

By considering the patient's constitution, age, anatomic location, meridian depths, disease nature, and even the season, the acupuncturist crafts a treatment tailored to the individual's unique Qi landscape.

5 Basic Needling Manipulations

In acupuncture practice, two fundamental maneuvers, Lifting and Thrusting, and Rotating and Twisting, stand as pillars in this symphony, each playing a unique role in harmonizing Qi flow.

Lifting and Thrusting (See Fig. 3.6)

Lifting and Thrusting Manipulation (Ti Cha Fa) involves a delicate yet powerful rhythmic motion. To initiate this technique, the acupuncturist gently lifts the needle upward, creating a subtle separation of tissues and Qi pathways. Following the lift, a controlled thrust ensues, stimulating the Qi flow and promoting its circulation along meridians.

Lifting and Thrusting is effective for clearing stagnant Qi, alleviating pain, and enhancing Qi circulation. It is suitable for points exhibiting signs of blockage or stagnation. The technique's controlled nature makes it an excellent choice for sensitive points or patients.

Fig. 3.6 Lifting and thrusting

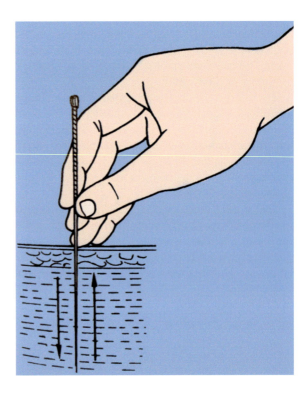

Basic Needling

The frequency of lifting and thrusting is typically approximately 60 times per minute, maintaining a rhythm that optimizes Qi movement. The needle should be kept straight during the motion, ensuring an even movement pattern. The lifting movement range should not be too large. The duration of each lifting and thrusting cycle is approximately 3–5 min, allowing sufficient time for Qi stimulation and response [5].

While lifting and thrusting is generally safe, practitioners must exercise caution around fragile tissues or points close to bones. Gentle, yet precise, movements are key to preventing discomfort or injury.

Rotating and Twisting (See Fig. 3.7)

Rotating and Twisting Manipulation (Nian Zhuan Fa) involves the rotation of the needle in a clockwise and then counterclockwise direction. This technique promotes lateral movement of Qi along meridians, enhancing the needle's interaction with the acupoints and meridians.

Rotating and twisting are valuable for harmonizing Qi flow, resolving stagnation, and promoting localized stimulation. This technique is often applied to points with underlying energy imbalances or tension [1].

Rotating and twisting can be applied in a single cycle or intermittently, depending on the intended Qi response. Frequent rotation can enhance Qi movement, while

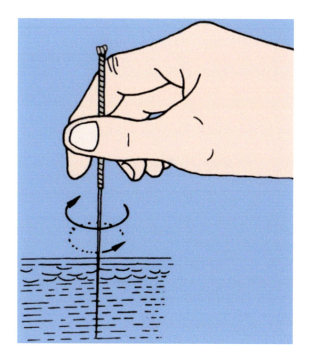

Fig. 3.7 Rotating and twisting

occasional use maintains a balanced approach. The technique should be gentle and controlled to prevent discomfort.

For rotating and twisting, the movement angle should ideally range between 180 and 360°. This ensures that the needle does not become lodged or cause discomfort. Twisting the needle in one direction should be avoided to prevent potential issues.

6 Auxiliary Needling Manipulations

6.1 Sparrow Pecking Technique

Named for the likeness of a sparrow pecking (Que Zhuo Fa) at corn, this technique was aptly named by Dr. Dan'an Cheng (承淡安). Its core function lies in facilitating Qi's arrival and promoting its circulation. Additionally, it augments the needling sensation, fostering a deeper connection with the patient's energy.

Precisely insert the needle to the designated depth. Employ a rapid, subtle thrusting motion akin to a sparrow's feeding rhythm. In this motion, the wrist subtly swing. The frequency, ranging between 150 and 300 times per minute, remains consistent. The needle's depth is retained throughout.

Distinguished from traditional lifting and thrusting, sparrow pecking employs smaller, rapid vibrations while maintaining a fixed position. This technique is suitable for regions with thin tissues, adjacent vessels, or muscle tendons where vigorous lifting and thrusting may be unsuitable.

Sparrow pecking is ideally suited for acupuncture points with thin tissues or proximity to vessels or muscle tendons. It substitutes robust lifting and thrusting in such areas. For instance, it finds application in headache management, targeting points such as BaiHui (DU20) and Touwei (ST8).

6.2 Vibrating Technique

The vibrating technique (Zhen Fa) derived from Bian Que's Spiritual Guide to Acupuncture and Moxibustion is a dynamic fusion of needle movement and energy flow. Its purpose is to usher in Qi's arrival, promote the flow of Qi, and support the deficiencies [5].

Precisely insert the needle. Should Qi be sluggish, hold the needle with the thumb and index finger. Swiftly rotate, lift, and thrust the needle, employing small amplitudes and high frequencies. Finger power dominates this technique to achieve a gentle stimulation.

Distinguished from shaking, vibrating involves quick, subtle rotations, lifts, and thrusts with limited amplitude. Unlike its counterpart, which employs forceful actions, vibrating harnesses the power of the practitioner's fingers for a mild yet potent stimulus.

Basic Needling

Vibrating resonates with muscles and nerves, rendering it versatile for various points across the body. It finds application in treating conditions ranging from indigestion with Pi Shu (BL-20) and Wei Shu (BL-21) to rhinitis with Ying Xiang (LI-20) and Cuan Zhu (BL-2).

6.3 Flying Technique

Inspired by a phoenix's wingspan, the flying technique (Fei Fa) symbolizes the spread of energies and converges with the technique of Phoenix Spreading Wings. This technique stimulate the flow of Qi and im in Qi's circulation, heightening sensations.

Ensure accurate needle insertion. Secure the needle's handle with thumb and index finger. The needle handle was gently twirled 1–3 times, swiftly releasing it. Simultaneously, spread your fingers akin to a bird's wingspan. The needle may tremor subtly on the point.

For optimal efficacy, keep the needle's rotation amplitude within 360°, avoiding excessive twirling. The direction of rotation holds no bearing on technique success.

The flying technique finds a wide berth across acupuncture points. Its versatility shines in addressing urination irregularities with Guan Yuan (RN-4), Qi Hai (RN-6), and Zhong Ji (RN-3).

6.4 Flicking Technique

Flicking is a technique that entails tapping the needle handle gently. The goal is to harmonize Qi flow, invigorate the needling sensation, and enhance the reinforcing and reducing effects.

Insert the needle accurately, achieving the Qi sensation. Employ your index or middle finger together with the thumb to tap the needle's tail horizontally, prompting incremental depth. After the initial nudge, withdraw the needle partially and repeat the process [3].

Flicking thrives on gentle stimuli. Its target points often include sensitive or delicate areas, welcoming its tender impact and it can be used for acupoints like Ming Men (GV4) and Yao Yang Guan (GV3), for low back pain.

6.5 Twirling Technique

Twirling (Xuan Fa) is to twirl the needle unidirectionally, this technique intertwines muscle fibers around the needle, imparting tension that facilitates Qi's circulation. By doing so, it amplifies the reinforcing and reducing effects while enhancing the needling sensation.

Insert the needle accurately and attain the Qi sensation (De Qi). Twirl the needle in a single direction, aligning with its purpose. Referring to "The Great Compendium of Acupuncture and Moxibustion", the direction of twirling forward or backward is defined as reinforcing or reducing. This motion was repeated three to five times during needle retention.

Differing intensities of twirling produce distinct sensations. Light twirling, with slow rotations within 180°, evokes gentle local sensation. Conversely, heavy twirling with rapid rotations encompassing 360° elicits strong needling sensations.

Twirling's applicability spans the head, neck, limbs, abdomen, and more. Points such as Jian Yu (LI-15), Qu Chi (LI-11), Huan Tiao (GB-30), Nei Guan (PC-6), and Ju Que (RN-14) were used for palpitations.

6.6 Scraping Technique: (see Fig. 3.8)

With the needle is in place, its depth is precise, and the operation begins. Scraping (Gua Fa) unfolds with one hand, where the thumb meets the needle's end, and the nail index or middle finger glides in fluid motion from zenith to nadir or in reverse.

In an alternative approach, the handle is gripped by the thumb and middle finger, while the index finger manipulates the nail. In this hand configuration, one thumb supports the end of the needle, while the other thumb, along with arched index fingers, encircles the body of the needle.

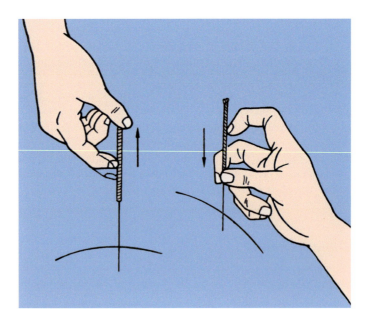

Fig. 3.8 Scraping technique

Basic Needling

Scraping can be applied on points surrounding eyes and ears, even fingers and toes—where the tissue is delicately thin, such as Ting Gong (SI-19), Ting Hui (GB-2), and Yi Feng (SJ-17), to alleviates deafness and tinnitus [1].

6.7 Shaking Technique

Within the hands of the practitioner, the needle finds a balance between the thumb and index finger. As it ascends from deep to shallow realms, a gentle cadence takes form. The needle is swayed in four directions—up, down, left, and right. In this way, the hole widens, a gateway for pathogenic factors to escape. The methods of reduction follow, maintaining this open passage [1].

In the acupuncture clinical practice, shaking (Yao Fa) is used for excess heat syndrome. For example, Qu Chi (LI-11) and Da Zhui (DU-14) reduce heat and fire. Tai Yang (Ex-HN-5), He Gu (LI-4), and Tai Chong (LV-3) relieve acute conjunctivitis.

6.8 Tapping Technique

Guided by intention, the needle reaches the acupuncture point. Once Qi's presence is palpable, the technique of tapping (Kou Fa) begins. Fingers become gentle drummers, tapping the needle's tail vertically. Each beat carries the needle deeper, layer by layer, until a certain depth is reached.

In the clinical practice, tapping technique is applied in the arms and legs, where tissues stand strong, such as Huan Tiao (GB-30) to Feng Shi (GB-31), Yang Ling Quan (GB-34), Wei Zhong (BL-40), and Cheng Shan (BL-57), tapping alleviates sciatic pain's grip.

7 De Qi

7.1 The Definition of De Qi

De Qi, a fundamental concept in acupuncture, involves the interaction between patient and practitioner during the needling process. Translated as "obtaining the qi" or "arrival of qi," De Qi encompasses subjective sensations, bodily responses, and the acupuncturist's perception. It is considered as the sign of effective stimulation of needles.

Essentially, De Qi marks the moment when the acupuncture needle engages with the meridians, evoking sensations ranging from tingling, warmth, heaviness, soreness, and fullness to distension and occasionally, mild ache (in Chinese they are called Suan, Ma, Zhang, Zhong, Tong).

7.2 The Significance of De Qi

The significance of De Qi extends beyond a mere physiological response; it acts as a gateway to therapeutic efficacy. When De Qi is appropriately achieved, it marks the activation of the body's innate regulatory mechanisms, fostering physiological responses. One of its primary roles lies in enhancing the flow of Qi and blood through the meridians, opening blockages, and restoring balance. This, in turn, stimulates the body's self-healing capacities.

From the viewpoint of modern medical science, De Qi's profound effects also touch upon the autonomic nervous system. As De Qi takes hold, it triggers parasympathetic responses, leading to a state of deep relaxation. This relaxation, in turn, fosters a harmonious balance between the sympathetic and parasympathetic nervous systems, creating an optimal environment for healing.

Acupuncturists often strive to attain De Qi, as it is believed that its absence might limit the potential healing effects of acupuncture treatment. Traditionally, it is believed that for acupuncture treatment, if the De Qi arrives late, the therapeutic effect comes later as well. If the De Qi arrives quickly, the therapeutic effect comes sooner. If Qi does not arrive, there is no treatment effect.

7.3 Factors that May Influence De Qi

De Qi's manifestation is influenced by multiple factors.

- One pivotal aspect is the acupuncturist's skill and technique. Skillful needle manipulation, with a focus on gentle twirling, lifting, and thrusting, enhances the likelihood of eliciting a balanced De Qi response.
- The depth, angle, and manipulation of the needle contribute to the quality and intensity of De Qi.
- The patient's constitution also shapes the De Qi experience. Factors such as sensitivity, pain threshold, and the body's energetic state play a role. Patients with heightened sensitivity might experience De Qi more intensely, while those with more robust constitutions might require more substantial stimulation.
- The choice of acupuncture points plays a role in influencing De Qi. Certain points are inherently more responsive, while others might require specific techniques to elicit De Qi effectively.

- The patient-practitioner rapport contributes to the De Qi experience. An environment of trust, relaxation, and open communication can facilitate the patient's perception of sensations and contribute to a more profound De Qi experience.

8 Tonifying and Reducing Techniques in Acupuncture

Both tonifying and reducing manipulations play integral roles in acupuncture therapy, contributing to the restoration of balance within the body's meridian system. Skillfully adapting these techniques to the patient's constitution, deficiency or excess type, and acupoint selection is crucial for achieving optimal therapeutic outcomes in acupuncture practice.

8.1 Tonifying Manipulations

Definition

Tonifying manipulations in acupuncture are specialized needling techniques designed to enhance the body's antipathogenic Qi, stimulate the function of deficient organs, restore balance within the meridian system, and harmonize the imbalance of two internal organs. These techniques aim to invigorate Qi and reinforce the body's resistance against ailments.

How to Operate the Needles

Tonifying manipulations are characterized by their gentle and nurturing approach and needling techniques that are slow, deliberate, and subtle to ensure harmonious stimulation of the acupuncture points. The manipulation involves inserting the needle to the desired depth and then employing gentle lifting, thrusting, and rotating motions. The needle is manipulated with care, emphasizing minimal discomfort for the patient.

Influential Factors

Several factors influence the efficacy of tonifying manipulations:

- Patient Constitution: The patient's overall constitution, including physical and mind strength, guides the acupuncturist in tailoring the intensity of tonifying manipulations.
- Excess or deficiency of the disease: Diseases in deficiency pattern, such as Qi deficiency, blood deficiency, Yin deficiency or Yang deficiency, are relatively easier to achieve tonification effect, by selecting appropriate points for tonification and determining the suitable stimulating quantity of manipulation.
- Needle Gauge and Length: The choice of needle gauge and length affects the sensation experienced by the patient and the depth of needle insertion. Fine-gauge needles are often preferred for tonifying manipulations due to their gentle nature.

- Acupoint Selection: The selection of acupuncture points is crucial. Points associated with deficient organs and meridians, Ren Mai, Du Mai, Bladder meridian are chosen to ensure targeted tonification.

8.2 Reducing Manipulations

Definition

Reducing manipulations in acupuncture are specialized techniques aimed at dispersing excess Qi, eliminating pathogens, and mitigating hyperactive functions. These manipulations serve to restore balance by reducing excesses and restoring optimal Qi flow.

How to Operate the Needles

Reducing manipulations are characterized by their swift, forceful, and prolonged actions on the acupuncture points. Acupuncturists employ techniques that involve rapid lifting, thrusting, and rotating movements. The intention is to provoke a stronger response from the body's Qi to alleviate excess conditions.

Influential Factors

Several factors influence the effectiveness of reducing manipulations:

- Patient Sensitivity: The patient's sensitivity to needling and their overall constitution guide the acupuncturist in determining the intensity of reducing manipulations.
- Excess or deficiency of the disease: Identifying the nature of excess, whether it is excess heat, dampness, or stagnation, assists in selecting appropriate points and manipulating techniques.
- Needle Gauge and Length: The choice of needle gauge and length influences the intensity of sensation and depth of needle insertion. Thicker needles may be chosen to elicit a stronger response.
- Acupoint Selection: Selecting acupuncture points associated with the excess condition is vital to achieving the desired outcome of reducing manipulations, often choosing acupoints from yang meridians, Lower He-Sea points, Ying-Spring points etc.

8.3 Common Practical Tonifying and Reducing Manipulations

A. Tonifying and Reducing by Rotating and Twisting (Nian Zhuan Bu Xie) [2]

Tonifying

When aiming to tonify the body's insufficiency, acupuncture practitioners employ a rotating and twisting technique. After achieving the De Qi sensation, the needle is gently and slowly rotated within a small range and for a short duration. This gentle rotation stimulates the acupuncture point and promotes the flow of Qi and blood, enhancing the body's vitality.

Reducing

Conversely, the reducing technique focuses on calming hyperfunctioning areas or dispersing excess pathogenic factors. This involves rapid and forceful rotation of the needle within a larger range and for a longer duration. This vigorous rotation helps disperse stagnation, clear excess, and regulate the body's energetic balance.

B. **Tonifying and Reducing by Lifting and Thrusting (Ti Cha Bu Xie)** [5]

Tonifying

In the tonification process, the needle is manipulated to strengthen weak or deficient areas. To achieve this, the needle is thrust deeply and lifted gently. This action stimulates the acupuncture point and tonifies the body's Qi, nourishing the affected area.

Reducing

For reduction, where the goal is to reduce excess or pathogenic factors, the needle is lifted vigorously and thrust gently. This combination of actions helps disperse accumulated Qi and promote the flow of Qi, aiding in the elimination of excess or harmful substances such as dampness, phlegm, blood stasis.

C. **Tonifying and Reducing Obtained by Rapid and Slow Insertion and Withdrawal (Xu Ji Bu Xie)**

Tonifying

A gradual approach characterizes tonification, involving slow insertion of the needle with minimal rotation. This gentle insertion technique allows the body to slowly adjust to the needle's presence. During withdrawal, the process is rapid, which helps stimulate the point and maintain the tonification effect.

Reducing

To achieve reduction, the needle is inserted rapidly with more rotation. This approach encourages a strong response from the body, promoting the movement of Qi and facilitating the elimination of excess or harmful energy. During withdrawal, the process is slower to further enhance the reduction effect.

D. **Tonifying and Reducing Achieved by Directing Needle Tip (Ying Sui Bu Xie)** [3]

Tonifying

When tonifying, the needle tip's movement follows the meridian's natural course. This technique aligns with the body's Qi flow, allowing the tonification effect to reach the target Zang Fu organs and meridians.

Reducing

In contrast, during reduction, the needle tip is directed against the meridian's course. This opposing movement aims to dispel the Qi stagnation and reduce the excess pathogenic factors or pathogenic products.

E. **Tonifying and Reducing Method by Means of Patient's Respiration (Hu Xi Bu Xie)**

Tonifying

In tonification, the needle is inserted when the patient inhales, aligning the Qi's flow with the body's natural rhythm. This method enhances the tonifying effect by synchronizing with the body's internal processes.

Reducing

For reduction, the needle is inserted during exhalation. This technique complements the body's natural movement of energy, assisting in the expulsion of excess or harmful factors.

F. **Tonifying and Reducing Achieved by Keeping Puncture-Hole Open or Closed (Kai He Bu Xie)**

Tonifying

The tonification technique involves applying pressure to the puncture hole immediately upon needle withdrawal. This action encourages the body to absorb the stimulation of needles and effects of the acupuncture treatment, reinforcing the tonification process.

Reducing

In reduction, the needle is manipulated to shake and enlarge the puncture hole upon withdrawal. This helps release any accumulated pathogenic factors or excessive pathogenic products, aiding in the reduction effect.

G. **Even Tonifying and Reducing (Ping Bu Ping Xie)**

In this comprehensive approach, practitioners combine various techniques to achieve balanced tonification and reduction effects. After achieving De Qi, practitioners execute moderate-speed lifting, thrusting, twisting, and rotating actions before withdrawing the needle. This synergistic approach maximizes the therapeutic impact by addressing both tonification and reduction needs simultaneously.

H. **Setting the Mountain on Fire (Shao Shan Huo): A Complex Manipulation of Tonifying and Reducing** [1]

"Setting the mountain on fire" is an acupuncture technique that tonifies methods to address conditions of a deficient-cold nature, such as wind-cold-damp obstructive

Basic Needling

joint pain. This method involves a precise sequence of needle insertion, rotation, and thrusting, meticulously tailored to promote healing and balance.

Procedure:

1. Begin by inserting the needle superficially to approximately one-third of the needed depth, representing the "Heaven" level.
2. Once the De Qi sensation is achieved, rotate the needle using the reinforcing technique.
3. Thrust the needle to the medium region, reaching approximately two-thirds of the needed depth, symbolizing the "Man" level.
4. Rotate the needle again using the reinforcing technique upon sensing the needle sensation.
5. Thrust the needle to the deep region, representing the "Earth" level, while applying reinforcing rotation.
6. After De Qi, slowly lift the needle back to the superficial region.
7. Repeat this sequence thrice, progressing from superficial to deep and back, reinforcing with rotation at each stage.
8. Finally, thrust the needle to the needed depth and retain it. Employ reinforcing by means of the patient's breathing during the operation for added effect.

9. **Penetrating Heaven's Coolness (Tou Tian Liang): A Complex Manipulation of Tonifying and Reducing** [1]

"Penetrating the heaven's coolness" is an acupuncture technique designed to address conditions of excess heat nature, including acute carbuncles and Bi syndrome of the heat type. This complex manipulation combines tonifying and reducing approaches to restore balance and promote healing.

Procedure:

1. Thrust the needle deeply to the needed depth, entering the "deep region—Earth".
2. Upon achieving the De Qi sensation, rotate the needle using the reducing technique.
3. Lift the needle rapidly back to the medium region—Man, applying reducing rotation after De Qi.
4. Continue by lifting the needle swiftly to the superficial region—Heaven, rotating with the reducing technique after De Qi.
5. Finally, thrust the needle slowly into the deep region—Earth, employing reducing rotation after De Qi.
6. Repeat this sequence thrice, consistently transitioning from deep to superficial regions—Heaven while maintaining reduced rotation.
7. Rapidly lift the needle to the superficial region- Heaven and retain it to conclude the manipulation.
8. Utilize the reducing method by means of the patient's respiration during the procedure for enhanced effectiveness.

9 Stimulation Quantity and Therapeutic Effects of Acupuncture

The concept of stimulation quantity forms a fundamental aspect of acupuncture, delineating the relationship between the degree of needle manipulation and the therapeutic effects achieved. In acupuncture practice, achieving the optimal balance of stimulation is crucial for achieving the desired therapeutic outcomes. This balance is determined by factors such as needle depth, manipulation techniques, and duration of retention.

The Interplay of Stimulation Quantity

A. **Mild stimulation** (Qing Ci Ji): Gentle needling techniques with minimal manipulation evoke a mild response from the body. This type of stimulation is often utilized in tonifying treatments, where the goal is to nourish and harmonize the body. Mild stimulation techniques are applied in cases of deficiency or sensitive patients, providing a gentle boost to the body's inherent healing capacities.
B. **Moderate Stimulation** (Zhōng Ci Ji): A moderate level of stimulation involves a combination of techniques that invoke a balanced response from the body. This level of manipulation is commonly used in treating a wide range of conditions, promoting Qi and blood circulation, alleviating stagnation, and encouraging the body's self-regulatory mechanisms. The therapeutic effects obtained from moderate stimulation are versatile and adaptable to various clinical scenarios.
C. **Strong Stimulation** (Zhòng Ci Ji): Employing vigorous and forceful manipulation techniques generates a strong stimulation response. These techniques are often chosen for reducing treatments aimed at dispersing excess or stagnation. Strong stimulation can provoke a more intense physiological response, promoting the clearance of pathogenic factors and encouraging the body to rebalance itself.

Tonification and Reduction: For tonifying treatments, a milder form of stimulation is preferred to invigorate the body, enhance its antipathogenic Qi, and reinforce deficiency. Reductive effects, on the other hand, are achieved through stronger stimulation methods that disperse excessive, alleviate pain, and promote harmonization.

Harmonization and Dispersal: Conditions characterized by imbalances, such as disharmony of the heart and kidney and disharmony of the liver and spleen, require a harmonizing effect, which is achieved through moderate stimulation to promote equilibrium and address underlying disharmony. Conversely, conditions marked by stagnation or excess benefit from stronger stimulation techniques that help disperse accumulations, relieve obstructions, and restore the free flow of Qi.

Enhancing Circulation and Nourishment: Stimulation quantity directly influences the circulation of Qi and blood. Mild and moderate stimulation facilitate gentle circulation, whereas strong stimulation can break through stagnation and enhance blood flow to nourish tissues and internal organs as well as pacify the mind and emotions.

10 Retaining and Withdrawing the Needle in Acupuncture

Retaining the Needle

Retaining the needle: it indicates of leaving the inserted needle within the acupuncture point. This approach extends the therapeutic interaction, fortifying the impact of the treatment while allowing for ongoing manipulation. Typically, the needle is retained for 15–30 min following the De Qi sensation. However, certain conditions warrant extended retention periods, sometimes spanning over an hour. For instance, acute abdominal pain, or stubborn cold-induced pain exemplify scenarios where prolonged retention is applied. During this span, periodic manipulation sustains and enhances the treatment's influence, mostly 3–5 times needling manipulating. If the De Qi sensation is not immediate, patient quiet fosters the arrival of Qi. The duration of needle retention depend on the patient constitution and the nature of the disease [2].

Manipulative Techniques During Retention

During the retention phase, reinforcing and reducing methods are employed to optimize treatment outcomes. Manipulating the needle at intervals serves to bolster and consolidate the therapeutic effects. This dynamics exchange between the practitioner, patient, and needles.

Withdrawing the Needle

Withdrawing the needle: gently pressing the skin surrounding the point, followed by gentle rotation of the needle. Gradually lifting the needle to the subcutaneous level ensures minimal discomfort. A swift withdrawal followed, accompanied by a sterile cotton ball to prevent bleeding. Should strategies involving rapid or slow insertion and withdrawal or maintaining the puncture hole be employed, needle withdrawal adheres to these principles. Diligence in counting needles ensures that none are inadvertently left behind. It is advisable to stay in the acupuncture bed for 3–5 min and then get up, and a brief resting period allows the patient to assimilate the treatment before departing.

Review Questions

1. What are the distinguishing features between the Puncturing hand and Pressing hand techniques in acupuncture needle insertion?
2. How do the depth, angle, and direction of needle insertion vary based on factors such as patient constitution, anatomical location, and disease nature?
3. What role does De Qi play in the therapeutic efficacy of acupuncture, and how is it achieved?

4. Explain the differences between tonifying and reducing techniques in acupuncture and how they adapt to a patient's condition.

References

1. Qiu ML. Chinese acupuncture and moxibustion. 1st ed. London: Churchill Liverstone; 1993.
2. Wang H, Du YH. Zhen Jiu Xue. 3rd ed. Beijing: China TCM Publishing House; 2012.
3. Liang FR, Wang H. Zhen Jiu Xue. 4th ed. Beijing: China TCM Publishing House; 2018.
4. Liu Y. Diagrams of acupuncture. 1st ed. Shanghai: Shanghai Scien&Tech Pulishing House; 2003.
5. Yang JS. Zhen Jiu Xue. 1st ed. Beijing: People's Publishing House; 1989.

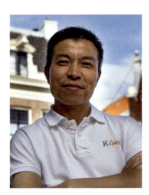

Prof. Dr. Weixiang Wang (王维祥) A PhD graduate of Nanjing University of Chinese Medicine (NJUCM), has played a pivotal role in advancing TCM in the Netherlands. Formerly serving at the Second Clinical College of NJUCM until 2003, he co-founded the European Academy of Traditional Medical Science and currently act as the academic dean of the Dutch Acupuncture Academy (DAA). With a rich background, Dr. Wang has led the Dutch Association of TCM (NVTCG Zhong) as chairman for six years, contributing an additional three years as a board member. Additionally, he serves as an executive member of the European Association of TCM (ETCMA). Driven by a commitment to elevate educational standards and integrate TCM into healthcare systems, his lectures on the integrative practice of TCM are highly sought-after in academic institutions and TCM congresses. An accomplished author, Dr. Wang has written and co-authored 11 TCM books in China since the commencement of his TCM career in 1989. Currently practicing at Klinic in Amsterdam, he holds the prestigious position of president for one of the most influential TCM events, the International Dutch TCM Congress (DTCMC).

Prevention and Management of Possible Accidents in Acupuncture Practice

Lin Chen

Learning Objectives

1. Identify potential accidents during acupuncture practice, such as fainting, stuck or bent needles, hematomas, and rare internal organ injuries.
2. Understand the manifestations and management strategies for each type of accident to ensure prompt and effective responses.
3. Apply preventive measures, including meticulous needle insertion, patient assessment, and maintaining a hygienic environment, to minimize risks and enhance patient safety during acupuncture sessions.

Acupuncture, known for its therapeutic effects, requires a careful approach to ensure the safety of both the practitioner and the patient. Practitioners should have a thorough understanding of potential accidents and the precautionary measures to prevent or effectively manage them.

Accidents that can occur in acupuncture practice encompass a range of scenarios, from mild discomfort to more serious complications. Fainting during acupuncture, although relatively rare, is one such occurrence that demands attention. Stuck, bent, or broken needles, while infrequent, can also arise and warrant careful consideration. Hematomas and injuries to internal organs, although uncommon, highlight the importance of skilful techniques and precise needle placement.

To ensure a safe and effective acupuncture practice, practitioners must be equipped with the knowledge and skills to prevent and manage these potential accidents. Diligent needle insertion techniques, thorough patient assessment, and close monitoring during treatment sessions are essential steps to mitigate risks. Additionally, understanding the patient's medical history, informing them about potential sensations, and maintaining a hygienic environment contribute to a safer acupuncture experience.

L. Chen (✉)
Klinic, Oude Waal 6h, 1011 BX Amsterdam, The Netherlands
e-mail: jadechenlin@gmail.com

1 Loss of Consciousness During Acupuncture [1]

Acupuncture offers numerous health benefits by harmonizing the body's yin and yang energies. While generally safe, uncommon incidents such as loss of consciousness during acupuncture, commonly referred to as acupuncture fainting, can occur. Understanding the factors contributing to this phenomenon, recognizing its manifestations, implementing effective management strategies, and prioritizing preventive measures are all essential for providing patients with a secure and comfortable acupuncture experience.

Loss of consciousness during acupuncture can be attributed to various triggers. Delicate constitution, nervousness, fatigue, hunger, excessive sweating, severe diarrhoea, improper positioning, and overly forceful needle manipulation are among the factors that can contribute to this reaction.

The signs of loss of consciousness during acupuncture are distinctive and encompass sudden fatigue, dizziness, vertigo, pallid complexion, restlessness, nausea, profuse sweating, palpitations, cold extremities, a drop in blood pressure, a deep and feeble pulse, fainting, collapsing, bluish lips and nails, involuntary bowel or urinary movements, and an extremely weak pulse.

Swift and effective management is crucial when loss of consciousness occurs during acupuncture. The practitioner should promptly withdraw all needles. The patient should be assisted in reclining and kept warm. In less severe instances, offering the patient warm water or water with sugar can help alleviate the symptoms. Typically, the symptoms will naturally abate. In more severe cases, along with the aforementioned steps, specific acupuncture points such as Shuigou (Du-26), Suliao (Du-25), Neiguan (Pc-6), and Zusanli (St-36) can be needled, and moxibustion can be applied to Baihui (Du-20), Guanyuan (Ren-4), and Qihai (RN-6). These measures are generally effective in eliciting a response from the patient.

Should the patient remain unconscious despite these efforts, displaying weak respiration and a faint pulse, further medical intervention or emergency measures should be considered.

Preventing loss of consciousness during acupuncture is paramount. Patients who are new to acupuncture, oversensitive, or have a delicate constitution should be provided with a clear explanation of the procedure to alleviate any apprehensions. Opting for a comfortable position, such as lying down, is advisable. Using fewer acupuncture points and employing gentle techniques are prudent choices, especially for patients who may be hungry, fatigued, or thirsty.

Throughout the procedure, the practitioner should attentively observe the patient's mental state and inquire about any discomfort. Being attuned to the initial indications of potential loss of consciousness empowers the practitioner to take swift preventive actions.

While occurrences of loss of consciousness during acupuncture are infrequent, practitioners should be well prepared to address them appropriately. By understanding the causes, recognizing the signs, implementing effective management strategies, and prioritizing preventive measures, practitioners can ensure the safety of the patients during the acupuncture sessions.

2 Stuck Needles in Acupuncture [1, 2]

While the safety of acupuncture is widely acknowledged, occasional situations such as needles becoming lodged during or after acupuncture sessions can emerge. It is imperative to grasp the underlying causes of stuck needles, discern their indications, implement adept management strategies, and emphasize proactive precautions. Doing so not only guarantees smooth and soothing acupuncture treatment but also underscores the practitioner's commitment to patient care and safety.

Stuck needles, also referred to as trapped needles, occur when the practitioner encounters resistance while manipulating the needle or during its retention. This sensation of being stuck around the needle can hinder its rotation, lifting, thrusting, or withdrawal. Such instances may stem from factors such as patient nervousness, strong muscle contractions upon needle insertion, imperfect manipulation techniques, or excessively prolonged needle retention.

When needles become stuck, both the practitioner and the patient may experience distinct signs. The practitioner might find it challenging to perform the intended needle movements or withdraw the needles, while the patient could feel intense pain or discomfort at the needle site.

Addressing stuck needles requires prompt and skillful intervention. If the needle is stuck due to muscle contractions, allowing some time for the muscle to relax might be effective. Alternatively, gently massaging the surrounding skin, carefully plucking the needle handle, or inserting another needle nearby to disperse qi and blood can release muscle tension.

If the needle becomes trapped due to imperfect manipulation, such as twirling in a single direction, corrective actions are necessary. Twirling the needle in the opposite direction while simultaneously plucking and scraping the handle can help release the muscle fibres and facilitate the needle's movement.

Preventing stuck needles hinges on careful measures taken during acupuncture procedures. Patients who are more sensitive should be encouraged to relax before and during the session. Practitioners must exercise caution to avoid rotating the needle solely in one direction during manipulation. Incorporating a combination of twirling, lifting, and thrusting movements during needle manipulation can help prevent entanglement with muscle fibres.

3 Bent Needles [1]

The occurrence of bent needles can present an uncommon yet noteworthy challenge in acupuncture practice. This occurrence, although infrequent, demands a comprehensive understanding of its causes, identification of related signs, implementation of effective management techniques, and adoption of preventive measures.

The phenomenon of bent needles stems from a constellation of factors that can disrupt the intended trajectory of an acupuncture session. Factors may include insufficiently refined manipulation techniques, overly forceful or hasty actions, inadvertent contact with dense tissues, abrupt alterations in the patient's position, or even external pressures exerted on the needle itself.

Recognizing a bent needle involves a convergence of tactile feedback and patient response. An acupuncturist may sense resistance or an abnormal curvature during manipulation, hindering the needle's intended movements. Meanwhile, the patient may experience discomfort or pain, signaling a departure from the expected sensations associated with acupuncture.

In the presence of a bent needle, a judicious approach to management is paramount. Immediate cessation of further attempts to lift, thrust, or rotate the needle is recommended to prevent exacerbation of the issue. The degree of curvature informs the subsequent steps. Slightly bent needles should be cautiously withdrawn at a steady pace to minimize patient discomfort. In instances of acute bending, the withdrawal should follow the trajectory of the curve, ensuring a methodical and gentle extraction. When positional changes result in bending, restoring the patient's original posture and alleviating local muscle tension can facilitate safe needle removal.

Preventing bent needles hinges on a fusion of procedural precision and precautionary measures. Rigorous adherence to appropriate insertion techniques and the application of controlled finger pressure (Pressing hand) helps avert unintended bending. Caution should be exercised to avoid undue haste or forcefulness in needle manipulation. The selection of an optimal patient position and the advice for the patient to remain motionless during the needle retention phase play pivotal roles in preventing abrupt curvatures. Furthermore, guarding the needle against external pressures safeguards its integrity and effectiveness throughout the acupuncture session.

4 Broken Needles [2]

The concept of broken needles represents an infrequent yet important concern. Amid needle insertion and manipulation, the possibility of needle fracturing inside the body underscores the importance of meticulous preparation and attentive practice.

Broken needles, an uncommon but potential outcome in acupuncture, trace their origins to an array of factors that can disrupt the fluidity of a session. Causes encompass the use of subpar quality needles or needles with compromised bases, inserting the needle's entire body into the point, exerting excessive force during lifting, thrusting, or rotating maneuvers that lead to sudden muscle contractions, abrupt alterations in patient positioning, or mishandling of needles that are already bent or stuck.

The manifestation of a broken needle manifests as an interruption in the anticipated needle manipulation or during the withdrawal phase. The needle body may fracture within the tissues, leaving part of the needle embedded beneath the skin's surface, sometimes with a portion of the needle exposed. This irregularity requires prompt recognition and immediate intervention.

Encountering a broken needle necessitates a composed and calculated response. The practitioner's composure is essential, ensuring that the patient remains in their original position to prevent further embedding of the broken part. If the broken segment protrudes from the skin, it can be carefully removed using forceps or fingers. When the broken part lies level with or just beneath the skin, the gentle application of pressure around the point with the thumb and index finger reveals the broken end for extraction using forceps. For instance, when the fragment is embedded deeply in muscle or tissue, the use of X-ray technology to locate the piece followed by surgical removal becomes necessary.

Preventing the occurrence of broken needles demands a meticulous approach and unwavering attention to detail. Preliminary inspection of the needle's quality prior to treatment and its adherence to specifications mitigates potential risks. Avoiding overly vigorous manipulation and maintaining patient stillness during needle manipulation or retention are paramount. Ensuring that the entire needle body is not fully inserted into the body, leaving part exposed above the skin, offers a safety mechanism for potential removal in the event of breakage. Immediate withdrawal in the case of a bent needle is essential. Vigilance against forceful insertion or manipulation is crucial, and correct protocols should be promptly followed in cases of accidents, such as discovering a stuck needle.

5 Hematoma [3]

The emergence of a hematoma stands as a potential occurrence warranting attention. Amid needle insertion and the body's response, the formation of a hematoma—a localized swelling stemming from cutaneous bleeding—underscores the significance of skilful practice.

Hematomas, although infrequent, emerge as a consequence of specific factors within the acupuncture process. These may arise from inadvertent skin and muscle injuries or the unintentional puncturing of blood vessels, particularly when employing a hooked needle. Understanding these causes underscores the importance of precision and care in acupuncture practice.

The presence of a hematoma becomes evident through the manifestations it brings forth. Upon withdrawing the needle, the patient may experience localized swelling, accompanied by a sense of distension and discomfort. As the hematoma evolves, the skin's appearance may transform, taking on hues of blue or purplish tones, underscoring the body's response to localized bleeding.

Mild cases of hematoma may resolve on their own. However, when confronted with pronounced swelling, intense pain, or a hematoma encompassing a substantial skin area impeding functional activities, a dual approach is employed. Initiating with a cold compress aids in halting further bleeding, followed by the application of a warm compress or gentle massage to disperse the stagnant blood and alleviate discomfort.

Preventing hematomas involves a comprehensive effort based on vigilance and careful practice. Thoroughly examining needles before use and maintaining awareness of regional anatomy helps prevent potential blood vessel injuries. Taking swift action upon needle withdrawal, such as applying pressure with a sterilized cotton ball, contributes to minimizing the likelihood of hematoma formation. This proactive approach helps avoid unnecessary complications and improves the overall acupuncture experience.

6 Injuries to the Internal Organs

Talking about adverse injuries in acupuncture, among these considerations is the possibility of rare inadvertent internal organ injuries, which underscores the importance of a practitioner's awareness. Injury to internal organs, such as the lungs, urinary bladder, liver, spleen, intestines, and more, is exceptionally rare when administered by qualified acupuncture practitioners.

Injuries to internal organs during acupuncture sessions can stem from a variety of sources. These may include improper needle depth that inadvertently reaches internal structures, forceful manipulation causing organ displacement or puncture, or selecting points in close proximity to vital organs without meticulous precision.

Signs of internal organ injuries in acupuncture can vary, manifesting as sudden, sharp pain, discomfort, or localized tenderness around the treated area. In severe cases, symptoms might include referred pain, changes in organ function, or unusual sensations indicating potential internal disturbances.

Swift recognition and response are paramount when an internal organ injury is suspected. If a patient experiences unusual discomfort or sharp pain during treatment, the practitioner should immediately withdraw the needle and assess the situation. Depending on the severity, referral to a medical professional or call emergency help might be necessary for further evaluation and management.

Preventing injuries to internal organs necessitates meticulous practice. Acupuncturists should have a comprehensive understanding of human anatomy, particularly organ locations and vulnerabilities. Points on chest, abdominal, back and near vital organs should be treated with heightened caution and skill, utilizing shallow insertions and minimal manipulation. Ensuring patient comfort and cooperation is essential to minimize involuntary muscle contractions that might lead to complications.

7 Precautions in Acupuncture [2–4]

When practicing acupuncture, attention and consideration should be paid to the following aspects to ensure a harmonious integration of the operation of the treatment and therapeutic results.

Patient's State: Acupuncture potency is optimized when patients are neither overly hungry, exhausted, nor anxious. For those with weakened qi and blood, a gentle supine position and tender needling approach are recommended.

Pregnancy Considerations: The first three months of pregnancy merit abstaining from puncturing the abdomen and lumbosacral area. Points such as Kun Lun BL-60, Zhi Yin BL-67, Jian Jing GB-21, Yang Ling Quan BL-34, He Gu LI-4, San Yin Jiao SP-6 etc. that invigorate Qi and blood circulation should be avoided throughout pregnancy especially for the first trimester.

Infant Care: Infants' fontanelles must be closed before needling their vertex. This cautious approach respects their delicate physiology.

Hemorrhage Risk: Patients prone to spontaneous or prolonged bleeding, take blood thinners, after chemotherapy etc. should get enough attention.

Local Conditions: Areas afflicted by infections, ulcers, scars, or tumors are avoided during acupuncture.

Organ-Proximity Points: Points near vital organs demand meticulous handling. Deep or perpendicular needling near organs, especially in patients with organ enlargement (for example the enlargement of liver and spleen) or conditions such as pulmonary emphysema, is approached with caution to avert inadvertent injuries.

Sensitive Points: Precise needling techniques are employed around the eyes, sexual organs and upper segments of the conjunction between cervical vertebrae and head.

Urinary Retention: Careful needle control in patients with urinary retention prevents potential bladder complications and supports effective treatment. It is advisable to remind the patient to urinate before the acupuncture treatment starts.

Medication Usage: Awareness of patient medications fosters a comprehensive understanding of potential interactions, enhancing treatment safety and efficacy. Please advise the patient taking HRT to consult with the gynaecologist before acupuncture intervention applied.

Integration with Ongoing Therapies: Patients receiving multiple therapies, like physiotherapy, benefit from a unified approach Collaborating with other healthcare providers ensures that acupuncture complements, rather than conflicts with, concurrent treatments.

Medical Devices: Caution is exercised when patients have implanted medical devices, such as heart pacemakers. Ensuring that acupuncture does not interfere with these devices is vital for patient well-being and overall safety.

Patient-Specific Considerations: Patients with distinct medical histories and conditions necessitate personalized strategies. An individualized approach to acupuncture enhances safety and efficacy.

Quality Needle Inspection: Thorough examination of needles prior to use safeguards against subpar quality, reducing the risk of complications during treatment.

Hygienic Environment: Maintaining a clean and sterile environment during acupuncture sessions minimizes the risk of infection and supports optimal healing.

Patient Communication: Clear communication with patients about potential sensations and expected outcomes fosters trust and reduces anxiety, contributing to a positive experience.

Documentation: Maintaining accurate records of each acupuncture session aids in tracking progress, identifying patterns, and ensuring a comprehensive understanding of patient history.

Informed Consent: Ensuring that patients are well informed about the acupuncture procedure, its potential benefits, and any associated risks empowers them to make informed decisions about their health.

Review Questions

1. What are the potential accidents that may occur during acupuncture practice, and what measures can practitioners take to mitigate their impact?
2. Describe the causes, manifestations, and management strategies for fainting during acupuncture sessions.
3. Explain the preventive measures and management techniques related to incidents such as stuck needles, bent needles, hematomas, and internal organ injuries during acupuncture practice.

References

1. Qiu ML. Chinese acupuncture and moxibustion. 1st ed. London: Churchill Liverstone; 1993.
2. Yang JS. Zhen Jiu Xue. 1st ed. Beijing: People's Publishing House; 1989.
3. Liang FR, Wang H. Zhen Jiu Xue. 4th ed. Beijing: China TCM Publishing House; 2018.
4. Wang H, Du YH. Zhen Jiu Xue. 3rd ed. Beijing: China TCM Publishing House; 2012.

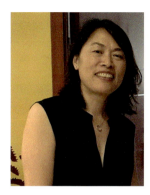
Dr. Lin Chen (陈琳) a Master of Medicine from Nanjing University of Chinese Medicine, formerly served as the Vice-director doctor at Jiangsu Provincial Hospital of Chinese Medicine, also known as the first affiliated hospital of Nanjing University of Chinese Medicine. Dedicated to integrating Chinese Medicine with Western Medicine, Dr. Chen has garnered invaluable insights from traditional Chinese Medicine through collaborations with esteemed practitioners such as Dr. Guicheng Xia, a globally influential TCM gynecologist. After two decades of service in Nanjing, she embarked on a new chapter in Europe, settling in the Netherlands. Dr. Chen currently practices at Klinic in Amsterdam, specializing in, but not limited to, areas such as infertility, IVF support, post-partum depression, Premenstrual Tension Syndrome (PMT), Menopause Syndrome, urinary tract infections, and various gynecological and hormonal disorders. Her commitment to holistic healthcare reflects a wealth of experience and a passion for improving women's health and well-being.

Classical Needling: Huang Di Nei Jing and Nanjing

Linjun Xia and Yun Ding

Learning Objectives

1. Understand the foundational contributions of Huang Di Nei Jing and Nan Jing to classical acupuncture techniques.
2. Familiarize yourself with the nine types of needling and twelve needling methods from Huang Di Nei Jing.
3. Comprehend the reinforcing and reducing principles and various needling methods introduced in Nan Jing.
4. Recognize the significance of directional reinforcement and reduction, lifting-thrusting, and nutrient-defense methods.
5. Recognize the ongoing influence of classical needling techniques on modern acupuncture practices.

Over two millennia ago, a significant milestone in the development of acupuncture techniques was marked with the creation of foundational texts like the "Nei Jing" and "Nan Jing." These ancient texts laid the groundwork for the art of acupuncture, providing essential knowledge and insights into this healing practice.

As time progressed, during the Yuan and Ming Dynasties, the field of acupuncture underwent further refinement and expansion. Notable works from this era, such as "Zhen Jing Zhi Nan," "Jin Zhen Fu," and "Zhen Jiu Da Cheng," emerged as classical texts that comprehensively documented various acupuncture methods. These texts played a pivotal role in fully shaping the rich tapestry of acupuncture techniques and principles.

Moreover, the Yuan and Ming Dynasties saw the flourishing and dissemination of different schools of acupuncture techniques. These schools were instrumental in carrying forward the traditions, knowledge, and expertise associated with acupuncture. They contributed to the evolution and diversification of acupuncture practices,

L. Xia (✉) · Y. Ding
Dong-Ou Bt China Naturheilzentrum, Kolbai K.u.2, Mosonmagyaróvár 9200, Hungary
e-mail: drxialj@163.com

ensuring that this ancient healing art continued to thrive and adapt to the changing times.

The enduring legacy of these classical acupuncture methods and the transmission of knowledge through different schools have played a crucial role in preserving and advancing acupuncture as a vital component of traditional Chinese medicine. These historical foundations continue to influence modern acupuncture practices and contribute to its ongoing development as a respected therapeutic modality.

Needling Methods from Huang Di Nei Jing《黄帝内经》针法

The "Huang Di Nei Jing" a seminal text in the realm of traditional Chinese medicine, particularly acupuncture, features a comprehensive discussion on needling methods [1]. This discussion primarily unfolds within the chapter known as "Lingshu·Guanzhen." Within this chapter, several key needling techniques are elaborated upon, each with specific applications and therapeutic goals.

1 Nine Types of Needling "九刺"

The "Huang Di Nei Jing" presents a set of "nine types of needling" [2] (see Fig. 1) designed to address nine distinct variations or changes within the body. Each type of needling is associated with a specific needle technique tailored to respond to these variations. This nuanced approach underscores the sophistication and precision inherent in acupuncture practice.

1.1 Transport Needling—"Shu Ci"

The acupuncture method for treating diseases of the five zang-organs, as described, involves a targeted selection of acupoints on the relevant meridians, specifically utilizing the Ying (brook point) and Shu (stream point) points. Additionally, acupoints associated with the Wu Zang Shu (five zang-organs) on the back (Bladder Meridian) are employed in this therapeutic approach. The coordination of these acupoints enables practitioners to address imbalances or ailments associated with the five zang-organs effectively.

Ying (Brook Point) and Shu (Stream Point) Selection: The choice of Ying and Shu points is determined by the specific zang-organ being targeted for treatment. Each zang-organ corresponds to a particular meridian, and the Ying and Shu points along these meridians are chosen to harmonize and balance the associated organ's function, such as Xing Jian (LV-2) and Tai Chong (LV-3).

Back-Shu points: The acupoints on the back mentioned, such as Gan Shu (BL-18), is associated with Liver and it plays a crucial role in regulating liver's function. By stimulating these 3 points, we aim to address liver disorders as well as the emotional disorders related to liver.

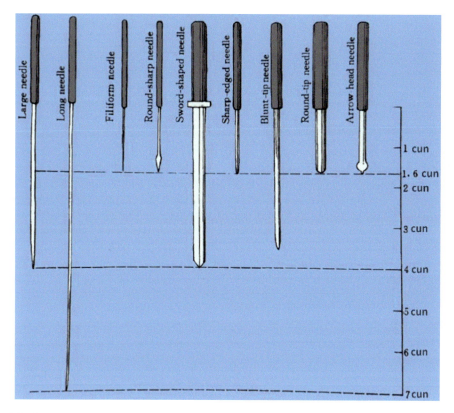

Fig. 1 Ancient nine needles

1.2 Distal Needling—"Yuan Dao Ci"

This is a needling technique used for treating diseases of the six Fu organs. In this method, the principle of treating diseases of upper body by needling acupoints in the lower part of the body, and selecting points along the meridians at a distance. Specifically, Distal Needling involves choosing points below the six Fu organs along the Foot Taiyang meridians, such as Zusanli (ST-36) on the Stomach meridian, Weizhong (BL-40) on the Bladder meridian, and Yanglingquan (GB34) on the Gallbladder meridian.

The uniqueness of this method lies in its selection of points that are farther from the disease site, influencing the entire body through the conduction of the meridian system.

1.3 Channel Needling—"Jing Ci"

This is a targeted acupuncture approach tailored to tackle ailments that directly impact the meridian itself. In the application of this technique, as needles are inserted into locations along the meridian pathways where there is a blockage to the free flow of qi and blood. This could manifest as stagnation, blood stasis, creating hardened areas or tender points.

The choice of acupoints and needling techniques in Channel needling is influenced by the nature of the obstruction—whether it be stagnation, blood stasis, or other forms of aggregation. The goal is not only to address the immediate symptoms but also to enhance the overall balance of the Qi flow.

1.4 Collateral Needling "Luo Ci"

This is a needle therapy employed to treat excessive and heat syndromes through the method of needling and bloodletting from the collaterals. In this technique, practitioners superficially needle the fine collaterals on the body's surface, inducing controlled bleeding. Instruments such as three-edged needles for bloodletting or cupping to needle the collaterals fall within this category. The primary objective is to regulate the circulation of qi and blood, alleviating symptoms associated with excessive and heat syndromes.

The choice of specific collaterals and the depth of needling may vary based on the individual's condition and the nature of the syndrome being treated.

1.5 Intermuscular Needling—"Fen Ci"

This is a needle technique specifically applied for treating muscle disorders. In this method, needles are inserted deeply into the spaces between muscles, aiming to regulate their meridian qi and dispel pathogenic factors. This approach is commonly used in clinical settings to address conditions where pathogenic factors are lodged within the muscles, such as treat arthralgia syndrome, pain, or chronic injuries.

By penetrating the muscles deeply, Intermuscular Needling seeks to influence the flow of meridian qi within the muscle layers. This, in turn, aids in dispelling pathogenic factors and promoting the body's natural healing processes. In clinical applications, the depth and precision of needling are adapted based on the individual's specific condition and the nature of the muscle disorder being addressed.

1.6 Drainage Needling—"Da Xie Ci"

This is a needle technique that utilizes a needle, specifically a lancet needle (Pi Zhen), as a substitute for a knife to incise and drain, facilitating the rupture of abscesses and the discharge of pus. This method is predominantly employed in clinical settings for procedures such as incising and draining abscesses, promoting the discharge of pus, bloodletting, and inducing drainage for conditions related to excess fluids.

The choice of specific acupoints, depth of needling, and other considerations are adapted based on the individual's condition and the nature of the pathology being treated.

1.7 Skin Needling "Mao Ci"

This is a needle technique where the skin is superficially needled for the treatment of chronic diseases and skin conditions. This method is akin to modern skin needling practices using instruments like "plum blossom needles" (Mei Hua Zhen) and "seven-star needles" (Qi Xing Zhen). During this process, the needling is akin to the pecking of a sparrow, involving gentle and continuous tapping. Depending on the size of the lesion, the practitioner repeats the needling until the skin exhibits slight congestion, without inducing bleeding.

In clinical applications, Skin needling is primarily used to address chronic diseases and various skin conditions. Common ailments treated using this method include headaches, hypertension, menstrual pain, intercostal neuralgia, neurodermatitis, pruritus, paralysis, and alopecia areata, among others.

1.8 Contralateral Channel Needling—"Hu Ci"

This is a needling technique that involves selecting acupuncture points on the contralateral side for treatment. In other words, if there is an ailment on the left side of the body, acupuncture points on the right side are chosen for needling, and vice versa. This method is primarily employed in clinical settings to address limb pain and functional disorders, including conditions such as hemiplegia after a stroke, facial asymmetry, shoulder stiffness, migraines, intercostal neuralgia, sciatic nerve pain, and more.

The concept behind Contralateral Channel Needling is rooted in the idea of balancing and harmonizing the body's energy by targeting acupuncture points on the opposite side. This technique is particularly useful for addressing asymmetrical conditions or disorders affecting one side of the body.

1.9 Red-Hot Needling—"Cui Ci"

This is a technique where a needle is heated until it becomes red-hot and is swiftly inserted into the body surface, followed by an immediate withdrawal. This method is comparable to modern fire needling practice. In clinical applications, Red-hot Needling is primarily used for treating conditions such as cold-induced arthritis, scrofula, and moist gangrene, among other ailments.

This technique is believed to have a warming effect on the body, dispersing cold and dampness, and promoting the flow of Qi and blood. The selection of acupoints and the depth of needling are adapted based on the specific diagnosis and the nature of the ailment being treated.

2 Twelve Needling Methods (十二刺)

Another significant aspect of needling techniques discussed in the "Huang Di Nei Jing" pertains to the "twelve needling methods." [2] These methods are devised to correspond to the twelve meridians of the body. By adapting the needling approach to the specific meridian affected, practitioners can effectively target various diseases and imbalances associated with those meridians. This demonstrates the intricate relationship between meridians and acupuncture treatment strategies.

2.1 Paired needling—"Ou Ci"

This is a technique in traditional Chinese acupuncture therapy. It involves locating specific tender points on the front chest and back, followed by symmetric needling on both the chest and back. This approach, referred to as paired needling or "Yin-Yang needling," later evolved into methods known as Front-Back point pairing method and Shu(back transport point)—Mu(Frontal alarm point) point pairing method, becoming significant techniques in treating diseases of Zang Fu organs. The practice aims to balance the body's Yin and Yang energies by stimulating tender points symmetrically, contributing to the maintenance of overall health.

2.2 Successive trigger needling—"Bao Ci"

This is an acupuncture technique that involves inserting the needle directly into painful areas identified by the patient. Following the application of needling techniques, the practitioner proceeds to locate other additional tender points. The needle is then withdrawn and reinserted in a successive manner, repeating this process on the Ashi points. The goal is to elicit a needling response, and this method is primarily employed in the treatment of migratory pain (Xing-Bi syndrome). It emphasizes a dynamic approach to address the evolving discomfort reported by the patient during the session.

2.3 Rehablitating needling—"Hui Ci"

This is a nuanced acupuncture technique designed to address conditions characterized by muscle rigidity, spasms, and pain. The process begins with the practitioner inserting the needle in proximity to the affected muscle, and after De Qi, let the patient do joint functional activities, and then change the needle direction continuously. This method is also called "multi-directional needling method". This interactive approach is essential in adapting the treatment to the patient's response.

This dynamic method aims to promote the smooth flow of Qi and Blood along the meridians, promoting balance and relieving muscular tension. It is particularly employed as an effective therapeutic approach for addressing conditions associated with muscle tightness, providing relief and improving joint functionality.

2.4 Triple needling—"Qi Ci"

This is an acupuncture technique where the practitioner inserts three needles simultaneously into the central point of the affected muscle, with one needle in the center and one on each side. This method, also known as "three-needling", is primarily employed in the treatment of conditions characterized by localized and deep-seated pain and cold, particularly when the affected area is relatively small. The simultaneous application of three needles aims to address specific points within the diseased muscle, providing a targeted and effective therapeutic approach.

2.5 Central-square needling—"Yang Ci" (see Fig. 2)

Central-square needling, aka Surrounded needling. It is an acupuncture technique involving the insertion of five needles. The practitioner starts by inserting a needle at the central point of the acupuncture site, followed by another four needles shallow

Fig. 2 Yang Ci

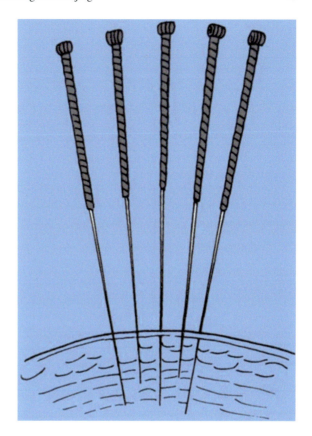

insertions above, below, to the left, and to the right. This method, primarily used in the treatment of conditions characterized by a large area of shallow cold-induced pain, aims to address specific points while covering a broader surface. The technique is tailored to treat the arthralgia syndrome where the affected area has a substantial but superficial extent of cold stagnation.

2.6 Direct subcutaneous needling—"Zhi Zhen Ci"

This is an acupuncture technique where the practitioner first pinches and lifts the skin at the acupuncture point before inserting the needle along the subcutaneous layer. This method involves a relatively shallow insertion of the needle and is primarily employed in the treatment of conditions caused by the invasion of external cold into the superficial region. The technique is specifically designed to address symptoms resulting from the influence of cold pathogenic factor on the skin and muscles.

2.7 Transport needling—"Shu Ci"

This is an acupuncture technique involving the vertical insertion of the needle into the acupuncture point to wait for the arrival of Qi. Once Qi is obtained, the needle is gradually withdrawn. The method emphasizes deep insertion followed by slow withdrawal, aiming to draw Yang from Yin and transport heat pathogens out. It is primarily used in the treatment of conditions characterized by excess Qi and heat. This technique is tailored to address imbalances in the body where excessive heat is prevalent.

2.8 Short needling—"Duan Ci"

This is an acupuncture technique where the needle is slowly inserted, gently shaking, and rotated slightly as it goes deeper, especially near the bone. The term "short" implies proximity, hence the name "short needling" indicating the needle is inserted to the short distance to the bone. This method is primarily used to treat deep-seated conditions such as bone rheumatism.

The aim of this technique is to stimulate specific acupuncture points, regulate the flow of qi and blood, and enhance the body's self-healing abilities, thereby alleviating deep-seated pain, especially related to bone ailments such as Bone-Bi sydrome.

2.9 Superficial needling—"Fu Ci"

This is an acupuncture technique where the needle is inserted shallowly, obliquely targeting the superficial layers of muscles. This approach is similar to modern wrist and ankle needling techniques. The primary application of this method is in the treatment of superficial muscle disorders, such as muscle stiffness accompanied by cold sensations, muscular spasms and numbness.

2.10 Yin needling—"Yin Ci"

This is an acupuncture technique where needles are simultaneously inserted into acupuncture points along both sides of the Yin meridians. During this method, reinforcing techniques are applied to enhance the needle sensation, aiming to improve the overall therapeutic effect. The primary application of Yin needling is in the treatment of conditions characterized by an excess of Yin leading to extreme cold-type pathologies.

2.11 Accompanied needling—"Bang Zhen Ci" (see Fig. 3)

This is an acupuncture technique where two needles are inserted into an acupuncture point. Initially, one needle is inserted directly into the selected acupoint, followed by the insertion of a second needle at a nearby location in an oblique direction, aligning the two needles side by side. This method is primarily employed in the treatment of conditions characterized by pronounced tenderness, immobility, and persistent pain, often associated with chronic obstructive diseases such as Tong-Bi Syndrome.

2.12 Repeated shallow needling—"Zan Ci"

This is an acupuncture technique where the needle is inserted straight into the skin and then withdrawn quickly, repeatedly, to create a series of shallow punctures. The aim is to make a superficial puncture and cause minor bleeding in the target area. This method is primarily used in the treatment of conditions such as abscesses, erysipelas, traumatic blood stasis, subcutaneous hematoma, and various skin disorders. The repeated shallow needling technique is applied to promote blood circulation, disperse blood stasis, and encourage the body's natural healing processes.

Fig. 3 Bang Zhen Ci

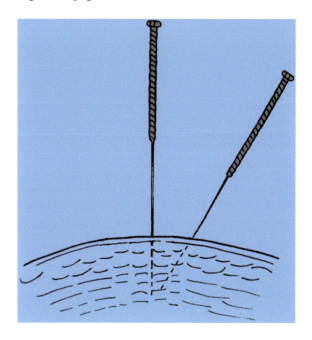

3 Five Needling Techniques "五刺"

The "Huang Di Nei Jing" also delves into "five needling techniques" tailored for addressing issues related to the five zang-organs [2]. Each technique is customized to target lesions or imbalances associated with a specific zang-organ, aligning with the traditional Chinese medicine concept of the zang-fu organs' roles in health and pathology.

3.1 Half Needling—"Ban Ci"

This is an acupuncture technique where the needle is inserted shallowly into the skin, reaching only a superficial depth. The needle is withdrawn quickly, resembling the action of plucking a hair. Because the insertion is extremely shallow and does not penetrate deeply, it is termed "half needling." This method is primarily used to disperse pathogenic factors in the superficial layers of the body.

Clinically, it is often employed in the treatment of conditions related to wind-cold affecting the surface, as well as disorders associated with the lungs, such as fever, cough, and wheezing. Additionally, half needling can be used in the treatment of certain skin disorders. TCM holds the lungs manifesting on the skin and body hair, Half Needling is associating with the lung meridians.

3.2 Leopard-Spot Needling—"Bao Wen Ci"

This is an acupuncture technique centered around acupuncture points, where the practitioner deliberately performs scattered needle insertions to induce bleeding.

The term "leopard-spot" is used because the resulting blood spots resemble the spots on a leopard. This needling technique is often associated with the heart meridian, as the heart governs blood vessels, and the method is believed to be effective in treating conditions characterized by redness, swelling, heat, and pain.

The rationale behind leopard-spot needling lies in its ability to promote blood circulation, dispel blood stasis, and address conditions associated with heat and inflammation. The scattered needle insertions are thought to stimulate the movement of qi and blood, encouraging the body's natural healing processes.

3.3 Joint Needling—"Guan Ci"

This is an acupuncture technique that involves inserting needles into the tendons and muscles around joints. This method is particularly applied near the joints where tendons and muscles converge. The name "joint needling" is derived from the proximity of tendons and muscles to the joints, as the terminations of the muscles and tendons are concentrated around the joints. This technique is often used to treat conditions related to sinew and tendon disorders.

The rationale behind joint needling is based on the idea that since tendons converge at the joints, needling in these areas can effectively address disorders related to sinews and tendons, such as conditions associated with stiffness and pain. Given that the liver is believed to govern the tendons in traditional Chinese medicine, joint needling is often associated with the liver meridian.

It's essential to note that joint needling involves deeper needle insertions, and caution must be taken to avoid damaging blood vessels and causing excessive bleeding.

3.4 He Gu Needling—"He Gu Ci" (See Fig. 4)

This is an acupuncture technique that is used in relatively thick muscles. After the needle is inserted, retreat to the superficial layer and then puncture obliquely to both

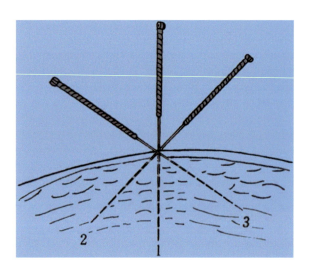

Fig. 4 He Gu Ci

sides in turn, shaped like the fork of a chicken's claw. "The assembly of muscles is the valley", so it is also called triple directional needling. It is clinically used to treat arthralgia syndrome.

In clinical practice, He Gu needling is often employed for the treatment of conditions related to Bi syndrome, which includes disorders characterized by pain and stiffness. By needling in multiple directions within the muscle, practitioners aim to promote the flow of qi and blood, dispel stagnation, and address issues associated with muscle and joint discomfort. He Gu needling is closely associating with the Spleen meridians.

3.5 Transport Needling—"Shu Ci"

This is an acupuncture technique characterized by inserting needles directly into the body, as deep as the bone, and then removing them directly. This method is similar to the "short needling" and "transport needling" techniques found among the twelve needling methods. "Shu" implies the transmission or connection between the interior and exterior, hence the term "transport needling."

Transport Needling is closely associating with the kidney meridians, therefore in clinical practice, it is primarily used for conditions related to bone rheumatism, including deep-seated ailments. By directly needling into the bones, this technique aims to address disorders involving the skeletal system, promoting the flow of qi and blood to alleviate pain and restore balance.

Needling Methods from "Nan Jing" 《难经》

"Nanjing," also known as the "Classic of Difficulties," stands as a pivotal work in the realm of traditional Chinese medicine, following in the esteemed footsteps of the seminal "Neijing" (Huangdi Neijing or Yellow Emperor's Inner Canon). While "Neijing" laid the foundation for traditional Chinese medical theory, "Nanjing" emerges as another cornerstone, focusing specifically on acupuncture techniques.

The structure of "Nanjing" is organized around the exploration of difficulties, starting with "Sixty-Nine Difficulties" and extending to the expanded version, "Eighty Difficulties." These difficulties encompass a range of challenges and intricacies encountered in the practice of acupuncture. This progression signifies the evolving nature of acupuncture practice and the growing complexity of the field [3].

Nanjing" not only preserves tradition but also inspires innovation. Practitioners, armed with insights from this classic work, are empowered to adapt and evolve acupuncture techniques to meet the demands of modern healthcare. The book becomes a source of inspiration for pushing the boundaries of traditional practices while staying grounded in the foundational principles set forth by ancient scholars. In conclusion, "Nanjing" holds a special place in the history of acupuncture, guiding practitioners from the roots of the practice to its expanding horizons today. It acts as a beacon of ancient wisdom, influencing how we approach acupuncture in the present day [4].

1. **Mother–child reinforcement and reduction** 母子补泻 [5]

The "Nanjing · Sixty-Nine Difficulties" proposes the acupuncture reinforcing and reducing principle of "tonify the mother in case of deficiency and reduce the child in case of excess." Under the guidance of this treatment principle, "Nanjing" outlines four methods of tonifying and reducing [5]:

The first method involves reinforcing and reducing based on the distinct mother–child relationships among the twelve meridians

The guiding principle in acupuncture, as described in the "Nanjing · Sixty-Nine Difficulties," revolves around the dynamic relationship akin to that of a mother and child within the twelve meridians. Applying the same analogy to the interplay of the five elements among these meridians, the strategy adapts based on whether the condition involves deficiency or excess.

In instances of deficiency, where there is a lack or imbalance, the approach is to supplement by focusing on the primary points of the mother meridian. For instance, in the case of lung deficiency syndrome, acupuncture may target nourishing Taibai (SP-3) at the Shu-Stream point (earth) of the spleen meridian.

Conversely, when dealing with excess, characterized by an abundance or stagnation, the emphasis shifts to purifying the main points of the son meridian. For example, in liver excess syndrome, acupuncture might involve purifying the kidney meridian He-Sea point (water), such as Yingu (KI-10).

The second method is to conduct the mother–child reinforcing and reducing of this meridian according to the five-element attributes of the five transport points of the diseased meridians

This technique involves considering the five-element attributes of the transport points within the affected meridian to address imbalances. Taking the example of the lung meridian, which is associated with the metal element, the application varies based on whether the condition involves deficiency or excess.

In cases of lung deficiency, the strategy is to nourish the meridian by focusing on its mother point, Taiyuan (LU9), associated with the spleen earth element. This approach aligns with the broader principle of tonifying the mother to address deficiency syndromes.

On the other hand, when dealing with lung excess conditions, the emphasis shifts to reducing the meridian by targeting its child point, Chize (LU5), linked to the kidney water element. This practice adheres to the principle of draining the child to alleviate excess syndromes.

The third method involves needling the Jing-well point (mother acupoint, wood) and purging the Ying-spring point (child acupoint, fire)

This means that in cases where the excessive heat syndrome requires needling the Jing-well point, it can be challenging due to the distribution of Jing-well points on the ends of the fingers (toes) and the limited qi in the meridian. Following the principle of "excess pattern will purify its son," the Ying-Spring point is used instead.

For instance, if there is an excess pattern in the stomach meridian, and the Jing-well point Lidui (ST45) should be purged, the Ying-Spring point Neiting (ST44) acupoint can be purged as an alternative.

The fourth method involves needling the Jing-well point (child point, wood) and supplementing the he-sea point (mother point, water)

Similarly to the previous methods, this means that when the Jing-Well point needs to be replenished, the He-Sea point can be supplemented, following the principle of "when deficient replenishes its mother." For instance, if there is insufficient heart yin, and the Jing-Well point Shaochong (HT9) needs to be replenished, its He-Sea point Shaohai (HT3) can be supplemented.

2. **Reducing the south and tonifying the north** 泻南补北 [5]

"Nanjing · Seventy-Five Difficulties" introduces the concept of "The east is strong, the west is empty. Purging the south and tonifying the north." This method serves as a dual-purpose approach, addressing liver hyperactivity and lung deficiency, while extending the principle of "replenishing the mother and purging the son." In this context, the east symbolizes wood, representing the liver, and the west symbolizes metal, representing the lungs. The phrase "the east is strong, the west is empty" reflects the imbalance where the liver (wood) is in excess, and the lungs (metal) are deficient, portraying a dynamic of "wood counter-restricting metal."

Furthermore, the instruction to "purge the south (heart) and nourish the north (kidney)" is a strategy to balance water and control fire. In other words, it involves nourishing the kidneys and purifying the heart. The elemental associations are significant here, with fire in the south representing the heart and water in the north representing the kidneys.

For instance, insomnia resulting from the hyperactivity of heart and liver fire, coupled with disharmony between the heart and kidneys, can be effectively addressed using the acupuncture technique of "purging the south and nourishing the north." Specific acupoints such as Taichong (LR3), Shenmen (HT7), Neiguan (PC6), and Shaohai (HT3) are selected for the purging method, aiming to clear the excessive fire in the heart and liver. Simultaneously, Taixi (KI3), Fuliu (KI7), Sanyinjiao (SP6), and Zhaohai (KI6) acupoints are employed for the nourishing method, replenishing the water element in the kidneys.

By incorporating complementary points such as Anmian (EX-HN0), Baihui (DU20), and Sishencong (EX-HN1), and skillfully applying tonification and reduction techniques, the treatment not only calms the mind but also promotes restful sleep. This holistic approach helps the body regain a harmonious "yin-yang balance," facilitating the restoration of normal sleep patterns.

3. **Directional reinforcement and reduction** 迎随补泻 [5]

This method was first observed in the "Neijing," indicating that draining excess should employ methods that oppose the flow of meridian qi, while tonifying deficiencies should utilize methods that follow the meridian qi. However, the "Nanjing" provides further clarification. In "Nanjing · Seventy-Two Difficulties," it points out that the circulation activities of defensive qi, nutrient qi and blood, their depth, intensity, and the direction of meridians exhibit variations, including both smooth and reverse flows. Therefore, the practice of supplementing and reducing based on the superficial and deep aspects of each meridian's qi and blood, the timing of fluctuations, and the directional flow falls under the category of directional reinforcement and reduction.

In "Nanjing · Seventy-Nine Difficulties," this concept is further expanded as "seizing while welcoming is draining its child, aiding while following is tonifying its mother." This represents a comprehensive approach that combines the welcoming and following reinforcement and reduction method with the mother–child tonifying and reducing method based on the five transport points. This method, originated in the "Nanjing," continues to guide clinical practice to this day.

4. **Lifting-thrusting reinforcement and reduction** 提插补泻 [5]

In building upon the respiratory reinforcement and reduction method established in the "Neijing," the "Nanjing" introduces the rudiments of the lifting and thrusting reinforcement and reduction method. The operative technique involves "get the arrival of qi, then pushing inward, called reinforcement; moving and extending it, called reduction" (see "Nanjing · Seventy-Eight Difficulties"). Subsequent generations have interpreted this as applying firm pressure during a slow lift for reinforcement and applying firm lift during a slow pressure for reduction, using this as the foundation.

5. **Nutrient-defense reinforcement and reduction** 营卫补泻 [5]

"Nanjing" establishes methods for reinforcing and reducing Ying and Wei (deep and shallow) based on the theory in the "Neijing" that states "Ying circulates within the vessels, Wei circulates outside the vessels." Due to the different distribution and pathways of Ying and Wei qi, the depth of acupuncture should naturally vary when regulating them. "Nanjing · Seventy-One Difficulties" emphasizes, "puncturing Ying does not harm Wei, puncturing Wei does not harm Ying." Furthermore, "Nanjing · Seventy-Six Difficulties" states, "When it is time to reinforce, draw qi from Wei; when it is time to reduce, place qi in Rong" (Wei and Rong refer to the Ying and Wei phases). This fundamentally guides practitioners to determine the depth of needling based on the specific condition of the illness.

Review Questions

1. How did the Huang Di Nei Jing and Nan Jing contribute to the development of classical acupuncture techniques?
2. Explain the significance of the nine types of needling and twelve needling methods outlined in Huang Di Nei Jing.
3. What are the reinforcing and reducing principles introduced in Nan Jing, and how do they guide acupuncture practice?
4. Discuss the directional reinforcement and reduction method and its relevance in acupuncture.

5. How does Nan Jing's lifting-thrusting reinforcement and reduction method influence needling techniques?
6. How do classical needling techniques continue to impact modern acupuncture practices?

References

1. Wang B (Tang Dynasty). Huangdi Neijing. Beijing: Traditional Chinese Medicine Ancient Books Publishing House; 2003.
2. Yin Y, Ran X. Comparison of the classification of acupuncture techniques in "Lingshu official acupuncture". Shanghai J Acupuncture. 2006;4.
3. Wang J, et al. (Ming Dynasty). Lu Guang et al. (Three Kingdoms period), Annotations of Nanjing. Beijing: People's Health Publishing House; 1963.
4. Chai T. The contribution of Nanjing to acupuncture. J Guangzhou Univer Chin Med. 2000;17:289.
5. Niu B. Translation and annotation of Nanjing. Beijing: Traditional Chinese Medicine Ancient Books Publishing House; 2004.

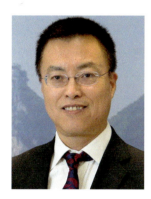

Prof. Dr. Linjun Xia, Ph.D. (夏林军) graduated from Changchun University of Chinese Medicine and Heilongjiang University of Chinese Medicine. A disciple of Professor Zhang Jin, a representative of the World intangible cultural heritage of Chinese medicine acupuncture.

He is currently a guest professor at Hungary Semmelweis University; Vice president of Hungarian TCM Association; Vice president of Specialty Committee of Chinese Medicine Manipulations (WFCMS); Member of the editorial board of the World Journal of Traditional Chinese Medicine (WJTCM).

With more than 30 years of clinical experience, he specializes in acupuncture techniques. Participated in the compilation of "Acupuncture", "Basic theory of Traditional Chinese Medicine" and many other works. He published more than 40 academic papers. For example, "Flying Meridian and Moving the Qi acupuncture technique of and its clinical application" and so on.

In 2022, he was honored with the World Integrative Medicine Top Ten Acupuncture Expert Award.

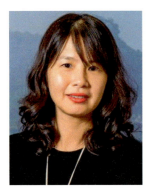

Dr. Yun Ding (丁芸) graduated from Zhongshan University of Medical Science in 1998 and completed his master degree in the same University. After graduating, she worked at the affiliated Stomatology Hospital of Zhongshan Medical University and the affiliated Stomatology Hospital of Kunming Medical University. She attained the position of Associate Professor in 2009.

In 2012, she undertook a year and a half of further studies at the University of Toronto Faculty of Dentistry as visiting professor. She have led various research projects and published numerous academic papers.

Since 2013, she has been studying TCM with Professor Xia in Hungary. From 2018she works as a guest professor of Shenzhou University of TCM. From 2021, She works as member of councel of the Central and Eastern European Federation of Chinese Medicine Societies. From 2022, she serve as the executive director of the Professional Committee on Target Differentiation and Treatment of the World Federation of Societies of TCM.

Jinzhenfu Needling Methods and Needling Technique on Reinforcement and Reduction

Linjun Xia and Yun Ding

Learning Objectives

1. Understand the historical significance of Jinzhenfu and its impact on acupuncture techniques.
2. Recognize and differentiate between the 14 single-needle techniques discussed in the chapter.
3. Explore compound needling techniques such as Setting Fire on the Mountain and Coolness through Penetrating heaven.
4. Comprehend the principles behind needling techniques for reinforcement and reduction.
5. Identify factors influencing the effectiveness of acupuncture, including the patient's functional status and acupoint specificity.
6. Learn the precautions and considerations for implementing tonification and reduction techniques.

1 Golden Needle Ode—Jinzhenfu《金针赋》Needling Methods

The 'Golden Needle Ode' was authored by Quan Shixin, a disciple of Ni Mengzhong and Peng Jiusi. Quan Shixin belonged to the school of Dou Hanqing (1195–1280), being a successor to his teachings. In the year 1439 (Ming Dynasty, Zhengtong Era, fourth year), Quan Shixin composed the 'Golden Needle Ode'. Building upon the foundation of the 14 single-technique methods established by the Dou school, Quan introduced compound needling techniques such as 'setting fire on the mountain' and

L. Xia (✉) · Y. Ding
Dong-Ou Bt China Naturheilzentrum, Kolbai K.U.2, Mosonmagyaróvár 9200, Hungary
e-mail: drxialj@163.com

'coolness through penetrating heaven. He systematically organised the procedures, clarified their therapeutic focus, identified key technical aspects, making this book the first specialised work on acupuncture techniques. Since the publication of the;Golden Needle Ode', ancient acupuncture techniques have taken shape as a comprehensive system, and various schools of acupuncture methods have flourished [1].

In 2008, the Chinese government initiated the development of the national standard text 'technical specifications for acupuncture and moxibustion', completing it by the end of 2013. The operational standards for the 'basic techniques of filiform needling' were based on the needling techniques outlined in the 'Golden Needle Ode'.

Single Needling Techniques (14 Types) [2]

1.1. **Type 1: ZAO爪: Locating the Acupoint with a Finger Nail**

   Pressing acupuncture points with a fingernail is a common method used to locate acupuncture points for more accurate needling. This technique typically involves using the fingernails of the fingers to determine the specific location of acupuncture points by feeling the surrounding tissues. During the process of pressing acupuncture points, based on experience, acupuncturists can sense specific changes in the tissues, aiding in ensuring the selection of accurate acupuncture points for needling. This method provides an intuitive, tool-free means of precisely locating acupuncture points in clinical practice.

1.2. **Type 2: QIE切: Pressing with a Thumb Nail**

   Using the thumbnail vertically on the acupuncture point for a cutting and pressing motion to disperse qi and blood, reducing the pain of needle insertion. In modern practice, a combination of type 1 Zao and type 2 Qie methods is commonly employed.

1.3. **Type 3: YAO摇: Rotating the Needle Handle**

   After the needle body is inserted to a certain depth, holding the needle handle and shaking the needle in a specific manner is a method to transmit the needle sensation through the joints.

   The rotating technique has three variations. Firstly, there is the shallow and broad rotation. When the meridian qi encounters resistance at the joint and the needle is inserted relatively superficially, practitioners use a technique involving shallow and broad rotation, known as the **green dragon rotates its tail** method. After which, there is the deep and small rotation. In situations where the meridian qi faces obstruction at the joint and the needle is inserted deeper, practitioners use a technique involving deep and small rotation, known as the **white tiger nods its head** method. The third method involves withdrawing the needle. During needle withdrawal, the practitioner holds the needle handle and rotates the needle while withdrawing, facilitating the release of stagnation during needle removal.

1.4. **Type 4: TUI退: Withdrawing Outwards**

This specific operating method involves withdrawing the needle from a deeper to shallower position. This technique is employed during needle withdrawal or when changing the direction of needle insertion.

1.5. **Type 5: DONG动: Lifting with Energy**

It is a method of withdrawing the needle from the acupoint with force, and it is a way to elicit a cooling response.

1.6. **Type 6: JIN进: Entering Inwards**

The acupuncture points are divided into three sections: Heaven, Man, and Earth. Inserting a needle within the boundaries of one or more of these sections is referred to as "entering" the point.

1.7. **Type 7: XUN循: Touching and Pressing Along the Meridian**

This method refers to following the course of the meridians, stimulating the flow of Qi along the pathways. Bend the index, middle and ring fingers of the right hand, keeping the finger pads perpendicular to the area being followed. Starting from the end point of a meridian (usually at the wrist or ankle joint), follow the course of the meridian in the direction of the heart, making several movements back and forth.

1.8. **Type 8: SHE摄: Hammer Down with the Fingers Along the Meridian**

This method involves using the nails to pinch and nip along the meridians, stimulating the flow of Qi. It is a technique employed when there is stagnation of Qi in the meridians. According to the 'Golden Needle Ode', which suggests "follow and gather", this method is often combined with the techniques of type 7 Xun; touching and pressing along the meridian.

1.9. **Type 9: CUO搓: Twisting the Needle**

Twisting the needle is considered one of the most crucial single-needle techniques. After swiftly inserting the needle, it is rotated continuously 360° in one direction, resembling the motion of twisting a thread. Care should be taken not to entangle the needle in the muscles during twisting, alternating between actual twisting and empty twisting. The hallmark of successful twisting is when lifting does not extract the needle, inserting does not penetrate further, and rotating does not turn the needle; the fullness of energy induces a natural swaying motion.

1.10. **Type 10: TAN弹: Flicking the Needle**

Flicking technique involves bouncing the needle handle and has two applications. Firstly, after the needle is inserted into the body, lightly tapping the needle handle with the fingertips induces a mild vibration in the lower part of the needle. This can alleviate the pain sensation after needle insertion and also has an invigorating effect. Secondly, it is used as a needle insertion method, where the needle is rapidly advanced by firmly tapping the needle handle during the insertion process.

1.11. **Type 11: PAN盘: Circling the Needle**

The Circling technique is a method used on the soft flesh of the abdomen to extract qi during acupuncture. After inserting the needle into abdominal acupoints, the needle is turned by inverting its body. The practitioner grips the needle tail with the thumbnails and index, middle fingers, applying wrist force to rotate the needle either clockwise or counterclockwise.

1.12. **Type 12: MEN扪: Sealing the Needle Hole**

Sealing method refers to holding a sterile dry cotton ball against the acupuncture point after removing the needle to prevent bleeding. It should not be rubbed or moved.

1.13. **Type 13: AN按: Pressing the Meridian**

Pressing the meridian involves using the fingers of assisting hand to apply pressure to the meridian above or below the acupuncture point. When combined with the twisting, lifting, and inserting actions of needling by puncturing hand, it helps control the direction of the needle sensation, either downward or upward. This method facilitates the transmission of stimulated meridian qi towards one end, promoting the flow of energy.

1.14. **Type14: TI提: Lifting the Needle**

Lifting the needle refers to the technique of lifting the needle upward with force when the needle is inserted into one of the three sections: Heaven, Man, or Earth. The lifting is done slowly and steadily, resembling the action of raising a soybean. Lifting the needle has a cooling effect and is considered a purging method. This technique is a crucial operational skill within the complex needling method known as "Penetrating the heaven with Coolness".

Compound Techniques 复式手法

A. **Setting Fire on the Mountain** 烧山火 [3]

The specific operating method involves quickly inserting the needle and using twirling, lifting-inserting, or twisting techniques to obtain a distending and sore needle sensation. Use pressing with the thumb next to the acupoint to guard the qi. Hold the needle handle tightly between the thumb and forefinger, inserting the needle downward. During needle insertion, the speed should be slow, and the force should be strong, which is considered traditionally as the quantity of Nine Yang. Alternatively, use the thumb to forcefully twist the needle forward, or apply force to push the needle handle downward. These methods can be combined using a combination of twisting and inserting techniques.

The classic technique involves operating within the depth range of the acupuncture point being needled, dividing the process into three layers: Heaven, Man, and Earth, with a sequence from superficial to deep. Modern medical practitioners also sometimes divide it into two layers or omit the layering approach.

The described technique can be repeated multiple times, advancing and retreating three times, until the patient experiences a sensation of warmth.

After completing the procedure, remove the needle and press a sterilized cotton ball against the needle hole, preventing the escape of true qi.

This method is often used to treat conditions such as stubborn numbness due to cold-induced obstruction and disorders related to deficient cold.

B. **Coolness Through Penetrating Heaven** 透天凉 [3]

The specific operating method involves quickly inserting the needle and using twirling, lifting-inserting, or twisting techniques to obtain a distending and sore needle sensation. Use pressing with the thumb next to the acupoint to guard the qi. Hold the needle handle tightly between the thumb and forefinger, inserting the needle downward. During needle insertion, the speed should be slow, and the force should be strong, which is considered traditionally as the quantity of Nine Yang. Alternatively, use the thumb to forcefully twist the needle forward, or apply force to push the needle handle downward. These methods can be combined using a combination of twisting and inserting techniques.

The classic technique involves operating within the depth range of the acupuncture point being needled, dividing the process into three layers: Heaven, Man, and Earth, with a sequence from superficial to deep. Modern medical practitioners also sometimes divide it into two layers or omit the layering approach. The described technique can be repeated multiple times, advancing and retreating three times, until the patient experiences a sensation of warmth.

After completing the procedure, remove the needle and press a sterilized cotton ball against the needle hole, preventing the escape of true qi.

This method is often used to treat conditions such as stubborn numbness due to cold-induced obstruction and disorders related to deficient cold.

The procedure involves quickly inserting the needle directly into the deep part of the acupuncture point. Use twisting, lifting-and-thrusting, or twirling methods to obtain the sensation of numbness, without the need for pressing on the needle. Hold the needle handle lightly between the thumb and forefinger, lifting the needle upwards. During lifting, maintain a slow speed and gentle force, representing the quantity of the six yin. Alternatively, gently twist the needle backward with the thumb or uniformly scrape the needle handle upwards.

The classical technique involves operating within the depth range of the needled acupuncture point, dividing the process into three layers: Earth, Man, and Heaven. The order typically involves first inserting the needle deeply and then more superficially. In modern practice, some practitioners opt for a two-layer approach or omit the layering altogether. These operations can be repeated several times, with a pattern of three withdrawals and three insertions, continuing until the patient experiences a sensation of coolness.

After the procedure is completed, gently withdraw the needle. Alternatively, withdraw the needle while simultaneously rotating it, aiming to disperse yang and alleviate heat. This method is often employed in the treatment of conditions such as Heat-Bi syndrome and acute inflammatory swellings with a heat component.

C. **Green Dragon Wagging Tail** 青龙摆尾 [4]

After obtaining the qi upon needle insertion, needle manipulation is carried out in the superficial layers. Using the thumb and index finger of the needling hand to grip the needle handle, akin to steering a boat, with a stable but gentle rocking motion, resembling the swaying of a dragon's tail. This technique can be repeated and is often applied when there is resistance to the transmission of needle sensation, such as when reaching the joints, or when qi is obtained in the superficial layers. Simultaneous application of the single needling techniques of Xun and She methods should be employed.

D. **White Tiger Shaking Head** 白虎摇头 [5]

First insert the needle, after obtaining qi in the deep layers, grip the needle handle with the thumb and index finger of the needling hand and perform a rotating motion. First, rotate from the lower right to the upper left, forming a half-circle; then, retreat from the upper left to the lower right, forming a semi-circle. Holding the needle handle with force towards the needle tip characterizes this deep and small rotating technique. When performing this technique, the hand resembles shaking a bell, with one shake and one swing, named after the tiger's head shaking. This method can be repeated and should be simultaneously combined with the techniques of Xun and She single needling techniques.

It is applied when there is resistance to the transmission of needle sensation (such as reaching the joints) and when obtaining qi in the deep layers.

E. **Black Turtle Probing Caves** 苍龟探穴 [6]

Method of Operation: The needle is slowly inserted, resembling a turtle entering the earth. After obtaining qi, the needle is withdrawn from the deep layer (Earth part) to the shallow layer (Heaven part) in one movement. Then, the needle tip direction is changed, and the needle is slanted in the upward, downward, leftward, and rightward directions. Each direction of needle insertion progresses gradually from shallow to deep, divided into three parts. When a new needle sensation is obtained, the needle is withdrawn to the shallow layer in one motion, and the direction is changed according to the above method for re-needling.

This method primarily aims to search for the qi along the meridian, while also having the function of promoting the flow of qi.

F. **Red Phoenix Welcomes Source** 赤凤迎源 [6]

When inserting the needle, first direct the deeper layer of the acupoint (Earth part), then raise it to the shallower layer of the acupoint (Heaven part). Insert the needle again into the deeper layer, and perform the twisting needle technique to stimulate qi. When qi is obtained under the needle and the needle moves on its own, use the thumb and index finger of the puncturing hand to perform the flying needle technique, with the two fingers twisting and releasing alternately, repeating this process resembling the wings of a phoenix spreading.

This method primarily aims to extract coolness using the flying needle technique, while also having the function of promoting the flow of qi.

2 Needling Technique on Reinforcement and Reduction 针刺补泻

The needling technique for reinforcement and reduction is a widely applied acupuncture method in clinical settings, exerting a regulatory influence on the body's balance between deficiency and excess. Acupuncture reinforcement serves to invigorate the body's antipathogenic Qi, restoring weakened functions, whereas reduction methods disperse pathogenic qi, bringing hyperactive functions back to normal. The primary techniques employed in clinical practice for needling reinforcement and reduction include:

2.1 Twisting and Rotating for Reinforcement and Reduction 捻转补泻 [7]

After obtaining the qi response in the acupuncture point, twisting and rotating the needle left and right is a method used for reinforcement and reduction.

Reinforcement: After the arrival of Qi, use the thumb and index finger to twirl the needle, applying strong pressure forward with the thumb and light pressure backward.

Reduction: After the arrival of Qi, use the thumb and index finger to twirl the needle, applying light pressure forward with the thumb and strong pressure backward.

2.2 Fast-Slow Needling Reinforcement and Reduction 徐疾补泻 [7] (See Fig. 6.1)

After obtaining the qi response in the acupuncture point, a method based on the speed of needle insertion and withdrawal (fast-slow) is employed for reinforcement and reduction.

Reinforcement: During needle insertion, the needle is slowly advanced with minimal twisting and quickly withdrawn.

Reduction: During needle insertion, the needle is rapidly advanced with more twisting, and it is slowly withdrawn.

Fig. 6.1 Fast-slow needling reinforcement and reduction

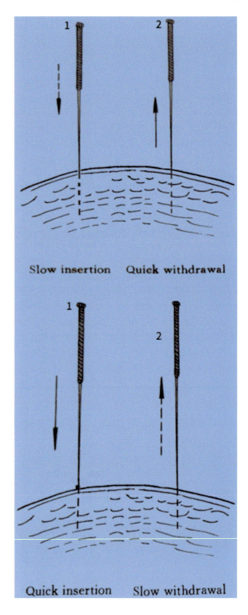

2.3 Lifting and Thrusting for Reinforcement and Reduction 提插补泻 *[7] (See Fig. 6.2)*

After obtaining the qi response in the acupuncture point, this method involves adjusting the strength, speed, and duration of lifting and thrusting for reinforcement and reduction.

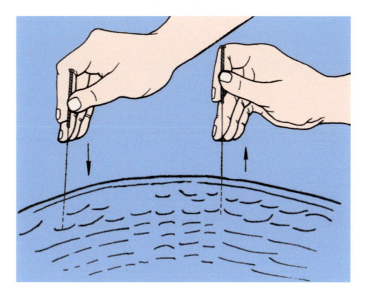

Fig. 6.2 Lifting and thrusting for reinforcement and reduction

Reinforcement: After obtaining the qi response, the needle is first lifted shallowly and then thrust deeply, with more emphasis on thrusting than lifting. The amplitude of lifting and thrusting is small, the frequency is slow, and the duration of the operation is short.

Reduction: After obtaining the qi response, the needle is first thrust deeply and then lifted shallowly, with more emphasis on lifting than thrusting. The amplitude of lifting and thrusting is large, the frequency is fast, and the duration of the operation is long.

2.4 *Respiratory Reinforcement and Reduction* 呼吸补泻 *[7] (See Fig. 6.3)*

This method involves needling and withdrawing the needle in coordination with the patient's breathing for reinforcement and reduction.

Reinforcement: Insert the needle during the patient's exhalation and withdraw during inhalation.

Reduction: Insert the needle during the patient's inhalation and withdraw during exhalation.

Fig. 6.3 Respiratory reinforcement and reduction

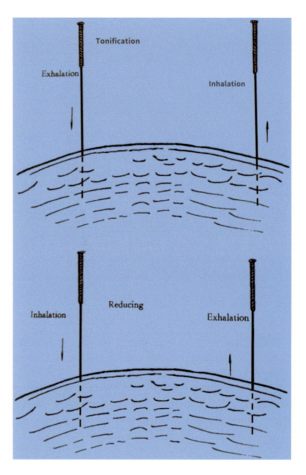

2.5 Opening and Closing Reinforcement and Reduction 开阖补泻 [7]

This method is based on whether to knead or press the needle hole after withdrawing the needle, using the openness or closure of the needle hole for reinforcement and reduction.

Reinforcement: Knead or press the needle hole quickly after withdrawing the needle.

Reduction: Shake the needle hole without immediately kneading or pressing it after withdrawing the needle.

2.6 Nine-Six Reinforcement and Reduction 九六补泻 [7] (See Illustration 6.4)

The term "nine-six" here refers to a concept from the "Yijing" (I Ching), broadly representing attributes such as yin, yang, hardness, and softness. The odd number nine represents yang and hardness, while the even number six represents yin and softness. Choosing the numbers nine and six reflects the ancient thinkers' quantification of acupuncture techniques. Here, "quantity" is not a specific measurement but rather a philosophical concept from the "Yijing," using nine and six to distinguish the magnitude of stimulation and the duration of stimulation time. The number six, representing yin, indicates light stimulation and a short stimulation time. The number nine, representing yang, indicates strong stimulation and a longer stimulation time (Fig. 6.4).

Therefore, the significance of Nine-Six Reinforcement and Reduction lies in the application of the numbers nine (yang) or six (yin) through methods such as twisting or lifting and thrusting. This approach aims to achieve the reinforcement or reduction effect in the three layers: Heaven, Man, and Earth. Reinforcement involves applying the method with the number nine (yang), while reduction involves applying the method with the number six (yin).

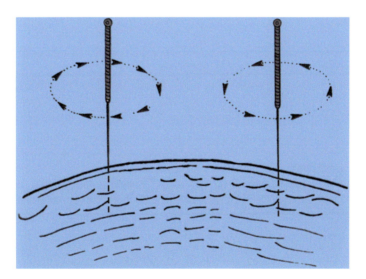

Fig. 6.4 Nine-six reinforcement and reduction

2.7 Even Reinforcement and Reduction (平补平泻) [7]

After obtaining the qi response upon needling, simply lift and thrust or twist the needle evenly before withdrawing it.

3 Factors Affecting the Reinforcement and Reduction Effect of Acupuncture

3.1 Patient's Functional Status

Needling can exert various adjustment effects (i.e., tonifying or reducing effects) depending on the patient's different pathological states. When the patient is in a weakened state, acupuncture can play a role in supporting and tonifying deficiencies. In cases of collapse or extreme weakness, needling can help restore yang and stabilize the patient. In situations of pathogenic excess, acupuncture can contribute to dispelling pathogenic factors and purging excess. The choice of needling technique is tailored to address the specific condition of the patient, aiming to restore balance and promote overall well-being.

3.2 Relative Specificity of Acupoints

The therapeutic functions of acupoints are not only general but also exhibit relative specificity. For instance, acupoints like Guanyuan RN-4, Qihai RN-6, and Mingmen DU-4 have the ability to inspire the body's antipathogenic Qi, promoting vigorous function and exerting a strengthening effect, making them suitable for tonifying deficiencies. On the other hand, there are acupoints such as Renzhong DU-26, Weizhong BL-40, and Shixuan (Extra point), which can disperse pathogenic factors, inhibit excessive bodily function, and are suitable for reducing excess conditions.

3.3 Selection and Application of Acupuncture Techniques

The choice and application of acupuncture techniques are crucial for facilitating the transformation of the body's deficiency and excess states. Tailoring the selection of tonification or reduction techniques to the nature and degree of the patient's deficiency or excess, and applying them appropriately, are essential steps to achieve the desired tonification or reduction effects. This approach enhances the overall therapeutic effectiveness of acupuncture treatments.

4 Precautions and Considerations

Before implementing tonification or reduction techniques, it is necessary to employ single-needle techniques to obtain qi beneath the needle. Without obtaining qi, it is impossible to regulate or direct qi to the affected area. In such cases, acupuncture tonification or reduction becomes ineffective.

The techniques of "Setting Fire on the Mountain" and "Coolness through Penetrating heaven" are often applied to acupoints located in areas with abundant musculature. These methods are not suitable for acupoints located in the extremities or areas with shallow muscle tissue.

Review Questions

1. What is the historical significance of the 'Golden Needle Ode' in acupuncture?
2. Describe the principles behind the compound needling techniques Setting Fire on the Mountain and Coolness through Penetrating heaven.
3. Enumerate and explain three single-needle techniques discussed in the chapter.
4. How do needling techniques for reinforcement and reduction contribute to balancing deficiency and excess in the body?
6. Discuss the factors influencing the effectiveness of reinforcement and reduction techniques in acupuncture.
7. Why is obtaining qi beneath the needle crucial before implementing tonification or reduction techniques?

References

1. Yang J (Ming Dynasty). ZhenJiu Da Cheng. Beijing: People's Medical Publishing House; 2006
2. Zhang J. Acupuncture Dacheng proof translation. 2nd ed. Beijing: People's Medical Publishing House; 2009.
3. Zhang J. The basis of the setting fire on the mountain and coolness through penetrating heaven techniques in the acupuncture technical operating standards. Heilongjiang Chin Med. 2008;1:9–10.
4. Xia L. Clinical observation on essential hypertension with "Green Dragon Wagging Tail and White Tiger Shaking Head" acupuncture technique in Europe. J Changchun Univ of Chinese Med. 2012;4:659–61.
5. Wang F, Wang C. Application research on the "flying meridian and moving the Qi" acupuncture technology. J Changchun Univ Chinese Med.2012;3
6. Xia L. Flying meridian & moving the Qi acupuncture technique and its clinical application. J Changchun Univ Chinese Med. 2018;5
7. National Acupuncture Standardization Technical Committee. National standard acupuncture technical operating code of the People's Republic of China Part 21: basic filiform acupuncture techniques. GB/T 21709.21-2013. Beijing: China Standards Press; 2013

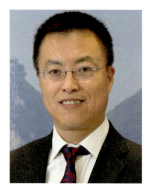

Prof. Dr. Linjun Xia (夏林军) PhD. graduated from Changchun University of Chinese Medicine and Heilongjiang University of Chinese Medicine. A disciple of Professor Zhang Jin, a representative of the World intangible cultural heritage of Chinese medicine acupuncture.

He is currently a guest professor at Hungary Semmelweis University; Vice president of Hungarian TCM Association; Vice president of Specialty Committee of Chinese Medicine Manipulations (WFCMS);Member of the editorial board of the World Journal of Traditional Chinese Medicine (WJTCM).

With more than 30 years of clinical experience, he specializes in acupuncture techniques. Participated in the compilation of "Acupuncture", "Basic theory of Traditional Chinese Medicine" and many other works. He published more than 40 academic papers. For example, "Flying Meridian and Moving the Qi acupuncture technique of and its clinical application" and so on.

In 2022, he was honored with the World Integrative Medicine Top Ten Acupuncture Expert Award.

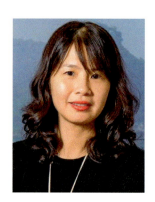

Dr. Yun Ding (丁芸) graduated from Zhongshan University of Medical Science in 1998 and completed his master degree in the same University. After graduating, she worked at the affiliated Stomatology Hospital of Zhongshan Medical University and the affiliated Stomatology Hospital of Kunming Medical University. She attained the position of Associate Professor in 2009.

In 2012, she undertook a year and a half of further studies at the University of Toronto Faculty of Dentistry as visiting professor. She have led various research projects and published numerous academic papers.

Since 2013, she has been studying TCM with Professor Xia in Hungary. From 2018she works as a guest professor of Shenzhou University of TCM. From 2021, She works as member of councel of the Central and Eastern European Federation of Chinese Medicine Societies. From 2022, she serve as the executive director of the Professional Committee on Target Differentiation and Treatment of the World Federation of Societies of TCM.

The Simple Burn-Penetrate Method in Acupuncture

Ying Wang

Learning Objectives

1. Understand the historical development of the traditional "burn-penetrate" method in acupuncture, tracing its roots back to the Ming Dynasty.
2. Identify and differentiate between the two main techniques within the traditional "burn-penetrate" method: "Burn Mountain Fire" and "Penetrate Sky Cool."
3. Comprehend the principles and procedures associated with each technique, including needle insertion depth, manipulation, and the intended effects on the body.
4. Explore the challenges and complexities faced by practitioners in mastering the traditional "burn-penetrate" method.
5. Understand the Four-Layer Theory of Acupoints and its role in the warming and cooling needling methods.

1 The History of the Traditional "Burn-Penetrate" Method in Acupuncture

The history of the traditional "burn-penetrate" method in acupuncture has deep roots, with early descriptions dating back to the Ming Dynasty. Xu Feng, in his work "Jin Zhen Fu," outlined the essential principles of this needling technique. He described two distinct methods: "Burn Mountain Fire" and "Penetrate Sky Cool."

1. "Burn Mountain Fire": This technique was employed to address conditions characterized by stubborn numbness and cold pain. The procedure involved inserting the needle from shallow to deep and moving it forward and backwards three times,

---

Y. Wang (✉)
Dr Ying Chinese Medical Centre, 50 London Road North, Lowestoft NR32 1EP, UK
e-mail: wangyingll@hotmail.com

using a yang number of 9. The needle was gently twisted, pulled up slowly, and pushed down firmly. Once the patient felt warmth, the needle was removed, and the point was closed quickly. The objective was to eliminate cold toxins from the body.
2. "Penetrate Sky Cool": This method aimed to treat conditions marked by hot muscles and a burning sensation in the bones. The procedure needed inserting the needle from deep to shallow and repeating the movement three times, using a yin number 6. Similar to the first technique, the needle was gently twisted and manipulated, with a particular emphasis on slow removal. This approach was intended to eliminate hot toxins from the body.

Both methods emphasized the importance of gentle needle twisting. The ancient texts stressed that these techniques had been established as effective criteria for treating various illnesses.

Yang Ji Zhou, another renowned acupuncturist from the Ming Dynasty, further elaborated on these methods in his book "Zhen Jiu Da Cheng" (The Great Compendium of Acupuncture). He provided additional details on the practices, offering insight into the manipulation of the needle. These early descriptions laid the foundation for the development and understanding of the "burn-penetrate" method in acupuncture, a tradition that has continued to evolve and adapt over the centuries.

"Mouth formula: 'Penetrate Sky Cool' can effectively eliminate hot toxins. Perform three retreats and one advance with the needle. You will experience a cooling sensation throughout the body and take five breaths by inhaling through the mouth and exhaling through the nose. When commencing acupuncture, insert the needle at the one Cun position and perform six needle manipulations, as six is associated with the Yin aspect. The 'five Fen values' represent starting from deep to shallow positions at the end. If Qi is obtained, withdraw the needle to the five Fen area, perform three advances and three retreats, and gently pull and slowly push down the needle. If you feel the needle tip becomes heavy and tight, withdraw the needle slowly; this will generate a cooling Qi, leading to the natural elimination of the hot ailment. If the desired effect is not achieved, simply repeat the previous process and attempt the procedure again" [1].

From ancient texts, it is evident that the manipulation of the traditional "burn-penetration" method comprises several replenishing and reducing techniques. These techniques include lifting and inserting, clockwise and anti-clockwise twisting, the use of yang number 9 or yin number 6, synchronized breathing with inhales and exhales, consideration of gender differences, and precise opening and closing of acupuncture points. However, these complex manoeuvres often lead to disappointment for many practitioners, as achieving the desired warm or cool results remains elusive. The intricate and abstract nature of these paired techniques makes them challenging to replicate for most learners. Unfortunately, this method remains the exclusive domain of a select few experts even today.

From ancient sources, it becomes evident that the manipulation of the traditional "burn-penetration" method encompasses various replenishing and reducing techniques. These techniques involve actions such as lifting and inserting, clockwise or anti-clockwise twisting, the utilization of yang number 9 or yin number 6, synchronization with inhalation and exhalation, consideration of gender distinctions, and precise opening and closing of acupuncture points.

However, these intricate procedures often lead to disappointment for the majority of practitioners who struggle to achieve the desired warm or cool outcomes. Due to the abstract and unverifiable nature of these paired techniques, they prove exceptionally challenging for most learners to replicate. Regrettably, even today, this method remains understood by only a select few experts.

How can we induce sensations of warmth and coolness within our bodies? When we trace back to historical records related to warming, tonifying, cooling, and reducing acupuncture, we find the earliest mention in "Huang Di Nei Jing Ling Shu Nine Needles and Twelve Origins First (The Yellow Emperor's Classic of Internal Medicine—Spiritual Axis)." It states, "The essence of deficiency and excess, nine needles are the best. When reinforcing and reducing, acupuncture was employed to achieve this. For reduction, the needle should be inserted and then released, expelling the Yang toxin, which leads to reduction. Pressing and guiding the needle induces internal warmth, preventing blood dispersion and preserving Qi" [2].

A similar description can be found in "Nan Jing Seventy-Eighth Difficulty" (The Classic Difficulties), which states, "De Qi, pushing the needle inwards, constitutes reinforcement; moving and outstretching, it signifies reduction" [3].

2 The Improved Method: The Simple Burn-Penetrate Method

When we refer to the original classic texts, such as Ling Shu and Nan Jing, it becomes apparent that inducing heating and cooling reactions in the body need not be as complex as described in works like "Jīn Zhen Fu" and "Zhen Jiu Da Cheng." Two educators, Guo Song Peng and Li Yu Jie, conducted a study of the traditional burn-penetrating needling method and drew upon the wisdom of past physicians who employed this technique. Their clinical practice confirmed that the primary acupuncture actions responsible for generating sensations of heat and coolness in the human body are the act of pressing down and lifting up [4].

Pressing down the needle can elicit feelings of warmth in a specific body part, a remote area, or even throughout the entire body. Conversely, pulling or lifting the needle up can create a sensation of coolness in the same regions. For the first time, these intricate procedures have been simplified. Furthermore, the two educators introduced a groundbreaking concept: they suggested that lifting the needle could be utilized to produce a cooling effect [5], further streamlining the process of creating cool sensations in the body.

3 The Four-Layer Theory of Acupoints

Traditionally, in the practice of acupuncture and moxibustion, acupoints have been categorized into three layers: heaven, man, and earth. However, through clinical research, Guo Song Peng and Li Yu Jie discovered that people often overlook the significance of the skin during acupuncture procedures, focusing solely on the subcutaneous tissue structure. However, the skin plays an integral role that cannot be disregarded in acupuncture. As a result, they jointly introduced the concept of "extremely superficial skin" and reclassified acupuncture points into four distinct three-dimensional structures [5].

Ultra-Superficial Layer: This layer is situated between the epidermis and dermis.

Superficial Layer: Found between the dermis and muscle.

Middle Layer: Located within the muscle.

Deep Layer: Situated deep to the bone.

This classification method underscores the vital role of the skin layer in the acupuncture process. In theory, warm and cooling sensations can be achieved in each layer. However, it is in the first two layers that cooling sensations are most easily induced.

4 Operation of the Warm Method

In this method, we typically use needles that are 0.25- or 0.30-mm-thick for needling. Depending on the depth of the acupoints, the method can be categorized as follows:

Ultrasupficial Intradermal Warm Needling Method: After identifying the acupoint, one hand is used to insert the needle. The needle tip is placed on the skin's surface and then gently pressed down, allowing the needle tip to slowly enter the skin without penetrating the dermis. When the needle tip encounters a sense of resistance, it is stopped at this point, referred to as the "origin of induction." The needle tip is maintained at the origin of induction, and gentle pressure is applied, creating a small depression in the skin. The pressing force is maintained, preventing the needle tip and needle body from advancing further until a warming sensation is felt in the body (see Fig. 7.1).

Superficial Subcutaneous Warm Needling Method

Upon identifying the acupoint, swiftly pierce the skin with the needle, and then gradually advance the needle downwards beneath the skin's surface. When the needle tip encounters a sense of resistance, it stops at that depth. Maintain the needle tip at the induction point, applying gentle yet firm pressure. This action will create a small depression on the skin's surface. Ensure that the pressing force is sustained while

Fig. 7.1 Operation of the warm method

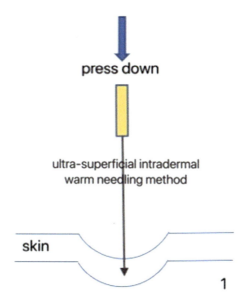

simultaneously preventing the needle tip and needle body from progressing deeper. Continue this process until a warming sensation is felt in the body. (see Fig. 7.2).

Middle-Layer Warm Needling Method

Upon identifying the acupuncture point, the needle was swiftly inserted through the subcutaneous and muscle layers. Once within the muscle layer, transition to a slower needle insertion. When you sense the needle tip encountering resistance, halt at that depth. Maintain the needle tip at the origin of induction, applying gentle pressure. This action will create a small depression on the skin's surface. Ensure that the pressing force is sustained while simultaneously preventing the needle tip and needle body from advancing deeper. Continue this process until a warming sensation is felt in the body (see Fig. 7.2).

Deep Warm Needling Method

Upon identifying the acupuncture point, the needle was inserted directly and rapidly until it reached the bone surface. Then, the needle tip was gently pressed down to stimulate the periosteum. At this point, the skin will also produce a small depression. Maintain this pressure and wait until a warming sensation is felt in the body (see Fig. 7.2).

Fig. 7.2 Superficial subcutaneous warm needling method

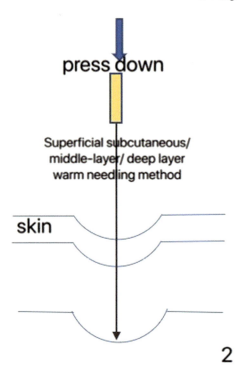

5 Operation of the Cool Method

For the cooling needling method, we apply distinct techniques based on the body's various layers. In the ultrasuperficial and superficial layers, we utilized 0.25 * 25 mm needles, employing the method of lifting the needles. In the middle and deep layers, we adopted the technique of pulling the needle. Depending on the specific body areas, needles measuring 0.30 * 40 mm or longer can be employed.

Lifting Up Needle Method:

Insert the needle quickly into the skin or subcutaneously at an angle of 45–75°, ensuring that there is no pain sensation. Directly use the needle tip to lift a small portion of the skin, creating a slight mound (similar to conducting a penicillin skin test). Maintain this raised state by applying gentle pressure and wait until a cooling or calming sensation is experienced in the body (see Figs. 7.3 and 7.4).

Pulling Up Needle Method:

Swiftly insert the needle into the subcutaneous layer, reaching the middle or deep layer that requires treatment. After obtaining Qi, the stuck needle technique is utilized to ensure that the muscle fibres encircle the needle body and anchor it securely. Then, gently pull the needle upwards while ensuring that it does not come out completely. This action will create a small mound on the skin. Wait until the body experiences a cooling or calming sensation (see Fig. 7.5).

Fig. 7.3 Lifting up needle method

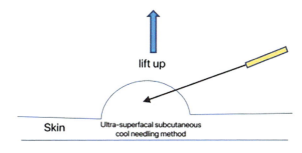

Fig. 7.4 Lifting up needle method

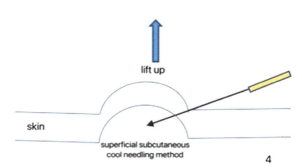

Fig. 7.5 Pulling up needle method

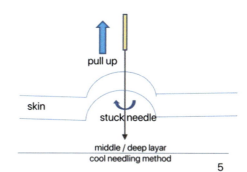

6 Successful Rate Increase

The following precautions are crucial, as they determine whether individuals can fully grasp the key aspects of the heating and cooling needling method. This is also a critical consideration for a successful procedure.

Selecting the appropriate type of acupuncture needles:

- We typically use 0.25 * 25 mm needles for the lifting method. Needles that are too thin and long may not effectively lift the skin. Conversely, overly thick needles can cause discomfort to the patient.

- For the pulling-up and pressing-down methods, we usually use 0.25- or 0.30-mm-thick needles. Thinner needles may not allow successful pulling up or pressing down. Thicker needles can induce pain in the patient.
- Patient comfort is essential during acupuncture. Pain experienced by the patient can mask temperature changes and lead to procedure failure.

Fixing the needle tip at the origin of induction during the warm method is crucial.

- Techniques such as sticking the needle, twisting the needle 180–360° in the same direction, or adding extra twists can help entangle the needle body with muscle fibres, increasing friction. It is important to note that the stuck needle technique is an auxiliary technique, not an accident.

When performing the press-down warm method, it is vital to maintain a stable state by balancing downwards pressure from the needle-holding finger and upwards force from the wrist.

- A slight downforce, slightly greater than uplift, is needed. This creates a small depression in the skin without allowing the needle tip to penetrate the origin induction plane, avoiding failure.

When practicing the cool pulling-up method, the stuck needle technique is utilized to fix the needles within muscle fibres.

- Maintain a dynamic balance between finger lifting force and wrist downwards pressure. A slightly greater upwards force from the fingers than a downwards force from the wrist ensures that skin mounds appear without risking procedure failure by pulling the needle out of the skin.

Both the doctor and patient should remain calm and breathe naturally during the operation.

7 Clinical Application

This warming acupuncture method can be applied to treat various conditions characterized by cold, dampness, deficiency, and blood stasis syndromes. Combining this warming acupuncture method with conventional acupuncture often yields more effective outcomes.

For instance, in cases of neck pain and eye conditions, selecting the Feng Chi point (GB20) and employing the warming acupuncture method can provide relief. When the needle tip encounters resistance, it is gently pressed down. After a brief period, the patient will experience localized warmth, which may even extend to the eyes, bringing comfort and relaxation to the neck and eyes.

For various types of joint pain, points located on or near the affected joints can be treated using the warming acupuncture method.

In the case of shoulder pain, locally affected meridians such as LI-15 Jianyu, SJ-14 Jianliao, and SI-9 Jianzhen points can be selected, along with distant points such as LI-4 Hegu, SJ-3 Zhongzhu, and SI-3 Houxi. Applying the warming acupuncture method to these points, whether near or far, can provide warmth and comfort to the entire shoulder and upper arm, effectively alleviating pain.

To address scapular pain, directly applying the deep layer warming acupuncture method to the SI-11 Tianzong point can relieve discomfort throughout the scapular area.

For lower back issues, using the warming acupuncture method on the BL-23 Shenshu and DU-4 Mingmen points can strengthen the lower back, invigorate kidney function, and alleviate pain.

In cases of sciatica, employing the warming acupuncture method on the GB-30 Huantiao point can generate a warm sensation, which travels from the buttocks down to the lower limbs, providing relief.

For various gynecological conditions, such as irregular menstruation, dysmenorrhea, ovarian cysts, uterine fibroids, endometriosis, and infertility, the warming acupuncture method can be applied to the REN-4 Guanyuan and REN-6 Qihai points. This approach warms the lower abdomen, dispels cold toxins, promotes blood circulation, and alleviates stasis to relieve pain.

To address extreme edema or water retention, points such as SP-6 Sanyinjiao, SP-9 Yinlingquan, SP-3 Taibai, ST-28 Shuidao, and LU-5 Chize can be chosen to nourish the spleen, dispel dampness, and promote water circulation. Incorporating the warming acupuncture method at these points enhances the effectiveness of the treatment.

For patients with weakened body conditions, applying the warming acupuncture method to the REN-4 Guanyuan, REN-6 Qihai, KD-3 Taixi, and BL-23 Shenshu points can warm and nourish the kidneys. Points such as REN-12 Zhongwan, ST-36 Zusanli, and SP-9 Sanyinjiao can be selected to warm and nourish the spleen and stomach, ultimately boosting the body's energy.

The cooling needling method is ideal for cases of heat syndromes and restlessness.

For instance:

- In cases of fever, using the cooling needle method on LI-4 Hegu, LI-11 Quchi, SJ-5 Waiguan, Yin Tang (extra point), and DU-14 Dazhui points can help reduce heat, detoxify, and lower elevated body temperature.
- For headaches, specific acupoints can be selected depending on the type of headache. The ST-44 Neiting point can be used for Yangming meridian headaches, the Shaoyang meridian headache can be addressed using the Shao Yang meridian Zu Lin Qi point, Taiyang headaches may be treated with the BL-60 Kunlun point, and the Jue Yin headache can be alleviated by using the LIV-3 Taichong point. Adding the extra point Yin Tang to any headache type using the cooling acupuncture method can enhance the results.
- For depression and insomnia, you could also choose the extra point Yin Tang point to operate the cooling acupuncture method, promoting calmness and facilitating sleep.

- For skin diseases with red and itchy skin lesions, such as eczema, psoriasis, or shingles, acupuncture at LI-15 Quchi, LI-15 Jianliao, LU-5 Chize, and Ashi points around skin lesions can use this cooling acupuncture method to reduce swelling and relieve itching.
- Patients experiencing burning pain can quickly reduce the burning sensation by adding a local cooling acupuncture method compared with conventional acupuncture.

In clinical practice, two acupuncture methods can be simultaneously applied to the same patient based on their pathogenesis and physical condition. For instance, for patients with heat in the upper Jiao and cold in the lower Jiao, the warm method can be employed at the REN-4 Guanyuan point to warm the lower Jiao, while the cool method can be applied to the extra point Yin Tang to clear the heat in the upper Jiao. These treatments will achieve a balance of yin and yang in the body. For example, in the treatment of menopausal syndrome patients, using this combination of warming and cooling treatments can quickly alleviate the symptoms of hot flashes, night sweats, insomnia, and depression.

8 Mechanisms of the Burn-Penetrate Method in Acupuncture

The traditional operation mechanism of "burning mountain fire" and "cooling through the sky" can be summarized as follows: "burning mountain fire" involves "introducing yang into yin," while "cooling through the sky" entails "introducing yang (yang evil) out of yin."

In terms of modern human physiological functions, changes in skin temperature are directly linked to blood perfusion in the microvascular bed of the skin. The microcirculation comprises arterioles and venules with sympathetic and parasympathetic nerve endings. Mechanical changes caused by depressing and lifting the needle tip affect pressure and temperature receptors in the skin, leading to a series of reactions. This information is integrated and transmitted, and due to the synergistic effect of the brain's body temperature center and peripheral sympathetic and parasympathetic nerves, blood perfusion in the microcirculation increases or decreases, resulting in sensations of cold and heat and changes in local or whole-body temperature.

Based on our clinical observations, we have outlined the mechanism of the "burn-penetrating" acupuncture method.

The Acupuncture DreamWorks team has identified that acupuncture's ability to produce a cool-warm response is associated with the changing pressures applied to skin, muscle, blood vessels, fascia, and other related structural elements. We further believe that the human body's baroreceptors must play a role in the physiological, pathological, and transformative processes of this cooling-warming phenomenon. (The relationship between pressure and temperature was confirmed through research in the 2021 Medical Award) [6].

The pressure changes induced by acupuncture stimulate corresponding baroreceptors, leading to alterations in body temperature perception, encompassing objective cooling and warming as well as subjective feelings of warmth and coolness.

Objective cooling and warming are temperature changes that can be externally detected using a thermometer or infrared scanner. Subjective feelings refer to the patient's perception of their body feeling warm and comfortable or remarkably calm and cool, even if they cannot discern these temperature changes.

This shift between warmth and coolness further activates the body's innate self-healing capabilities. Considering this, everyone: our aim is not merely to cool or heat the patient during the procedure. Rather, our goal is for this temperature change to enhance the body's inherent self-healing function.

Building upon this theory, we simplified and refined the "Burn-Penetrate" technique to press down and lift up.

The research has revealed that the core element of the burn-penetrate method, which elicits warming and cooling responses, is the act of pushing down and lifting up.

Review Questions

1. What were the two distinct methods outlined in the traditional "burn-penetrate" method, and what conditions were each intended to address?
2. Describe the key steps involved in the "Burn Mountain Fire" technique, emphasizing needle manipulation and the intended outcome.
3. How does the "Penetrate Sky Cool" method differ from the "Burn Mountain Fire" technique, and what conditions is it designed to treat?
4. According to ancient texts, what were the challenges and disappointments faced by practitioners attempting to master the traditional "burn-penetrate" method?
5. Explain the Four-Layer Theory of Acupoints and its significance in the practice of acupuncture. How does it contribute to the understanding of warming and cooling sensations?

References

1. Cheng ZJ (Ming), Zhou YJ, Xian J. Supplementary reediting, Huang Long Xiang arrange. Beijing: People's Health Publishing House; 2017. pp. 150–151
2. Jing LS, Hua TD. Arrange. Beijing: People's Health Publishing House;2005. p. 2
3. Yi NJY, Xing LY, editors. Chief. Beijing: People's Health Publishing House;2013. p. 118
4. Qi LC. The improvement and clinic applications of burning mountain fire and penetrating sky cool. 2nd ed. National Medical Forum; 1994, pp. 32–33
5. Guo-Li. Acupuncture method in dermal to produce warm and cool effect on lesion and body/ Ying Wang. J Chinese Med Acup.2015;22(2):23–24
6. Zhen Y. The 2021 Nobel Prize focus on heat-sensitive channels, what enlightenment does it have on the interpretation of cold and heat theory in TCM. QH web; 2021-11-26
7. Wang Y. Simple "burn-penetrate" method in acupuncture. World Chin Med. 2(1):40–47

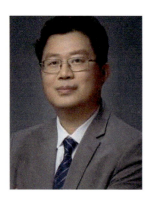

Ying Wang (王迎) graduated from the Acupuncture Department of Shandong University of Traditional Chinese Medicine in 1992. He was invited to the UK for work and teaching since 2001.

He is a professor of acupuncture at the UK Academy of Chinese Medicine. Served as the executive vice president of the Overseas Alumni Association of Shandong University of TCM, Distinguished expert of the French Association of TCM and from Swiss University of Chinese Medicine. The general manager of the overseas acupuncture technology development team "Acupuncture Dream Factory".

He dedicated himself to global promotion and training in abdominal diagnosis acupuncture. And published many articles.

Dao-Qi Needling Technique

Zunli Guo

Learning Objectives

1. Understand the fundamental principle of acupuncture, emphasizing the importance of achieving the Deqi sensation.
2. Comprehend the concept of "Qi Zhi Bing Suo" (气至病所), where the therapeutic effectiveness relies on the extension of Qi to affected areas.
3. Identify the purpose of the Dao-qi Needling technique in guiding Qi along meridian pathways.
4. Recognize the role of the Dao-qi Needling technique in restoring balance by harmonizing rebellious Qi.
5. Appreciate the suitability of the Dao-qi technique for addressing disorders of Qi, physical deficiencies, and conditions involving pathogenic Qi.

1 General Introduction to the Dao-Qi Needling Technique

The Dao-qi Needling technique finds its roots in the Huang Di Nei Jing, specifically in Lingshu, Chapter 34, known as Wu Luan—The Five Disturbances. This method is characterized by the deliberate approach of slow needle insertion and slow withdrawal, which is referred to as the Dao-qi Needling technique. Rather than focusing on visible supplementation and drainage, it concentrates on the subtle manipulation of Qi, a concept known as gathering the essence. In essence, this technique is not concerned with addressing excess or deficiency; its aim is to restore harmony to disturbed Qi that deviates from the norm [1].

The Dao-qi Needling technique involves the practice of slowly inserting and withdrawing the needle, ensuring the attainment of Deqi (a characteristic needle

Z. Guo (✉)
London Academy of Chinese Acupuncture, London, UK
e-mail: zguo176@hotmail.com

sensation). It incorporates gentle lifting with insertion, a minimal twisting range, and a slow frequency. The sensations experienced during needling spread along the meridian pathways, effectively releasing pathogenic Qi and facilitating the restoration of healthy Qi. This method is widely employed in the treatment of conditions arising from disturbances in Qi movement, where distinctions between deficiency and excess are unclear or both are present simultaneously. Its primary objective is to fortify the body and expel pathogenic Qi.

The fundamental technique of Dao-qi needling primarily comprises lifting with insertion and gentle twisting, with specific standards for the frequency, angle, and amplitude of these actions. Adhering to these standards is pivotal to the technique's success.

Key features of the Dao-qi Needling technique include a minimal selection of acupuncture points, a gentle and unhurried approach, a high level of patient compliance, and remarkable therapeutic outcomes. This technique has garnered recognition from acupuncturists and patients alike. Furthermore, it exhibits significant advantages in the treatment of chronic diseases and conditions related to emotions.

A detailed explanation of the Dao-qi Needling technique can be found in the 2014 publication by Dr. Tianjin Wang and colleges in the journal "Acupuncture in Medicine." The paper, titled "Acupuncture Combined with an Antidepressant for Patients with Depression in Hospital: A Pragmatic Randomized Controlled Trial," elaborates on the specific manipulations involved in the Dao-qi technique. It is believed to be the first text on this subject published in English in the Western world, focusing on the Dao-qi acupuncture technique and its intricate manipulations [2].

2 The Dao-Qi Needling Technique

The Purpose of Dao-qi

Dao-qi involves guiding Qi to flow within the meridians, not only delivering Qi to the affected areas but also ensuring smooth Qi circulation throughout the meridian system. Throughout the Dao-qi process, sensations along the meridians may arise, and these sensations can ultimately lead to the affected areas. Therefore, when inserting the needle, it is essential to first achieve the Deqi sensation and then manipulate the Qi.

Through the Dao-qi Needling technique, disorderly Qi located in the superficial layer gradually shifts into the deeper layers. Simultaneously, the disorderly Qi that should have remained in the superficial layer but had reversed into the deeper layers is progressively guided upwards to the superficial layer. The needle is slowly and gently inserted to direct the disorderly Qi, which resists the Yang, back toward the Yin. Similarly, the needle is slowly and gently withdrawn to guide the clear Qi, which opposes the Yin, back toward the Yang. This process allows the disorderly Qi, ranging from clear Qi and turbid Qi to Ying Qi and Wei Qi, which had deviated from

Dao-Qi Needling Technique

their intended positions, to return to their respective roles and fulfil their functions, ultimately eliminating the disorderly Qi.

The Mechanism of the Dao-qi Needling Technique

The most fundamental requirement of the Dao-qi Needling technique is to attune the mind. To better facilitate the prerequisites of spiritual healing, it is imperative to position the patient comfortably during acupuncture, allowing the patient's emotions and body to relax. The sensation experienced during needle insertion is known as Deqi. Slow and gentle needle insertion entails slowly twisting the needle from the superficial layer to the deeper layers, while slow and gentle needle withdrawal entails slowly twisting the needle from the deeper layers back to the superficial layer. Directing Qi to the affected area involves using acupuncture to prompt local or systemic Qi and blood responses, adjusting functions, and propagating the needle sensation to the site of the ailment, ultimately achieving an enhanced clinical curative effect.

The crux of the Dao-qi Needling technique lies in its deliberate and gentle approach, emphasizing precise control over the speed of needle twisting. Acupuncturists must strive for an optimal balance, avoiding excessive tonification or dispersion, ensuring that the stimulation intensity remains measured. This entails maintaining a deliberate slowness in the frequency of lifting, inserting, twisting, needle insertion and withdrawal. Gentleness dictates that the angle of twisting and the range of lifting and insertion should be minimal to induce a relatively mild and comfortable needle sensation. The acupuncturist's touch should be gentle, ensuring that patients do not experience pain during needle insertion or withdrawal but rather a subtle and comfortable sensation during the procedure.

The effectiveness of the Dao-qi Needling technique becomes evident beneath the needle, as it should possess a certain degree of tension while allowing for free lifting, insertion, and twisting. This sensation of unhindered operation manifests as consistent resistance during both upwards lifting and downwards insertion, as well as equivalent resistance during left twisting and right turning. Such consistent resistance ensures that the muscle fibres beneath the needle maintain a gentle and appropriate tension. The continuous and rhythmic twisting of the needle during the procedure enhances patient comfort. Sustaining a prolonged, stable, and faint sense of acquiring Qi and experiencing the needle sensation is paramount. Maintaining this connection to Qi throughout the process of guiding it is essential; losing this connection equates to losing the needle sensation and, consequently, diminishing the curative effect. Achieving this level of mastery necessitates that the practitioner possess a solid foundation in acupuncture techniques.

At its core, Qi-guiding acupuncture treatment demands the regulation and healing of the mind. To better fulfil the need for spiritual healing, the Dao-qi Needling technique should ensure that the patient assumes a comfortable acupuncture position, allowing them to relax both their emotions and body throughout the entire duration of the procedure. This commitment to maintaining patient comfort is essential for the success of the technique.

3 Key Points of Clinical Operation of the Dao-Qi Needling Technique

In Huang Di Nei Jing, Lingshu Chapter 71—Xieke (Retention of the Evil), it is emphasized that in the manipulation of pricking, one should maintain an upright and calm posture. Understanding the asthenia and sthenia of the disease is crucial before determining the speed of needle insertion. During insertion, the left-side hand should grip the patient's bone, while the right-side hand presses on the acupoint with a finger to prevent the needle from becoming entangled in muscle fibres. When pricking, it is essential to keep the needle straight and ensure a direct forward insertion. In invigorating, the needle held on the skin must be sealed. The technique of twisting the needle is applied to Dao-qi to prevent it from running rashly, thereby stabilizing the healthy qi.

These operational guidelines are derived from Huang Di Nei Jing and provide insights into the Dao-qi Needling technique and the results it achieves.

Accurate selection of acupoints is the basis for the success of the Dao-qi Needling technique. If acupoint selection is inaccurate or inappropriate, it is often difficult to obtain Deqi. When selecting acupoints, press repeatedly and do not deviate from their exact positions.

Acupuncture direction and depth are crucial factors. If the acupuncture direction, angle, or depth is incorrect, obtaining Deqi from the needle becomes challenging. In such cases, it should be readjusted, and exploration around the acupuncture point or Tian Di Ren three parts should be conducted until a satisfactory needle sensation is achieved.

Regarding the gesture for holding the needle, the thumb and index finger of the left hand should be pressed next to the point of insertion. The right hand's thumb and index finger should hold the upper 2/3 of the needle handle relative to each other, while the middle finger pad supports the lower 1/3 of the needle handle. After inserting the needle, based on the Deqi obtained through lifting with insertion and twisting, the thumb of the pricking hand was used for soft and slow lifting with insertion and twisting. This causes a heavy and tight sensation under the acupuncturist's fingers, unifying the heart, hand, and needle. The three fingers tighten the needle handle, following the mind. The sensation of tightness and astringency under the fingers becomes more apparent, experiencing the sensation around the patient's acupoint or along the meridian route.

The selection of needles is important. The commonly used needles have a diameter of 0.20–0.30 mm, and the length is determined based on the patient's body size and tolerance for Dao-qi.

In specific operations, the frequency of lifting with insertion and twisting is approximately 60–100 times per minute, with a twisting angle less than 90°. The lifting with the insertion range should not exceed 2 mm. Additionally, lifting with insertion and twisting should be performed slowly and softly, ensuring uniform force and equal amplitude and frequency. The speed should be slow with continuity. Adequate time should be allowed for manipulation, with approximately 1 min for acupuncture at matching points and approximately 2 min for the main acupoints. For intractable diseases, the Dao-qi Needling technique can take several minutes, enhancing the needle sensation during the process of needle retention.

During the Dao-qi Needling technique, acupuncturists should pay constant attention to the feeling under the needle and maintain communication with the patient to observe their reactions. As long as the patient experiences a slight and comfortable needling sensation, the technique is being performed effectively.

The Dao-qi Needling technique requires a slow, gentle, and even approach. Achieving the technique's requirements is possible only through low-frequency, small-angle, small-amplitude, and even lifting with insertion and twisting.

4 Common Acupoint Selection for Dao-Qi Needling Technique

The Dao-qi Needling technique is versatile and can be applied to various acupoints throughout the body, selected based on the specific needs of the disease. A concise overview of commonly used acupoints for the clinical Dao-qi Needling technique is provided below:

GV-14 Da Zhui

For this point, the patient assumes a prone or sitting position. Needle selection is based on the patient's body size and tolerance, commonly using a 0.25*40 mm needle. To initiate the Deqi sensation at the GV-14 Da Zhui point, the acupuncturist uses the Dao-qi Needling technique to guide the Qi and regulate the spirit.

The procedure involves the thumb and index finger of the left hand pressed next to the GV-14 Da Zhui point, while the right-side hand's thumb and index finger hold the upper 2/3 of the needle handle. The middle finger pad supports the lower 1/3 of the needle handle, and the three fingers cooperate. The needle is inserted at the GV-14 Da Zhui point, and the patient may experience the Deqi sensation after insertion to a depth of approximately 5–10 mm. Subsequently, lifting with insertion and twisting is performed evenly and slowly. The direction of the needle is adjusted after the Deqi sensation, and persistent twisting and lifting with inserting techniques are applied to reach a depth of 25–30 mm.

The sensation of the needle spreads along the governor meridian (Du Mai) to areas such as the shoulders, chest, and waist, with continuous twisting and lifting with insertion to stimulate the Qi during this period. Typically, this technique is employed for approximately 2 min. Following the Dao-qi Needling technique, the needle is retained for 20–30 min, and the Dao-qi Needling technique is applied once more in the middle of the needle retention process to enhance the needle sensation.

When performing acupuncture to regulate the spirit and guide Qi to the brain at the GV-14 Da Zhui point, it is essential not to insist on forcing Qi along the meridian route, especially during the first treatment. The acupuncturist should attentively monitor the sensation under the needle and stay in touch with the patient to observe their reactions throughout the Dao-qi Needling technique. The goal is for the patient to experience a slight and comfortable needling sensation.

Ba Liao Points (BL31, BL32, BL33, BL34)

The patient is positioned prone, and initially, the sacral area is explored with potential points (Chuai Xue) to locate the posterior sacral foramen. Starting from the lower part, the index finger of the left hand is pressed next to S4 (Xia Liao point BL34). The right-hand thumb and index finger hold the upper 2/3 of the needle handle, while the middle finger pad supports the lower 1/3, and the three fingers cooperate. The needle is inserted sequentially at S3 (Xia Liao point BL33), S3 (Zhong Liao point BL33), S2 (Ci Liao point BL32), and finally S1 (Shang Liao point BL31), with specific angles and sensations as described. The needle tip should face the midline of the spine crest.

For patients with hypertrophy or local subcutaneous fat, placing a pillow on the lower abdomen to raise the buttocks facilitates exposure of the sacrum. This method aids in locating acupoints and performing the procedure. If bony obstruction occurs, adjusting the needle tip and changing the insertion direction is advised until a sensation akin to falling is felt.

Upon entering the presacral foramen from the posterior sacral foramen, if there is a strong needling sensation radiating to the perineum and lower abdomen or a painful feeling, needle insertion should stop. If the patient experiences a strong needling sensation not radiating to the perineum and lower abdomen, the needle insertion angle and direction are adjusted, and the needle is slowly inserted until reaching the predetermined depth.

Following the completion of acupuncture, the Dao-qi Needling technique is employed with gentle, soft, and slow movements, using small doses, low frequency, and continuous lifting with insertion and twisting. The sensation of the needle induces a slight, radiating acupuncture or tingling sensation in the lower abdomen, anus, perineum, and pelvic cavity, possibly even an electric shock sensation.

Throughout the process, efforts are made to ensure the patient's comfort and minimize pain. The Dao-qi Needling technique is applied for approximately 2 min, followed by needle retention for 20–30 min based on the patient's tolerance or needs. In the middle of the needle retention process, the Dao-qi Needling technique is performed once more to enhance the needle sensation.

RN-4 Guan Yuan, RN-6 Qi Hai

The patient is in the supine position, and the choice of needles is tailored to the patient's body size and tolerance, with a commonly used needle size of 0.25*40 mm. Using the index finger of the left hand pressed next to the RN-4 Guan Yuan or RN-6 Qihai points, the right-hand thumb and index finger hold the upper 2/3 of the needle handle relative to each other, while the middle finger pad supports the lower 1/3 of the needle handle, and the three fingers cooperate with each other. During needle insertion, the thumb and index of the left-hand fingers are pressed, pushed, and kneaded around the RN-4 Guan Yuan or RN-6 Qihai points on the abdomen. The right-side hand fingers hold a 0.25*40 mm needle and insert it down approximately 10–30 mm, gently guiding the needle with the right-side hand fingers.

After achieving Deqi, the tip of the needle is inserted vertically into the back or adjusted to the lower abdomen and directed toward the uterus, based on the patient's sensitivity. Using the Dao-qi Needling technique, the needle is slowly, softly, and gently twirled, with the dose and frequency adapted to the patient's needs and comfort. This allows the needling sensation to radiate to the lower abdomen or reach the pelvic cavity. The Dao-qi Needling technique is applied for approximately 2 min, followed by needle retention for 20–30 min according to the patient's tolerance. In the middle of the needle retention process, the Dao-qi Needling technique is employed once more to enhance the needle sensation.

Considering the patient's specific needs and diseases, one acupoint is chosen as the main point and the other as the matching point. There are differences between them in the Dao-qi Needling technique, with the main acupoint requiring approximately 2 min and the matching point requiring approximately 1 min.

5 Indications for the Dao-Qi Needling Technique

The Dao-qi Needling technique is applicable to a wide range of diseases, as the lesion can involve any viscera in the whole body or even multiple viscera co-occur. The indication is the reverse disorder qi, meaning it is neither the excess of evil qi nor the deficiency of health qi. It is suitable for disordered qi with abnormal qi. The Dao-qi Needling technique restores the normal state by guiding the body's rebellious qi, adjusting the patient's health physiological function, and promoting psychological balance through physiological balance to achieve qi and spiritual peace. Because this kind of disease does not belong to the syndrome of excess and deficiency but is caused by the temporary confusion of qi mechanism, it is not aimed at the disease of excess and deficiency but mainly treats disorder qi [3].

The Dao-qi Needling technique is commonly used in mental disorders and nervous system diseases, such as depression and anxiety. Acupuncturists will be needed to carefully understand and feel the movement of qi at the operation site, making appropriate adjustments if necessary, during the Dao-qi Needling technique period. The patient will also be needed to carefully understand the various sensations and changes in the acupoint. Its change is not only a process of biological change but also a process of psychological change at the same time during the Dao-qi Needling technique.

As the Dao-qi Needling technique has a more definite curative effect in regulating and curing the spirit, it can be widely used in internal medicine, surgery, women and children, eye, ear, nose, throat, trauma, mental illness, etc.

6 Precautions for the Dao-Qi Needling Technique

Acupuncture has an effect on regulating and curing the spirit, encompassing both the patients' and the acupuncturist's spirits. It is crucial to emphasize the regulation and healing of the spirit during Dao-qi Needling technique treatments. Healing the spirit is key to the effectiveness of the Dao-qi Needling technique [3].

Treating the spirit of patients entails providing targeted psychological counselling before the treatment, fostering a positive attitude in patients towards their health, and creating a conducive psychological environment for acupuncture treatment to achieve the goal of treating both the mind and body.

Effective communication with the patient before treatment is advocated, including addressing doubts and fears about acupuncture. This helps patients relax physically and mentally, eliminating external interference and allowing them to focus on their experience under the needle.

Close cooperation between the acupuncturist and the patient during treatment is crucial. The acupuncturist must concentrate on the feeling under the needle, observe changes in Qi and blood from the patient, and make timely adjustments. Observing the patient's mental state and encouraging communication if there is any discomfort under the needle are essential. Conducting Qi is easier if the patient's mind is focused and the mood is comfortable, while a trance or divergent thoughts are not suitable for Dao-qi Needling technique treatment.

The Dao-qi Needling technique treatment is based on the individual state of the patient. Different physiques have varying tolerances, pain thresholds, and sensitivities to acupuncture. The state of Qi and blood in the patient's body also differs. Therefore, the Dao-qi Needling technique treatment should be flexible according to the patient's constitution, condition, and the acupuncturist's feeling under the needle.

In clinical practice, attention must be paid to these differences, and the amplitude, frequency, and angle of lifting, insertion, and twisting under the finger should be adjusted according to the individual. The acupuncture depth varies, generally focusing on the three parts of heaven, earth, and humanity. Specific depth needs to be determined based on individual conditions and the location of selected acupuncture points.

The Dao-qi Needling technique is mostly used for patients with complex conditions and a limited response to other conventional treatments. It may not be suitable for first-time patients or those sensitive to acupuncture, especially when dealing with high-risk areas such as the back-shu points, chest area, and front and neck points. If needed, these high-risk areas should only be treated by trained acupuncturists proficient in local anatomy and with extensive acupuncture experience.

Environmental factors are also crucial, with the treatment room ideally maintaining a suitable temperature, being quiet, and being free from excessive noise. Patients should be advised to rest, stay hydrated, replenish energy, and receive sun exposure after treatment. Immediate contact with the doctor is recommended if the patient feels unwell.

Choosing the right patient, considering their physical condition, and selecting the appropriate position are vital factors for the success of Dao-qi Needling technique treatment.

7 Clinical Research on the Dao-Qi Needling Technique

Research conducted by Wang TJ et al. utilized Du channel-based acupoints to treat hospitalized patients with depression through Qi-guiding acupuncture, achieving a more significant effect than antidepressants alone. Early acupuncture intervention, in particular, proved helpful for the treatment of depression and reduction of adverse reactions [4].

Tao and colleagues conducted a study comparing Qi-guiding acupuncture at governor points and common electroacupuncture to observe the clinical efficacy in treating lumbar disc herniation. The conclusion indicated that Qi-guiding needling at governor points is superior to electroacupuncture in treating lumbar disc herniation [5].

In another study [6], Xie et al. observed differences in the clinical curative effects of various acupuncture methods on dry eye syndrome. The conclusion revealed that both conventional electroacupuncture therapy and air-conducting acupuncture combined with electroacupuncture were effective for dry eye syndrome. Air-conducting acupuncture Fajia electroacupuncture was found to be more effective than conventional electroacupuncture in treating dry eye syndrome.

Yang et al. conducted a clinical observation on Ba Liao Acupoints Dao-qi Method combined with Needle-Warming Moxibustion in treating ulcerative colitis of the spleen and kidney. The study discussed the curative effect of Qi-guiding acupuncture at the Ba Liao point combined with warming needling moxibustion in the treatment of ulcerative colitis. It was found that this combined therapy had a significantly lower relapse rate and shorter healing time than only warming needling moxibustion therapy. The conclusion suggests that Qi-guiding acupuncture at the Ba Liao point combined with warming needling moxibustion is more effective in treating ulcerative colitis [7].

Wang et al. conducted a clinical observation on Governor Vessel Dao-qi Method for the treatment of dyssomnia in patients with depression. While seeking an effective method to treat sleep disorders in depression, Wang J observed that acupuncture combined with antidepressant drugs had a significantly different clinical curative effect in treating sleep disorders compared to antidepressant drugs alone. The conclusion indicates that Du Channel Guidance Acupuncture combined with antidepressant drugs can significantly improve depression and sleep disorders [8].

8 Summary

The Dao-qi Needling technique treatment employs a method characterized by slowness, gentleness, and softness as the needle technique. Tailored to the individual state of the patient and the specific condition and guided by the principles of dialectical treatment, the amount, intensity, and duration of stimulation needed for the Dao-qi Needling technique are flexibly controlled.

Acupuncturists must possess high-level skills, profound theoretical knowledge, solid foundational skills, and maintain good physical health to instill trust in the patient and effectively collaborate in the treatment. The application of the Dao-qi Needling technique involves a comprehensive adjustment of both the spirit and body. It is more than a mere physical stimulation process; it is a nuanced method requiring careful consideration of the core aspect of healing the spirit. This is particularly crucial in the treatment of mind regulation and qi guidance, involving the adjustment of the patient's emotional and bodily functional state to achieve noticeable effects. Despite its delicacy and time-consuming nature, the Dao-qi Needling technique offers significant advantages in treating chronic diseases and emotion-related conditions.

Review Questions

1. What are the fundamental principles underlying the Dao-qi Needling Technique, and how do they differentiate it from conventional acupuncture methods?
2. Explain the step-by-step process of using the Dao-qi Needling Technique on a specific acupoint, outlining the exact manipulations and sensations involved during the procedure.
3. Describe the key criteria for selecting appropriate acupoints for the Dao-qi Needling Technique. How does the correct selection of acupoints impact the effectiveness of this method?
4. What are the primary indications and patient considerations for applying the Dao-qi Needling Technique? Discuss the pivotal precautions and environmental factors necessary for successful treatment.

References and Key Reading Material

1. Unschuld PU. Huang Di Nei Jing Ling Shu: the ancient classic on needle therapy. California USA: University of California Press; 2016, ebook.
2. Wand B, Wu LS, Wu Q (Trans). Yellow Emperors cannon of internal medicine. Beijing: China Science and Technology Press; 1997.
3. Wang TJ. Acupuncture for brain-treatment for neurological and psychological disorders. Chan, Switzerland: Springer; 2021.
4. Wang TJ, Wang LL, Tao W, et al. Acupuncture combined with an antidepressant for patients with depression in hospital: a pragmatic randomized controlled trial. Acupuncture Med. 2014;32:308–12.

5. Tao Q, Zhang JF, Wu CH, et al. Clinical study of Qi-guiding acupuncture at Du Meridian points for treatment of Lumbar intervertebral disc herniation. Shanghai J Acupuncture Moxibustion. 2018;37:665–70.
6. Xie WZ, Zeng L, Tao Y, et al. Guiding-Qi acupuncture for dry eye syndrome. Chin Acupuncture Moxibustion. 2018;38:153–7.
7. Yang X, Li CR, Liu XY. Clinical observation of Ba Liao Acupoints Dao-qi method combined with needle-warming moxibustion in treating UC of Spleen and Lindey. J Clin Acupuncture Moxibustion. 2021;37(07):29–32.
8. Wang J, Jiang JF, Wang LL. Clinical observation on governor vessel Dao-qi method for treatment of dyssomnia in the patient of depression. Chin Acupuncture Moxibustion. 2006;26:328–30.

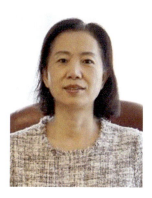

Dr. Zunli Guo (郭尊莉) has worked in a Chinese Medicine hospital for 10 years before moved to the UK. She has worked as practitioner of Chinese Medicine and acupuncture from 2002 till now. She established her Chinese Medicine centre since 2007.

Dr Guo has completed her master's degree of Traditional Chinese Medicine in the University of Middlesex UK in 2011. She completed her PhD study of acupuncture in Nanjing University of Chinese Medicine Nanjing China in 2021 and gained Doctor's degree of Medicine.

Dr Zunli Guo has talked as speakers in many seminars and conference in TCM and acupuncture. She is the executive director of the Academy of Scalp Acupuncture UK, and the senior member of the Chinese Acupuncture and Herbal Medicine Alliance UK.

Moxibustion and Cupping

Moxibustion

Phoebus Tian

Learning Objectives

> Understanding the history of moxibustion, including its origins and historical development in various cultures.
> Learning about different types of moxibustion and techniques, such as direct and indirect moxibustion, and the various methods used in these techniques.
> Exploring the clinical applications of moxibustion, focusing on how it's used in traditional Chinese medicine for treating various conditions.
> Understanding the contraindications for moxibustion.
> Investigating current research on moxibustion, including studies on its efficacy and potential health benefits.

1 History of Moxibustion

艾灸 in Chinese is a combination of two words, 艾 (Pinyin: Ai), meaning mugwort, 灸 (Pinyin: Jiu), meaning burn. Mugwort was first used as a tool to start fires with prisms made of ice in ancient times [29]. Studies of the earliest known form of Chinese writing, Oracle Bone Script (Jiagu Wen, 甲骨文), indicated that moxibustion might have been applied in the Shang period.

P. Tian (✉)
London Academy of Chinese Acupuncture, London, UK
e-mail: hello@phoebustian.com

In ancient times, mugwort (Artemisia vulgaris) was commonly used by the Greeks and Romans for its medicinal properties. The herb was believed to be a remedy for digestive disorders. In Europe, mugwort has been used in many cultural and religious practices. It was believed to have protective properties and was often used to ward off evil spirits. In traditional Chinese medicine, the species Artemisia argyi is more commonly used for moxibustion treatments.

Since the beginning of the twentieth century, a large number of bamboo slips and silk books have been unearthed from Mawangdui tombs of the Han (202 BC–220 AD) dynasty in China. These documents documented valuable medical materials and partially illustrated how Chinese medicine originated. The records of moxibustion showed that it had been developed into different modalities and utilized to treat many diseases at that time. Additionally, the indications and contraindications of moxibustion and the method of post moxibustion care were also discussed. Wushi'er Bingfang, or Recipes for Fifty-Two Ailments, discovered in 1973 in Mawangdui, is the earliest medical record of using mugwort for moxibustion. It also mentioned other martials for moxibustion but mugwort is more suitable.

The Huangdi Neijing, or Yellow Emperor's Classic of Internal Medicine, is one of the oldest and most fundamental works on TCM. It states that moxibustion originated in the north, and it also explains that moxibustion was used to disperse harmful accumulations that had been caused by food stagnation. The text also states that practitioners should use moxibustion for tonifying/reducing and adjust the moxibustion dosage and time according to the patients' situation.

Moxibustion flourished during the Tang dynasty (618–907). The Imperial Medical Academy of the Tang Dynasty appointed specialists to teach and use the therapy. During this period, moxibustion was much appreciated as a treatment method. Many doctors believed that acupuncture was not easy to master, while moxibustion was simple, easy to use, safe and easy to popularize.

Suppurative moxibustion became popular from the Song dynasty to the Qing dynasty (960–1912). The importance of moxibustion sores has been stressed by many medical practitioners, who regard moxibustion sores as the key to effectiveness.

In recent years, research has sought to better understand the mechanisms behind moxibustion and its potential clinical applications. Moxibustion has been found to affect the levels of proinflammatory and anti-inflammatory cytokines, possibly helping to reduce inflammation [28]. Min et al. [25] found that moxibustion may also affect the release of certain hormones in rats, such as corticosterone (CORT), adrenocorticotropic hormone (ACTH), and corticotropin-releasing hormone (CRH). Another study found that moxibustion can regulate T lymphocyte subsets and the activity of NK cells [20]. One team suggested that the effect of moxibustion appears to be determined by the activation of transient receptor potential vanilloids (TRPVs) [9].

2 Types of Moxibustion and Techniques

2.1 *Moxa Cone*

2.1.1 Direct Moxibustion

Direct moxibustion is a moxa cone (Fig. 9.1) that is directly used on the selected area and then ignited to create a superficial burn. Moxa cones are usually compacted forms of mugwort that are compressed into a cone shape. There are two types of direct moxibustion: scarring and nonscarring. If the skin is burned and a scar is left afterwards, it is called scarring moxibustion. If the skin is not burned, it is called nonscarring moxibustion Fig. 9.2.

Nonscarring Moxibustion

A small amount of Vaseline was applied to the acupuncture point to make the moxa cone adhere easily, and then a suitably sized moxa cone was placed on the acupuncture

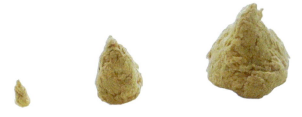

Fig. 9.1 Moxa cones

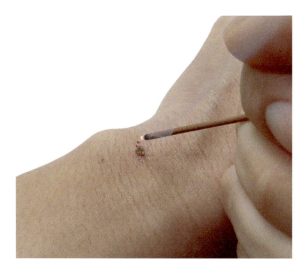

Fig. 9.2 Direct moxibustion

point and lit. When the cone was two-fifths or one-fourth burned and the patient felt slight burning pain, the cone was replaced and relit. When using rice grain moxa, the practitioner can extinguish the cone with a tweezer handle and then continue until the required number of cones is completed. Moxibustion should be applied until the skin is red and not blistered.

Scarring Moxibustion

When moxibustion was applied, a suitably sized moxa cone was placed on the acupuncture point, and the cone was ignited with fire. Each moxa cone must be burned out, and the ashes must be removed before continuing with the next cone until the required number of cones is completed. The fire burns the skin during moxibustion and can cause severe pain, which can be relieved by gently patting the area around the acupuncture point. The moxibustion site will become pus-filled and form a moxibustion ulcer approximately 1 week later, and the ulcer will heal on its own in approximately 5–6 weeks, leaving a scar after the nodules fall off. It is often used clinically to treat chronic diseases such as asthma.

Scarring moxibustion is the most potent form of moxibustion. *Zhen jiu zi sheng jing* (The Classic of Supplementing Life with Acupuncture and moxibustion) mentioned, "If moxa causes a blister, the disease will be cured; if moxa does not form a blister, the disease will not be cured". It is used less frequently than non-scarring techniques due to the discomfort and potential for scarring. Practitioners who use this method believe that the scar formation is integral to the healing process, offering a deeper and longer-lasting effect compared to non-scarring methods.

> **Cautions**
> Avoid direct moxibustion on face, joints and thin skin areas. Scarring moxibustion should be done with professional medical care.

2.1.2 Indirect Moxa

This is a method in which insulated materials are placed between the moxa cone and the skin.

Ginger Moxibustion

Fresh ginger was cut into thin slices 2–3 cm in diameter and 0.2–0.3 cm thick, and several holes were pierced in the middle with a needle. Place the ginger on the skin, put a moxa cone on the ginger and then ignite. When the moxa cone is burnt out,

Fig. 9.3 Garlic moxibustion

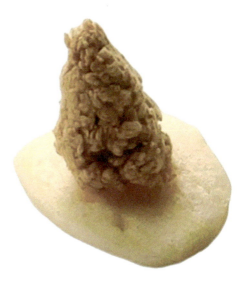

replace it with another cone. Generally, 5–10 cones of moxa are required for the skin to be red and not blistered. If the patient feels unbearably hot, lift the ginger upwards or move it slowly. This method is mostly used for vomiting, abdominal pain, diarrhoea, wind-cold and damp paralysis and external symptoms caused by cold.

Garlic Moxibustion

Fresh garlic was cut into thin slices of 0.3–0.5 cm, punctured with a needle and placed on the skin. Put the moxa on top and ignite. Usually, 5–7 cones of moxa are required for the skin to be red and moist. Replace garlic slices after 3 to 5 cones. This method is mostly used to treat tuberculosis, lumps in the abdomen, and encapsulated abscesses Fig. 9.3.

Salt Moxibustion

Place some salt (usually at Ren-8 Shenque) between the moxa cone and the skin. Place one slice of ginger on top of slat before moxa to avoid burns. If the patient felt a little burning pain, the cone was replaced. This method has the function of returning Yang. It is often used to treat acute cold abdominal pain, vomiting and diarrhoea, dysentery, urinary discomfort and stroke Fig. 9.4.

Fig. 9.4 Salt moxibustion

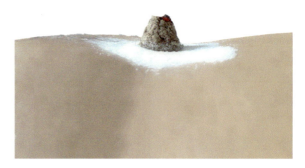

Monkshood Moxibustion

Monkshood (*Fuzi,* Radix Aconiti Lateralis Praeparata) is a Chinese medicinal herb. It can restore *Yang* from collapse, reinforce Fire and strengthen *Yang*, dispel cold. Chop and grind the monkshood, mix it with Huangjiu (a type of alcoholic beverage) and make a cake approximately 0.4 cm thick. Puncture some holes in the cake with a needle and placed it on the acupuncture point with moxa cones on top. Monkshood has a strong warming property. It is suitable for treating *Yang* deficiency, impotence, and ulcers that do not heal after a long period of time.

> **Cautions**
> Avoid direct moxibustion on face, joints and thin skin areas. Scarring moxibustion should be done with professional medical care.
> Garlic is irritating to the skin, use with caution for those with sensitive skins.

Direct moxibustion is more intense and potentially more effective for certain conditions, but it carries a higher risk of pain and skin damage. Indirect moxibustion is gentler, safer, and more widely used in modern practice.

2.2 Moxa Stick

2.2.1 Gentle Moxibustion

One end of the moxa stick was ignored and held at the acupuncture point or selected area, approximately 2–3 cm away from the skin, so that the patient felt warmth and no burning pain, generally 10–15 min per point, until the skin was slightly red. Gentle moxibustion is widely used clinically for various conditions.

Fig. 9.5 Sparrow-pecking moxibustion

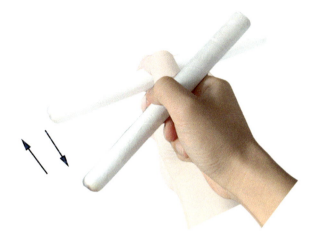

2.2.2 Sparrow-Pecking Moxibustion

Place an ignited moxa stick near the acupuncture point or selected area and move it up and down like a bird pecking Fig. 9.5.

2.2.3 Circling Moxibustion

Keep the end of an ignited moxa stick at a fixed distance from the acupuncture point or selected area and move it around in a continuous circle or a spiral pattern over the area until the skin is warm to touch Fig. 9.6.

2.2.4 Mild-Warm Moxibustion

Place several layers of cloth or paper on the selected area and then firmly press the ignited end of a moxa stick on the cloth or paper to allow the heat to penetrate the skin. Reignite the moxibustion after the fire is extinguished and the heat is reduced. Each point can press several times.

> **Cautions**
> When treating fainting or hypoesthesia patients and children, to prevent burns, the practitioner can place two fingers on the moxibustion area to feel the local heat level through the practitioner's fingers so that the distance and time of application can be adjusted.
>
> Press the paper or cloth tightly when applying mild-warm moxibustion, so they do not burn through and damage the skin.

Fig. 9.6 Circling moxibustion

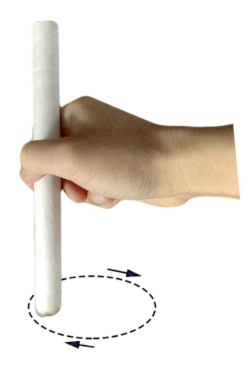

2.2.5 Warming Needle

The warming needle is a combination of acupuncture and moxibustion. Leave the needle at the appropriate depth after the needling. Use a 2 cm long moxa cone to warp the needle handle. The moxa cone should be 2–3 cm away from the skin and then the moxa should be lit from the lower end. Place a piece of cardboard on the acupoint area to reduce the heat and catch the ashes Fig. 9.7. It is commonly used for Bi syndromes and other cold illnesses.

Fig. 9.7 Warming needle

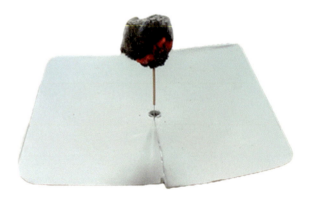

> **Cautions**
> Be aware of the falling ashes. Make sure to place a piece of cardboard with a small notch in the centre of the acupuncture site under the needle. Remind patients not to move during moxa.
> The length of needles should be long enough to hold the moxa cone stably and not too short to prevent burns.

2.3 Moxa Burner

There are three types of moxibustion devices commonly used in clinical practice: the moxibustion pot, the tiger warmer and the moxibustion box. The moxibustion pot is usually made of clay. It can hold heat longer than other materials. The tiger warmer is usually made of metal, so it can heat up quickly. The tiger warmer is more flexible to use in small areas. The moxibustion box can be made of metal and wood. It is more stable for use in larger body areas and suitable for longer moxibustion sessions.

2.4 Other Moxa

2.4.1 Juncus Moxibustion

Juncus moxibustion is a method in which the juncus (a plant commonly known as rushes) is dipped in vegetable oil and then burned directly on the acupoints. During the treatment, the juncus was dipped in an appropriate amount of oil to ensure that the oil was not dripping. Wipe the juncus if there is too much oil on the juncus surface. Ignite the juncus and quickly burn it on the skin; when the juncus burns on the skin, it can make a slight "clap" sound. After treatment, local skin may be flushed slightly, so attention should be given to avoid infection.

Juncus moxibustion is effective in clearing the Wind and resolving Phlegm and opening Orifices. *Ben cao gang mu* (Compendium of Materia Medica) mentions the use of juncus moxibustion for childhood wind epilepsy, childhood fright wind, and head wind.

2.4.2 Medicinal Moxa Stick

Medicinal moxa sticks refer to mugwort sticks supplemented with some Chinese medicinal herbs to assist moxa sticks in expanding the treatment range and enhancing the curative effect. There are two types of commonly used medicinal moxa sticks.

Thunder-Fire Moxa Stick

The moxa stick is made of fine powder of Chen Xiang (Lignum Aquilariae Resinatum), Mu Xiang (Radix Aucklandiae), Ru Xiang (Olibanum), Yin Chen (Herba Artemisiae Scopariae), Qiang Huo (Rhizoma et Radix Notopterygii), Gan Jiang (Rhizoma Zingiberis), Chuan Shan Jia (Squama Manitis), and She Xiang (Moschus).

Ignite the moxa stick and wrap several layers of red cotton cloth at the burning end of the moxa stick. Press it onto the skin. This was repeated several times. It is very similar to mild-warm moxibustion.

Taiyi Moxa Stick

The Taiyi moxa stick is an alternation of the thunder-fire moxa stick. The moxa stick is made of fine powder of Tan Xiang (Lignum Santali Albi), Shan Nai (Rhizoma Kaempferiae), Qiang Huo (Rhizoma et Radix Notopterygii), Gui Zhi (Ramulus Cinnamomi), Mu Xiang (Radix Aucklandiae), Xiong Huang (Realgar), Bai Zhi (Radix Angelicae Dahuricae) and Xi Xin (Radix et Rhizoma Asari).

It can be used as a normal moxa stick or the same technique as the thunder-fire moxa stick. It is used to treat wind-cold-damp Bi-syndrome, weakness, and other chronic cold-deficiency conditions.

> **Cautions**
> The cloth has to be thick enough, do not use synthetic fabric, as it may burn too quickly.
> Make sure the cloth is not burnt and can protect the skin.

2.4.3 Thermosensitive Moxibustion

Thermosensitive moxibustion is a new technique developed in recent years. It is one type of indirect moxibustion. Practitioners held the moxa stick above different acupuncture points on the targeted meridians. When patients feel the heat penetrating and spreading to the surrounding area or the heat sensation travelling in one direction while receiving moxa at specific points, these points are thermosensitive acupoints. Practitioners then continued the moxa treatment at these points until the patient nearly felt the disappearance of the heat sensitivity.

2.4.4 Blistering Moxibustion

It is a method to apply irritant herbs to acupuncture points or selected areas to produce blistering. There are dozens of natural moxibustion agents, including mashed garlic, *Xi Xin* (Radix et Rhizoma Asari), *Bai Jie Zi* (Semen Sinapis), and *Tian Nan Xing* (Rhizoma Arisaematis).

Blistering moxibustion is popular during the peak of the Yang season (San Fu "三伏" is a Chinese term that refers to a period of time in the traditional Chinese calendar that is divided into three parts, each lasting for ten days. They occur during the hottest and most humid months of the year, usually between July and August.) and the coldest time of the year (San Jiu "三九" is a Chinese term that refers to a period in the traditional Chinese calendar that is also divided into three parts, each lasting for nine days.). The method involves grinding these pungent and warm herbs into a powder and mixing them with ginger juice to make a paste. Then, the paste was applied to some acupuncture points. It is usually removed after 30 min-1 h for children and 1–2 h for adults. Redness, slight tenderness, swelling, itching or even blisters may occur at the patch site.

> **Cautions**
> Do not scratch the blister, as this may cause infection. If the blister breaks and exudes fluid, use antiseptic solution/saline to clean the lesion.
> Some of the herbs used contain toxicity and some have a strong irritating effect on the skin, so they should be used with caution or forbidden by pregnant women, the elderly and patients with skin allergies.

3 Clinical Applications

3.1 Moxibustion Functions

Moxibustion serves multiple functions aimed at enhancing health and well-being. Its primary role is to fortify Yang Qi, that governs warmth and activity in the body. It is especially effective in warming the body's meridians, the pathways through which Qi flows, and in expelling cold, making it ideal for conditions characterized by a deficiency of Yang Qi.

Additionally, moxibustion is adept at countering Wind and Dampness within the body, which in traditional Chinese medicine are often linked to a variety of conditions. It plays a crucial role in dispersing blockages and alleviating swelling, thereby contributing to the reduction of physical discomfort and inflammation.

One of the most significant benefits of moxibustion is its ability to enhancing circulation, and thereby providing relief from pain. This is particularly beneficial in conditions where pain is a predominant symptom. Moreover, it assists in unblocking meridians, ensuring a smooth and balanced flow of Qi.

Moxibustion is particularly useful in treating conditions marked by a deficiency of Qi, coldness, and pain. These include situations where the body's Yang Qi is weak, leading to discomfort or a sensation of coldness.

The application of moxibustion is guided by principles of meridian theory, which is a cornerstone of traditional Chinese medicine. This theory outlines the pathways through which Qi flows in the body. It's often personalized based on pulse and tongue diagnosis.

Due to its warming properties, moxibustion is frequently employed on local areas of the body that exhibit signs of coldness or blockages. By targeting these specific areas, it helps to restore balance and alleviate symptoms associated with cold and Yang deficiency.

3.2 Determining Moxibustion Dosage Based on Age, Constitution, and Moxibustion Location

The moxibustion dosage is determined by age. "Ling Shu·Jing Shui" says: "For the young and the old, the big and the small, the fat and the thin, use your heart to measure it".

Moxibustion methods include tonification and reduction: "Ling Shu·Bei Shu" points out: "If the Qi is abundant, reduce it; if it is deficient, tonify it. To tonify with fire, do not extinguish the fire, but let it extinguish naturally. To reduce with fire, quickly blow the fire, and let the fire extinguish."

3.3 Contraindications for Moxibustion

"Nei Jing" points out that there are some contraindications for moxibustion:

(1) Those with both Yin and Yang deficiency should not receive moxibustion, as stated in "Ling Shu·Zhong Shi": "Both Yin and Yang are deficient, tonifying Yang will exhaust Yin, and reducing Yin will cause Yang collapse. In this case, you can use herbal medicine, but you cannot drink strong doses. Moxibustion is not allowed for such cases."
(2) Those with both Yin and Yang overflowing should not receive moxibustion, as stated in "Ling Shu·Zhong Shi": "When the Renying (carotid artery) pulse and the pulse are both three times more abundant, it is called Yin and Yang overflowing. If you do not open it, the blood vessels will be blocked. Qi cannot flow freely and is stagnant within the body, which damages the internal organs.

If this condition is treated with moxibustion, it may transform into another disease."
(3) Moxibustion is prohibited for patients with excess flow of Yang Qi upwards. In "Su Wen·Fu Zhong Lun", it says: "Moxa aggravates the Yang condition, which causes it to further dominate the Yin."

4 Research

4.1 Asthma

One study aimed to compare the efficacy of scarring moxibustion in the treatment of bronchial asthma with modified nursing (inducing the formation of postmoxibustion sores) and conventional nursing (no formation of sores). Three hundred and seventy-two cases were randomly divided into the two groups. The modified nursing group showed a significantly higher total effective rate and an increase in C3 content in blood serum [16].

In another study, participants were divided into two groups: group A received heat-sensitive moxibustion, and group B received Seretide. The scores of the asthma control test, lung function, peak expiratory flow, and attack frequency were measured at different intervals during and after treatment. The results indicated that heat-sensitive moxibustion had a comparable curative effect to Seretide on asthma, and it significantly reduced the attack frequency [1, 3].

4.2 Breech Presentation

One review by Schlaeger et al. [15] found that moxibustion may be helpful in promoting cephalic version of breech presentation. However, more rigorous research is needed to establish its effectiveness and develop evidence-based protocols for its use.

A recent systematic review involving sixteen RCTs suggests that moxibustion at acupuncture point BL-67 Zhiyin has positive effects on correcting breech presentation [13].

4.3 Cancer

Han et al. [7] found that moxa can improve cancer-related fatigue even 4 weeks after treatment.

A randomized controlled trial of 60 patients showed that intradermal needling combined with heat-sensitive moxibustion can reduce the dose of opioids, improve the quality of life, relieve anxiety in patients with moderate to severe cancer pain, and reduce the incidence of common adverse reactions to opioids [8].

Zhang et al. [27] suggested that some limited evidence shows that moxibustion treatment may help to reduce the hematological and gastrointestinal toxicities of chemotherapy or radiotherapy, improving quality of life in people with cancer.

A study by Chen et al. [1, 3] reported that acupoint stimulation, including moxa, has a strong immunomodulatory effect on lung cancer patients, as demonstrated by the significant increase in IL-2, T-cell subtypes (CD3+ and CD4+ , but not CD8+ cells), and natural killer cells. It can improve the Karnofsky performance status, immediate tumour response, quality of life and pain control of cancer patients.

4.4 Endometriosis

A small-scale study by Chen et al. [2, 4] found that Herb-separated moxibustion (indirect moxa) can effectively improve dysmenorrhea symptoms and shorten dysmenorrhea days in patients with ovarian endometriosis.

Xue et al. [21] analysed data from the last 10 years and found that moxibustion has played a positive role in relieving dysmenorrhea, reducing pelvic masses, and improving pain thresholds and pregnancy rates in patients with endometriosis. However, more rigorously designed and large-scale RCTs are required to provide more robust evidence.

4.5 Irritable Bowel Syndrome

In a randomized controlled study of moxibustion for irritable bowel syndrome, Wang et al. [19] reported that mild moxibustion may be more effective than placebo moxibustion for the treatment of IBS-D, with effects lasting up to 12 weeks.

A systematic review by Dai et al. [5] showed that moxibustion is effective in treating IBS-D.

4.6 Rheumatoid Arthritis

One systematic literature review by Zhong et al. [28] concluded that moxibustion can protect the synovium of joints in animal models with rheumatoid arthritis by upregulating the levels of anti-inflammatory cytokines and downregulating the levels of proinflammatory cytokines. Moxibustion has the potential to relieve inflammation in rheumatoid arthritis.

A small-scale study by Gong et al. [6] found that moxibustion enhanced the anti-inflammatory and analgesic effects of conventional medicine and can enhance the effect of conventional medicine, downregulating HIF-1α/VEGF contents to inhibit angiogenesis.

4.7 Osteoarthritis

In a multicentre, randomized, controlled study of moxibustion for knee osteoarthritis, Kang et al. [10] found that while there was no significant degree of pain change in the usual care, electrical moxibustion and traditional indirect moxibustion showed a significant pain decrease after treatment. However, there was no significant difference between the two groups.

In the study carried out by Chen et al. [2, 4], serum TNF-α, IL-1β and MDA were reduced, and the activity of serum SOD was increased after 14 moxibustion treatments over a four-week period in knee osteoarthritis patients.

4.8 Primary Dysmenorrhea

In a randomized controlled trial, Yang et al. [24] found that moxibustion was as effective as drugs in alleviating menstrual pain-related symptoms, even three months after treatment, the effectiveness of moxibustion was sustained and started to be superior to the drug's effect.

In another study, Pan et al. [14] suggested that moxibustion can reduce the dose of drugs and any related adverse reactions. It was effective in reducing menstrual pain and improving the quality of life of women with primary dysmenorrhea.

5 Summery

Moxibustion has a long history in traditional Chinese medicine (TCM). The practice is said to have originated in the Shang Dynasty (seventeenth-eleventh century BC) and since then has been used to treat a variety of conditions. Today, moxibustion is used to help treat a wide range of conditions, such as pain relief, digestive issues, and gynecological disorders.

References

1. Chen HY, Li SG, Cho WC, Zhang ZJ. The role of acupoint stimulation as an adjunct therapy for lung cancer: a systematic review and meta-analysis. BMC Complement Altern Med. 2013;13:362.

2. Chen LF, Jin XF, Li BW, Zhan MJ, Hu HT. Herb-separated moxibustion on dysmenorrhea in ovarian endometriosis: a randomized controlled trial. Zhongguo Zhen Jiu. 2020;40(7):717–20.
3. Chen R, Chen M, Xiong J, Chi Z, Zhang B, Tian N, et al. Curative effect of heat-sensitive moxibustion on chronic persistent asthma: a multicenter randomized controlled trial. J Tradit Chin Med. 2013;33(5):584–91.
4. Chen Y, Wang RQ, Liu JX, Zhang ZD, Jia YJ, Lv JH, et al. Effect of moxibustion on inflammatory factors and oxidative stress factors in patients with knee osteoarthritis: a randomized controlled trial. Zhongguo Zhen Jiu. 2020;40(9):913–7.
5. Dai YQ, Weng H, Wang Q, Guo XJ, Wu Q, Zhou L, et al. Moxibustion for diarrhea-predominant irritable bowel syndrome: a systematic review and meta-analysis of randomized controlled trials. Complement Ther Clin Pract. 2022;46:101532.
6. Gong Y, Yu Z, Wang Y, Xiong Y, Zhou Y, Liao CX, et al. Effect of moxibustion on HIF-1α and VEGF levels in patients with rheumatoid arthritis. Pain Res Manag. 2019;2019:4705247.
7. Han K, Kim M, Kim EJ, Park YC, Kwon O, Kim AR, et al. Moxibustion for treating cancer-related fatigue: a multicenter, assessor-blinded, randomized controlled clinical trial. Cancer Med. 2021;10(14):4721–33.
8. Ji JF, Ge XX, Xu CM, Jiang Y, Gu JH, Wei GH, et al. Intradermal needling combined with heat-sensitive moxibustion for moderate to severe cancer pain. Zhongguo Zhen Jiu. 2021;41(7):725–9.
9. Jiang J, Wang X, Wu X, Yu Z. Analysis of factors influencing moxibustion efficacy by affecting heat-activated transient receptor potential vanilloid channels. J Tradit Chin Med. 2016;36(2):255–60.
10. Kang HR, Lee YS, Kim SH, Sung WS, Jung CY, Cho HS, et al. Effectiveness and safety of electrical moxibustion for knee osteoarthritis: a multicenter, randomized, assessor-blinded, parallel-group clinical trial. Complement Ther Med. 2020;53:102523.
11. Lee HG, Kim S, Jung DJ, Choi YM, Sin MS, Choi SW, et al. Single intramuscular-dose toxicity of water soluble Carthmi-Flos herbal acupuncture (WCF) in Sprague-Dawley rats. J Pharmacopuncture. 2014;17(1):27–34.
12. Lei Z, Rong-Lin C, Ling H. [Achievements of moxibustion therapy in Wushier Bingfang (prescriptions for fifty-two diseases) of Mawangdui silk manuscript]. Zhongguo Zhen Jiu. 2013;33(3).
13. Liao JA, Shao SC, Chang CT, Chai PY, Owang KL, Huang TH, et al. Correction of breech presentation with moxibustion and acupuncture: a systematic review and meta-analysis. Healthcare (Basel). 2021;9(6).
14. Pan S, Wang S, Li J, Yuan H, Xue X, Liu Y, et al. Moxibustion for primary dysmenorrhea: an adjuvant therapy for pain relief. Evid Based Complement Alternat Med. 2022;2022:6864195.
15. Schlaeger JM, Stoffel CL, Bussell JL, Cai HY, Takayama M, Yajima H, et al. Moxibustion for cephalic version of breech presentation. J Midwifery Womens Health. 2018;63(3):309–22.
16. Sha JM, Deng XJ, Shao ZC. Effect on therapeutic effect of inducing the formation of the post-moxibustion sore for bronchial asthma. Zhongguo Zhen Jiu. 2012;32(4):305–8.
17. Shi F. Shang Yi Jiu Ruo Kao [A study on medical moxibustion practices during the shang dynasty]. Cult Relics Central China. 2022;01:139–44.
18. Unschuld PU. Huang Di Nei Jing Ling Shu: the ancient classic on needle therapy. University of California Press; 2016.
19. Wang Z, Xu M, Shi Z, Bao C, Liu H, Zhou C, et al. Mild moxibustion for irritable bowel syndrome with diarrhea (IBS-D): a randomized controlled trial. J Ethnopharmacol. 2022;289: 115064.
20. Xia D, Chen P, Du P, Ding L, Liu A. Efficacy of acupoint catgut embedding combined with ginger-partitioned moxibustion on chronic fatigue syndrome of spleen-kidney Yang deficiency syndrome and its effects on T lymphocyte subsets and activity of NK cell. Zhongguo Zhen Jiu. 2017;37(8):814–8.
21. Xue Y, Wang H, Liu YJ, Zhao BX. Ai jiu zhi liao zi gong nei mo yi wei zheng de yan jiu jin zhan[A review of moxibustion for endometriosis]. World Chinese Med. 2022;17(06):891–4.

22. Yan H, Huang XH, Deng GF. Observation on therapeutic effect of acupuncture and moxibustion on disorders of myometrial gland. Zhongguo Zhen Jiu. 2008;28(8):579–81.
23. Yan Wei, Wang. Y. [Treatment of 200 cases of acute sialadenitis with juncus moxibustion]. China's Naturopathy. 2005(03):24–5 1007–5798 11-3684/R.
24. Yang M, Chen X, Bo L, Lao L, Chen J, Yu S, et al. Moxibustion for pain relief in patients with primary dysmenorrhea: a randomized controlled trial. PLoS ONE. 2017;12(2):e0170952.
25. Min YJ, Yao HH, Wang ZQ, Luo KT, Sun J, Yuan Z, et al. Efficacy of suspended moxibustion stimulating Shenshu (BL23) and Guanyuan (CV4) on the amygdala-HPA axis in rats with kidney-deficiency symptom pattern induced by hydrocortisone. J Tradit Chin Med. 2023;43(1):113–23
26. Zeng Y, Liu Y, Liu Q. [Clinical observation of 45 cases of herpes zoster treated with juncus moxibustion]. Yunnan J Traditional Chin Med Materia Medica. 2017;38(10):23–6 1007–2349 53-1120/R.
27. Zhang HW, Lin ZX, Cheung F, Cho WC, Tang JL. Moxibustion for alleviating side effects of chemotherapy or radiotherapy in people with cancer. Cochrane Database Syst Rev. 2018;11(11):Cd010559.
28. Zhong YM, Cheng B, Zhang LL, Lu WT, Shang YN, Zhou HY. Effect of moxibustion on inflammatory cytokines in animals with rheumatoid arthritis: a systematic review and meta-analysis. Evid Based Complement Alternat Med. 2020;2020:6108619.
29. Li JM. [Fire and the origins of moxibustion]. Studies in the History of Natural Sciences. 2002;21(4):320–331.

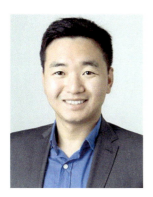

Phoebus Tian (田野) graduated from the Heilongjiang University of Chinese Medicine. After 2 years of working in a hospital orthopaedics unit, he was offered a teaching position at the London South Bank University. Phoebus's foundational training is in classical acupuncture, drawing from the ancient wisdom of Neijing and Nanjing. This traditional base is complemented by his proficiency in several specialized acupuncture styles.

Phoebus now works in a private clinic in Knightsbridge, London.

Cupping Therapy

Lin Chen

Learning Objectives

Understand the historical evolution and cultural importance of cupping therapy in Traditional Chinese Medicine.

Distinguishing Cup Types and Techniques.

Assess indications and contraindications.

Explore Clinical Applications.

1 History of Cupping Therapy

The history of cupping therapy is a journey that spans thousands of years and traverses various cultures. Originating in ancient civilizations and evolving over time, cupping therapy has left a lasting mark on traditional medicine systems and continues to intrigue modern practitioners and researchers.

Ancient Origins: The practice of cupping therapy dates back to ancient times and can be traced to multiple cultures across the globe. Its origins are embedded in the traditions of Egypt, Greece, China, and the Middle East.

Egypt: The ancient Egyptians were among the earliest practitioners of cupping therapy. Archaeological findings reveal cupping instruments made from materials such as metal and horns in ancient Egyptian tombs. Cupping was used for a variety of purposes, including treating ailments and enhancing general well-being.

L. Chen (✉)
Klinic, Oude Waal 6H, 1011 BX Amsterdam, The Netherlands
e-mail: jadechenlin@gmail.com

Greece and Rome: Cupping therapy was embraced in ancient Greece and Rome, where it was considered a common medical practice. Renowned Greek physician Hippocrates, often referred to as the "Father of Medicine," endorsed cupping therapy for various conditions. Greek philosopher Plato also mentioned cupping's benefits in his works.

China: Cupping therapy's deep-rooted connection with traditional Chinese medicine (TCM) is well documented. Chinese medical texts such as the Huangdi Neijing (Yellow Emperor's Inner Canon), dating back to approximately 300 BC, outline the principles and applications of cupping therapy. In China, cupping therapy is used to balance the body's vital energy, or qi, and to treat a wide range of ailments.

Middle East and Islamic Medicine: The practice of cupping therapy was transmitted to the Islamic world, where it became an integral part of traditional medical practices. Renowned Islamic physicians such as Avicenna mentioned cupping therapy in their medical writings, further promoting its use and understanding.

Medieval and Renaissance Periods: Cupping therapy continued to flourish during the medieval and Renaissance eras. It was embraced across various cultures and regions, with different societies adopting and adapting cupping techniques to suit their medical philosophies.

Nineteenth and Twentieth Centuries: As Western medicine and scientific advancements gained prominence, traditional practices such as cupping therapy faced some decline. However, cupping therapy persisted in some regions and continued to be a part of traditional medical systems.

Modern Revival: In the latter half of the twentieth century, cupping therapy experienced a resurgence in popularity, both within traditional medicine systems and among individuals seeking alternative and complementary therapies, although cupping therapy faced skepticism as modern medicine gained prominence. The spread of information through globalization and the internet contributed to the renewed interest in this ancient practice. It is embraced not only by traditional practitioners but also by modern health enthusiasts seeking holistic and non-invasive treatment options.

Today, cupping therapy is practiced worldwide, with diverse approaches and techniques. Traditional methods, such as fire cupping and wet cupping, are still used alongside modern adaptations such as silicone cups and vacuum devices. The integration of cupping therapy into modern healthcare settings, its use by athletes and celebrities, and ongoing research into its potential benefits continue to shape its role in contemporary health care practices.

2 Definition of Cupping Therapy

Cupping therapy, a therapeutic modality rooted in traditional medicine, involves the application of cups to the skin to create a vacuum effect that draws the skin and underlying tissues into the cups. This therapy has gained prominence in complementary and alternative medicine, particularly within acupuncture clinics, for its potential to address a range of health concerns. Cupping is based on the principle that stimulating specific points and meridians on the body's surface can promote healing, improve Qi and blood circulation, and alleviate various conditions.

Furthermore, cupping therapy is valued not only for its physical benefits but also for its capacity to address "Shen"—emotional and mental health. The relaxing sensation induced by cupping can alleviate stress and anxiety and promote a sense of calm.

3 Features of Cupping Therapy

Non-invasive and Gentle Approach: One of the most notable features of cupping therapy is its noninvasive and gentle approach to healing. Unlike surgical procedures or invasive interventions, cupping therapy involves the application of cups to the skin's surface. The cups create a vacuum effect that gently draws the skin upward, promoting blood circulation and the flow of Qi. This gentle suction is well tolerated by most individuals, making it particularly appealing to those who may be apprehensive about more aggressive treatment methods.

Therapeutic Effects on the Body: Cupping therapy's therapeutic effects on the body are multifaceted and impactful. By creating a localized vacuum, the cups stimulate blood flow to the area, which helps to alleviate muscle tension, reduce inflammation, and enhance the body's natural healing responses. This approach is particularly effective in addressing pain, stiffness, and discomfort.

Safety and Minimal Side Effects: Safety is a paramount concern in any therapeutic practice, as for acupuncturists, and cupping therapy boasts a favorable safety profile. Although it is necessary to be performed by trained practitioners, cupping is generally considered safe and well tolerated. The non-invasive nature of the therapy minimizes the risk of infection or complications associated with invasive procedures. Additionally, the therapeutic effects are localized to the treated area, reducing the likelihood of systemic side effects.

Affordability and Accessibility: The accessibility of cupping therapy is enhanced by its affordability and the simplicity of its tools. Cups used in therapy are often made from materials such as glass, bamboo, or plastic, making them cost-effective and widely available. This affordability makes cupping therapy accessible to individuals from various socioeconomic backgrounds, ensuring that more people can benefit from its healing effects.

4 Mechanism of Cupping Therapy

Cupping therapy, as an ancient practice deeply rooted in Traditional Chinese Medicine, has captured the fascination of practitioners and patients across time and cultures. In addition to the explanation of Chinese medicine, it is also very helpful to understand the mechanism in the view of modern medical science, such as how cupping therapy stimulates immunity, influences the brain and endocrine system, engages the nervous system, and even promotes the vitality of internal organs.

Enhancing Blood Circulation: Cupping therapy may enhance the blood circulation. The application of cups initiates localized negative pressure, resulting in vasodilation—the dilation of blood vessels—and an intensified blood flow to the treated area. This enhanced circulation brings a surge of oxygen, nutrients, and immune cells, all of which are crucial for tissue repair, pain reduction, and overall healing.

Promoting Lymphatic Drainage: The therapeutic scope of cupping therapy extends to the lymphatic system, which is responsible for eliminating waste, toxins, and excess fluid from tissues and can sometimes become sluggish, leading to oedema and compromised immune function. By generating pressure gradients, cupping therapy encourages lymphatic fluid to move toward the cups, facilitating waste removal and detoxification and thereby revitalizing tissues.

Stimulating Immunity: Cupping therapy influences the immune system. The suction triggers an immune response as the body recognizes the localized stress as a potential threat, prompting the release of immune cells to the area. This immune reaction bolsters the immune system's effectiveness, enhancing its defence against pathogens and potentially contributing to better overall immune function.

Modulating the Nervous System: Cupping therapy's engagement with the body is not limited to the physical aspects; it also profoundly interacts with the nervous system. The application of cups stimulates nerve endings situated in the skin and underlying tissues. This stimulation initiates a cascade of neural responses, including the release of neurotransmitters such as endorphins. These neurotransmitters contribute to pain relief, relaxation, and a heightened sense of well-being.

Promoting Organ Vitality: Cupping therapy is beneficial to internal organs such as the gastrointestinal tract, bladder, and hormone systems. The influence on blood circulation, lymphatic drainage, and meridian stimulation indirectly promotes the health and vitality of these organs. By improving circulation, cupping therapy aids in optimizing organ function, reducing stagnation, and supporting their natural detoxification processes. For example, in cases of gastrointestinal discomfort, cupping therapy may stimulate blood flow to the digestive organs, potentially aiding digestion and reducing discomfort.

Influencing the Brain and Endocrine System: Cupping therapy's impact transcends the physical to influence the brain and the endocrine system. The suction applied to the skin triggers sensory receptors, leading to the release of endorphins and other neuropeptides. This release induces relaxation, pain relief, and mood enhancement. Additionally, cupping therapy's effects on the skin may influence the hypothalamus–pituitary–adrenal (HPA) axis, modulating stress responses and hormonal balance. For instance, cupping therapy might contribute to a more balanced release of stress-related hormones.

5 Types of Cups and Cupping Therapies

Cupping therapy has manifested in various forms over time, each utilizing distinct cup types. These diverse cupping techniques, ranging from traditional methods to modern innovations, have expanded the therapeutic possibilities. In addition, it is often referred to as dry cupping, and wet cupping depends on whether bloodletting is combined.

Glass Cups: Glass cups, which are transparent vessels, offer practitioners a unique advantage - the ability to monitor the skin's reaction during treatment. Glass cups are often associated with the traditional practice of fire cupping, which involves briefly introducing a flame into the cup to create a vacuum before placing it on the skin. The transparency of glass cups allows practitioners to observe the colour changes in the patient's skin, aiding in the assessment of qi and blood flow and enabling adjustments to the treatment as needed.

Bamboo Cups: Bamboo cups are crafted from bamboo, a natural material that has been used for centuries. Bamboo cups are less commonly used in contemporary cupping practices. The lightweight nature of bamboo makes these cups easy for practitioners to handle. While their prevalence has diminished in modern times, bamboo cups remain being applied in some practice for herbal boiling cupping therapy.

Plastic Cups: Plastic cups for cupping therapy have evolved as a modern alternative in the twenty-first century, departing from conventional cupping materials and offering several notable advantages. Their adaptability to curved body regions and the absence of fire risk associated with traditional cupping methods underscore their appeal. These cups embody a secure, practical, and efficacious approach to cupping therapy. Some complaints on the plastic cups are related to the thin edge of the cup opening which is not as comfort as glass cups.

Silicone Cups: they have emerged as a contemporary innovation in cupping therapy in the twenty-first century. Silicone cups offer several distinct advantages. They are well regarded for their user-friendly nature, gentle suction, and ability to conform to diverse body shapes. Silicone cups have garnered significant attention and approval from both practitioners and patients due to their adaptability to curved body areas and their safety features, as they eliminate the fire risk associated with traditional fire cupping methods. These cups present a safe, convenient, and effective approach to cupping therapy, particularly suitable for home use.

Fire Cupping: Fire cupping is a traditional approach that employs glass cups to create a vacuum through the use of an open flame. The process involves briefly igniting a cotton ball soaked in alcohol inside the cup, which consumes the oxygen and creates a vacuum effect. The cup is then quickly placed on the patient's skin, allowing the cooling air inside to create suction [1].

Dry Cupping: Dry cupping involves creating a vacuum using cups made of materials such as glass, bamboo, or plastic. The cups are placed on specific acupuncture points or affected areas of the body. It is commonly employed for musculoskeletal issues, pain management, and relaxation promotion (see Fig. 1).

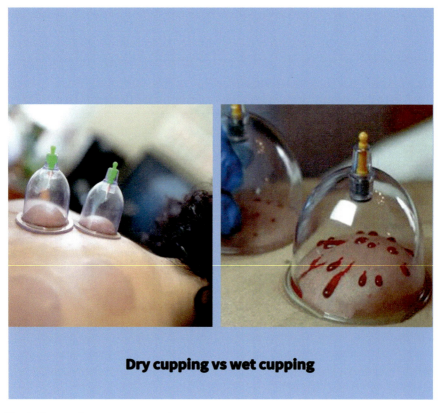

Fig. 1 Dry cupping versus wet cupping

Wet Cupping: Wet cupping takes dry cupping a step further by applying plum-blossom needling on the skin before applying the cups. The purpose is to extract a small amount of blood along with toxins from the body. This technique may purify the blood and remove blood stasis. Wet cupping is often utilized for detoxification, addressing chronic conditions such as chronic lower back pain and enhancing local circulation especially after some sport injuries (see Fig. 1).

6 Comparison of the Advantages and Disadvantages of Each Type of Cup Used in Cupping Therapy

6.1 Glass Cups

Advantages:

- Visibility: Glass cups are transparent, allowing practitioners to monitor the skin's reaction during treatment.
- Traditional appeal: Glass cups are associated with the traditional practice of fire cupping, which can appeal to individuals seeking an authentic experience.
- Customization: Practitioners can control the amount of heat applied to the cups, enabling customization of the level of suction.

Disadvantages:

- Fire Hazard: The use of an open flame for heating can pose a fire hazard and requires careful handling.
- Risk of Burns: There is a risk of burns if the cups are not properly heated or if they come into contact with the patient's skin before cooling down.

6.2 Bamboo Cups

Advantages:

- Historical Significance: Bamboo cups have historical significance and can offer a connection to traditional cupping practices.
- Lightweight: Bamboo cups are lightweight, making them easy for practitioners to handle.
- Can be boiled in herbal decoction and used as Water Cupping Therapy.
- Eco-Friendly: Bamboo is a renewable resource, making bamboo cups an environmentally friendly option.

Disadvantages:

- Limited Availability: Bamboo cups are less commonly used in modern cupping therapy, so they might be less readily available.
- Variable Suction: Achieving consistent suction can be challenging with bamboo cups, as they do not create a perfectly airtight seal.

6.3 Silicone Cups

Advantages:

- Flexibility: Silicone cups are flexible and can conform to various body contours, making them comfortable for patients.
- Ease of Use: Silicone cups do not require heating or an open flame, making them convenient for practitioners and home use.
- Variety of Sizes: Silicone cups come in various sizes, allowing practitioners to target specific areas effectively.

Disadvantages:

- Less Traditional: Silicone cups do not have the same traditional aesthetic as glass or bamboo cups, which may matter to some patients.
- Limited Heat Option: Silicone cups cannot be heated directly, which might limit the depth of suction in comparison to fire cupping.

6.4 Plastic Cups

Advantages:

- Lightweight: Like silicone cups, plastic cups are lightweight and easy to handle.
- Affordability: Plastic cups are often more affordable than other cup types.
- Transparent: Plastic cups can be transparent, enabling practitioners to monitor the skin's response.

Disadvantages:

- Perceived Quality: Some plastic cups might be perceived as lower quality or less traditional by patients.
- Variable Suction: Achieving consistent suction with plastic cups may require more careful handling.
- Thin and sharp edge may create some discomforts.

6.5 Vacuum Devices

Advantages:

- Precision: Vacuum devices allow practitioners to precisely control the level of suction applied.
- Ease of Use: Vacuum devices eliminate the need for manual suction or heating, streamlining the cupping process.

Disadvantages:

- Cost: Vacuum devices can be more expensive to acquire than traditional cups.
- Training: Proper training is essential to use vacuum devices effectively and safely.
- Discomfort: Some patients dislike its "artificial sucking power".

6.6 Fire Cupping Sets

Advantages:

- Traditional Appeal: Fire cupping sets offer an authentic traditional experience.
- Effective Suction: Fire cupping sets can create strong and consistent suction.

Disadvantages:

- Fire Hazard: The use of an open flame poses a fire hazard and requires careful handling.
- Risk of Burns: There is a risk of burns if the cups are not properly heated or if they come into contact with the patient's skin before cooling down.

When choosing a cupping method, practitioners and patients should carefully consider these advantages and disadvantages to ensure a safe and effective cupping therapy session to meet the individual preferences and health needs.

7 Operation Steps of Fire Cupping Therapy

It is crucial to emphasize that fire cupping therapy should only be performed by trained and qualified practitioners. Proper technique, hygiene, and patient comfort are of utmost importance during the procedure. Always prioritize the safety of the patient.

1. Preparation:
   - Gather Supplies: Collect the necessary supplies, including glass cups of various sizes, an alcohol-soaked cotton ball or alcohol swab, a lighter or flame source, and a clean towel.
2. Patient Preparation:
   - Explain the Procedure: Communicate with the patient about the procedure, its purpose, and what sensations they might experience, and consent of remaining of cupping marks for a week or so.
   - Ask about medical history: Inquire about the patient's medical history (whether taking blood thinner), any skin conditions, allergies, or concerns that might affect the suitability of fire cupping for them.
3. Setting Up the Cups:
   - Prepare the Cups: Ensure the cups are clean and free of debris. Place them within reach, along with the cotton ball and flame source.
   - Ignite the Cotton Ball: Light the cotton ball soaked in 96% alcohol. Hold it with a pair of forceps or tongs to prevent burns.
4. Creating Suction:
   - Introduce Flame: Hold the ignited cotton ball inside the cup briefly, allowing the heat to consume the oxygen within the cup (see Fig. 2).
   - Swift Application: Quickly remove the cotton ball and immediately place the cup, open side down, onto the patient's skin at the desired location. The skin will be drawn upward into the cup due to the vacuum created by the cooling air inside [2].
5. Observation and Monitoring:
   - Observe Reaction: Observe the patient's skin and their response to the suction. Some redness may occur as blood vessels dilate.

Fig. 2 Fire cupping

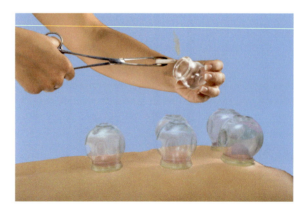

Cupping Therapy

- Communication: Keep communication open with the patient, asking about their comfort level and any sensations they might be experiencing.

6. Duration and Movement:

   - Duration: Cups are typically left in place for a few minutes, but the duration can vary based on the patient's response and the condition being treated.
   - Optional Sliding Cupping: If using the sliding cupping technique, apply a lubricant to the skin before placing the cups and gently move the cups along the meridian pathways or affected areas.

7. Removing the Cups:

   - Breaking the Seal: To remove the cups, break the vacuum seal by gently pressing on the skin near the cup's edge. This allows air to enter and release the suction.
   - Comfort: Ensure that the removal process is comfortable for the patient and does not cause unnecessary discomfort.

8. Post-treatment:

   - Observation: Observe the cupping marks that might develop on the patient's skin. These marks are temporary and normal aftereffects of the therapy.
   - Patient Care: The patient was advised to keep the cupped areas warm and avoid exposure to wind and cold immediately after the treatment.
   - Hydration: Encourage the patient to drink water to help flush out toxins that might have been brought to the surface during treatment.

9. Follow-Up:

   - Schedule: Discuss the recommended frequency of cupping sessions based on the patient's condition and response to the treatment.
   - Monitoring: Monitor the patient's progress and adjust the treatment plan as needed.

8 Moving Cupping

Moving cupping, a dynamic variation of traditional cupping therapy, introduces a unique approach to harnessing the therapeutic benefits of cupping. This technique involves applying gentle suction to the cup and allowing it to glide smoothly over the body's surface. As the cup moves, it creates a massage-like sensation that complements the traditional static cupping method (see Fig. 3).

Moving cupping involves the following steps:

1. **Preparation**: Similar to static cupping, prepare the patient by explaining the procedure and obtaining informed consent. Appropriate cups were selected based on the treatment plan and the patient's condition.

Fig. 3 Moving cupping

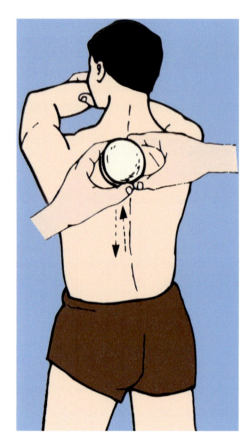

2. **Application of Oil**: To facilitate smooth movement, apply a thin layer of massage oil or cupping oil to the area where the cups will be placed. Some herbal oils made from Chinese herbal medicine can be used to promote blood circulation, or dispel the cold dampness etc. The oil reduces friction and enhances the gliding motion.
3. **Suction Application**: Gently create suction within the cup using the chosen method (fire, manual suction, or mechanical device). The suction should be light to ensure ease of movement.
4. **Placement of Cups**: Place the cups on the designated areas of the body. Depending on the treatment goals, cups can be placed along meridian lines, specific acupuncture points, or areas of tension.
5. **Gentle Glide**: Once the cups are in place, gently tilt the cups to create a slight vacuum, and then begin the gliding motion. With careful control, the cups were moved in a continuous motion over the oiled skin, following the natural contours of the body. The suction created by the gliding cups facilitates movement.

6. **Adjusting Pressure**: During the gliding process, assess the patient's comfort level and adjust the pressure as needed. Communicate with the patient to ensure that the pressure is within their tolerance.
7. **Duration**: The duration of moving cupping can vary depending on the treatment plan and the patient's response. It is advisable to start with shorter durations (5 min) and gradually increase (10–15 min) as the patient becomes accustomed to the sensation.
8. **Completion and Aftercare**: After the moving cupping session, the cups were gently lifted to release suction. Apply a soothing oil or moisturizer to the treated area to nourish the skin. Provide the patient with posttreatment care instructions, including staying hydrated and avoiding exposure to extreme temperatures.

9 Skin Reactions and Indications

After cupping therapy, patients often experience specific skin reactions that can provide valuable insights to both the practitioner and the patient. These skin reactions are a normal part of the healing process and can help guide the course of future treatments. Here are the common skin reactions after cupping therapy and their indications.

1. Cupping marks (Petechiae or ecchymosis):

Appearance: Cupping marks, also known as "sha" or "cupping bruises," appear as circular or oval patches on the skin. They range in color from pink to dark purple, depending on the intensity of the suction and the patient's individual response.

Indications:

- Blood Stagnation: Darker or more prominent cupping marks indicate deeper blood stagnation in the body. The appearance of these marks may suggest that there is an accumulation of blood or energy in the treated area.
- Qi Stagnation: Lighter or less prominent marks might indicate mild qi stagnation, suggesting that the flow of Qi in the treated area was somewhat obstructed.

2. Redness:

Appearance: Redness or erythema is common after cupping therapy, especially in areas with a significant amount of stagnation. The skin might appear pink or reddish, which is a sign of increased blood circulation.

Indications:

- Improved Blood Flow: Redness indicates improved blood circulation to the treated area. This suggests that the therapy has successfully increased blood flow and is helping to address stagnation.

3. Skin Elevations

Appearance: The skin beneath the cup might be slightly elevated or swollen. This is a result of suction and indicates that the therapy effectively lifted the skin and underlying tissues.

Indications:

- Stimulation of Energy Flow: The skin elevations signify that the suction has stimulated energy flow and increased circulation in the treated area.

4. Minor bruising:

Appearance: In some cases, cupping might lead to minor bruising, especially if the patient's skin is sensitive or if there is excessive suction.

Indications:

- Excessive Suction: Minor bruising indicates that the suction might have been too strong or applied for too long. This suggests the need to adjust the treatment intensity in subsequent sessions.

5. Warmth and Tingling:

Sensation: Patients might feel warmth, tingling, or a sensation of energy movement in the cupped area during or after the session.

Indications:

- Enhanced Qi Flow: Sensations of warmth and tingling indicate the improved flow of qi and blood in the treated area, suggesting that the therapy has successfully stimulated energy movement.

6. Temporary Discoloration:

Appearance: The skin under the cups might temporarily appear paler than the surrounding skin immediately after the cups are removed.

Indications:

- Temporary Lack of Blood Flow: This indicates that blood flow was drawn to the surface during the treatment, leaving the skin momentarily paler. It typically resolves quickly.

7. Absence of Reactions:

Indications:

- Balanced body: If there are minimal to no visible reactions or sensations, it may indicate balanced Qi flow in the treated area. This is a positive sign that the therapy is helping maintain the harmonization.

10 Indications and Contraindications [1–3]

It is important to note that while cupping therapy shows promise for these indications, individual responses can vary. Additionally, cupping therapy should be administered by qualified practitioners and tailored to each individual's unique needs.

1. **Musculoskeletal Pain**: Cupping therapy's ability to alleviate musculoskeletal pain is well recognized. By promoting blood circulation and relaxing muscle tension, it can effectively target conditions such as back pain, neck pain, shoulder pain, and even conditions such as Bi Syndrome, fibromyalgia. The suction effect created by the cups helps to increase blood flow to the affected area, facilitating the removal of metabolic waste and toxins that might contribute to pain and discomfort.
2. **Respiratory Issues**: Cupping therapy can be beneficial for respiratory ailments such as chronic coughs, asthma, and bronchitis. The technique aims to enhance lung function by stimulating Qi and blood flow to the chest and back, which can help to alleviate congestion, facilitate the movement of mucus, and improve breathing.
3. **Stress and Anxiety**: The relaxation-inducing effects of cupping therapy make it useful for managing stress, anxiety, and related symptoms. The gentle suction of the cups at specific points encourages relaxation and the release of endorphins, which are natural mood-enhancing and pain-relieving chemicals. This can promote a sense of calm and reduce stress-related tension.
4. **Sports Injuries**: Athletes often turn to cupping therapy to aid in injury recovery and improve athletic performance. By increasing blood circulation to injured muscles and tissues, cupping can help reduce inflammation, enhance nutrient delivery, and promote the removal of waste products. This can expedite the healing process and provide relief from pain caused by sports-related injuries.
5. **Digestive Disorders**: Cupping therapy's influence on energy flow can also extend to digestive health. It may help improve digestion by stimulating the stomach and spleen meridians and enhancing the movement of qi and blood in the digestive system. This can assist in alleviating conditions such as indigestion, bloating, and constipation.
6. **Cellulite Reduction**: While the efficacy of cupping therapy for cellulite reduction is debated, some practitioners believe that the technique's ability to stimulate blood flow and promote lymphatic drainage can contribute to improving the appearance of cellulite. By enhancing circulation to the affected areas, it is thought to reduce fluid retention and encourage the breakdown of fatty deposits.
7. **Immune System Support**: Cupping therapy is believed by some to boost the immune system. By increasing blood circulation and stimulating specific points related to immune function, it may enhance the body's ability to fight off infections and illnesses. Du Mai and Bladder meridians with moving cups are often recommended for this purpose.

8. **Skin Conditions**: Cupping therapy can be used to address certain skin conditions at certain stages, such as acne, eczema, and psoriasis in quiet stage. The increased blood flow to the skin's surface and the removal of toxins through the lymphatic system may help improve skin health and appearance. However, special attention needs to be paid to whether the local skin is inflamed or has open injuries. Do not apply the cupping on face unless for deviation of eyes and mouth and it is consent by the patient.
9. **Menstrual Disorders**: For women, cupping therapy can be applied to address menstrual disorders, such as irregular periods or menstrual pain. By promoting blood circulation in the pelvic area, cupping therapy might help regulate menstrual cycles and alleviate discomfort.

11 Contraindications [1]

1. **Skin Conditions**: Cupping therapy involves creating suction on the skin, which can worsen existing skin conditions such as eczema and psoriasis. In conditions such as eczema, the skin is already inflamed, sensitive, and prone to itching. The application of cups and subsequent suction can further irritate the skin, leading to increased inflammation and discomfort. Similarly, in the case of psoriasis, the raised and scaly skin patches can be aggravated by the pressure and suction exerted during cupping.
2. **Open Wounds or Cuts**: Cupping involves placing cups on the skin, which can lead to increased pressure on wounds, cuts, or abrasions. This pressure can delay the natural healing process of these areas and increase the risk of infection. Since the cups create a seal on the skin, they can trap bacteria and prevent proper air circulation, potentially leading to complications.
3. **Pregnancy**: During pregnancy, certain acupuncture points and areas of the body, such as the lower back and abdomen, lower back area, on top of shoulders are avoided due to their potential to stimulate uterine contractions. Cupping therapy involves suction and pressure, which could inadvertently stimulate these points and lead to uterine contractions, potentially causing harm to the pregnancy.
4. **Muscle Strain or Sprain**: While cupping therapy can be beneficial for muscular tension, it is not advisable during the acute phase of muscle strains or sprains. Applying suction to injured muscles can increase blood flow to the area, potentially exacerbating bleeding and pain. Once the acute phase has passed and healing has begun, cupping might be considered a complementary treatment.
5. **High Fever or Infections**: Cupping therapy promotes increased blood circulation, which can lead to an elevated body temperature. If a person already has a high fever, cupping therapy could intensify it, potentially causing discomfort or complications. Additionally, cupping should be avoided over areas with active infections, as increased blood flow can contribute to the spread of infectious agents.

6. **Blood Disorders**: Individuals with blood disorders, such as haemophilia or other clotting disorders, should avoid cupping therapy. The suction and pressure involved can lead to excessive bleeding or bruising, which could be dangerous for those with impaired blood clotting mechanisms.
7. **Severe Oedema**: Cupping therapy involves creating suction, which can further disrupt the delicate balance of fluids in the body. People with severe oedema are at risk of exacerbating their condition through the use of cupping, potentially leading to more discomfort and swelling.
8. **Cancer**: Cupping therapy's potential influence on blood circulation and immune responses makes it a consideration for those undergoing cancer treatments or with a history of cancer. Individuals with cancer should consult their oncologist before pursuing cupping therapy.
9. **Sunburned Skin**: Cupping therapy can involve some degree of pressure and friction, which can be painful and further damage sunburned or extremely sensitive skin. Applying cups over sunburned areas can cause additional discomfort and delay the healing process.
10. **Fragile or Aging Skin**: Elderly individuals often have thinner, more delicate skin that is prone to bruising and damage. The suction and pressure involved in cupping therapy can cause excessive bruising and skin trauma in such cases.
11. **Chronic Health Conditions**: Individuals with chronic health conditions, such as cardiovascular disease, diabetes, and hypertension, should exercise caution when considering cupping therapy. Cupping's effects on blood pressure and circulation could exacerbate these conditions or interact with medications.
12. **Medication Interactions**: Some medications influence blood clotting, skin sensitivity, or overall health. Patients taking medications such as blood thinner should consult their medication provider before undergoing cupping therapy to ensure that there are no adverse interactions between the therapy and their medications.

12 Combination of Cupping and Other TCM Therapies

1. Acupuncture and Cupping:

Acupuncture is often combined with cupping therapy. Cupping is employed before, after, or alongside acupuncture sessions. The synergy between these two therapies often complements each other's effects. While acupuncture targets specific meridians and points to regulate the body's energy flow, cupping helps to release muscle tension, enhance blood circulation, and alleviate stagnation in those areas. Their combined application is believed to enhance the overall therapeutic effects. For an individual experiencing chronic back pain, an acupuncturist might use acupuncture to target specific points, such as BL-25 Da Chang Shu. After the acupuncture session, cupping therapy could be applied to the area of BL-25 Da Chang Shu. The purpose is to further relax the muscles, enhance blood flow, and release tension in the affected area.

2. Tuina and Cupping:

Tuina, a form of Chinese therapeutic manipulation therapy, is frequently integrated with cupping therapy. Tuina's focus on manipulating soft tissue and acupressure techniques complements the effects of cupping. Practitioners might use Tuina manipulations, such as Rolling (Gun Fa) and Kneading (Rou Fa), to prepare the body by relaxing muscles and tendons before cupping. The combination often improves blood circulation, relieves muscle tension, and enhances the body's response to cupping therapy. Tuina can also be employed post-cupping to further relax the treated area and stimulate healing, but special attention should be given not to too hard manipulation force to prevent skin damage.

3. Herbal Medicine and Cupping:

Cupping therapy sometimes coincides with herbal medicine. Practitioners might suggest herbal formulas to be taken internally or applied topically to the cupping sites. These herbal remedies are believed to enhance the therapeutic effects of cupping, promote faster healing, and address specific health issues. They might target inflammation, support detoxification, or enhance the body's natural healing mechanisms, amplifying the benefits of cupping treatment. For instance, a patient seeking relief from chronic joint pain. In addition to cupping therapy applied to the affected joint, the practitioner might recommend an herbal liniment or poultice, such as a combination of warming herbs such as Sheng Jiang/ginger and Rou Gui/cinnamon, Hong Hua/safflower, to be topically applied after cupping. This external herbal remedy aims to support cupping treatment by further reducing inflammation and providing relief.

13 Precautions of Cupping Therapy

Cupping therapy, while offering numerous potential benefits, should be approached with care. Several precautions can ensure a safe and effective cupping experience:

1. Skin Sensitivity and Integrity: Ensure that the skin is free from lesions, cuts, or irritations in the area where cupping will be applied. Damaged or highly sensitive skin may not tolerate cupping well and could lead to discomfort or potential complications.
2. Avoid Bony Areas: Refrain from placing cups directly over bony prominences or sensitive areas such as the face, breasts, or genital regions. Cupping over these areas could lead to discomfort, bruising, or potential injury.
3. Fire Safety Measures: In traditional fire cupping, be vigilant about handling the flame and cups. Avoid accidental burns by ensuring a safe distance from the patient's skin when igniting the cups.

4. Duration and Intensity: Limit the duration of cupping and the level of suction applied, especially for first-time recipients or those with sensitive skin. Excessive suction or prolonged application might result in skin bruising, discomfort, or other adverse effects.
5. Hygiene and Sterility: Ensure that the equipment used is clean and sterile. Hygiene is crucial to prevent infections or complications posttreatment.

14 Challenges and Considerations

It is essential to acknowledge potential challenges and considerations that practitioners should be mindful of when integrating this modality into comprehensive treatment plans:

1. Personalized Responses:

Cupping therapy is not a one-size-fits-all approach. Patients may respond differently to therapy due to variations in their constitution, health status, and sensitivity. Some individuals might experience immediate relief and noticeable changes, while others might require more sessions to witness significant improvements. Practitioners need to carefully monitor and adjust the treatment plan based on each patient's unique responses.

2. Bruising and Sensitivity:

One of the visible aftereffects of cupping therapy is the possibility of bruising, especially in patients with more sensitive skin. While bruising is generally mild and temporary, it can be a concern for some patients. Practitioners should educate patients about the possibility of bruising and ensure that they are comfortable with the potential visual effects. Adjusting the intensity of suction and duration of cupping can help minimize bruising.

3. Contraindications:

Cupping therapy is not suitable for everyone. Practitioners must be diligent in assessing contraindications before applying cupping to a patient. Conditions such as skin infections, open wounds, pregnancy, certain blood disorders, and severe edema are situations where cupping therapy should be avoided [3].

4. Integration with complementary therapies:

Cupping therapy often works synergistically with other therapies, such as acupuncture, Tuina, and herbal medicine. However, the integration requires careful planning and coordination. Practitioners should have a solid understanding of how different therapies interact and complement each other. Collaborative efforts can lead to enhanced treatment outcomes, but a comprehensive approach should be thoughtfully designed to prevent overexertion or counterproductive effects.

5. Patient Education:

Educating patients about cupping therapy is crucial to manage expectations and dispel any misconceptions. Patients should understand the therapy mechanisms, the potential sensations during and after treatment, and the range of possible outcomes. Patient cooperation and informed consent are essential for a positive therapeutic experience.

6. Cultural and Emotional Considerations:

Cupping therapy can be unfamiliar to some patients, particularly those from cultures where it is not traditionally practiced. Practitioners should approach each patient with cultural sensitivity, explaining the therapy's principles and benefits in a way that resonates with their beliefs. Additionally, patients' emotional responses to the treatment should be considered, as some might experience strong sensations or emotional releases during or after cupping.

7. Practitioner Skill and Training:

Effective cupping therapy requires proper training and skill development. Practitioners need a deep understanding of cupping techniques, appropriate cup selection, suction intensity, and the therapy's potential effects on different health conditions. Inadequate training can lead to suboptimal results or even adverse effects. Ongoing professional development and staying updated on best practices are essential for safe and effective application.

Review Questions

1. Highlights how cupping therapy influences different bodily systems.
2. Describe the various cupping methods and the advantages and disadvantages associated with each type of cup material used in cupping therapy.
3. How does moving cupping differ from static cupping?
4. How do cupping marks, redness, and skin elevations serve as indicators of the effectiveness of cupping therapy?
5. What are the contraindications for cupping therapy?
6. Discuss the precautions that should be taken before administering cupping therapy, especially concerning skin sensitivity, fire safety, and hygiene.

References

1. Yang JS. Zhen Jiu Xue. 1st ed. Beijing: People's Publishing House; 1989.
2. Wang H, Du YH. Zhen Jiu Xue. 3rd ed. Beijing: China TCM publishing house; 2012.
3. Liang FR, Wang H. Zhen Jiu Xue. 4th ed. Beijing: China TCM publishing house; 2018.

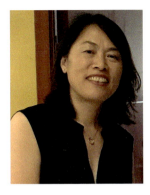

Dr. Lin Chen (陈琳) a Master of Medicine from Nanjing University of Chinese Medicine, formerly served as the Vice-director doctor at Jiangsu Provincial Hospital of Chinese Medicine, also known as the first affiliated hospital of Nanjing University of Chinese Medicine. Dedicated to integrating Chinese Medicine with Western Medicine, Dr. Chen has garnered invaluable insights from traditional Chinese Medicine through collaborations with esteemed practitioners such as Dr. Guicheng Xia, a globally influential TCM gynecologist. After two decades of service in Nanjing, she embarked on a new chapter in Europe, settling in the Netherlands. Dr. Chen currently practices at Klinic in Amsterdam, specializing in, but not limited to, areas such as infertility, IVF support, post-partum depression, Premenstrual Tension Syndrome (PMT), Menopause Syndrome, urinary tract infections, and various gynecological and hormonal disorders. Her commitment to holistic healthcare reflects a wealth of experience and a passion for improving women's health and well-being.

Micro Acupuncture Systems

Scalp Acupuncture

Tianjun Wang and Katherine Dandridge

Learning Objectives
- To understand the theoretical knowledge, history and development SA.
- To be able to locate SA areas accurately.
- To develop the skill of applying therapeutic SA techniques to those areas.
- To critically evaluate which of the SA areas are applicable in commonly seen clinical situations.
- To understand current SA evidence in clinical research.

1 General Introduction

Scalp Acupuncture (SA) is one of the foremost integrated modern acupuncture techniques. It is a combination of traditional Chinese acupuncture techniques and modern neurological knowledge. It originated from China in 1971 and continually develops and furthers understanding of the types of diseases and indications that it can treat [1].

The special function of SA is to impact the brain cortex functional zones through stimulating the corresponding scalp areas. Its main indications for treatment are brain related conditions including neurological diseases, psychological disorders and other related problems.

The theoretical basis of the TCM Brain theory developed initially from the era of the famous text; the Huangdi Neijing. There are many texts since that explain the TCM Brain functions, pathological changes and the channels of the Brain and its

---

T. Wang (✉)
London Academy of Chinese Acupuncture, UK, 70 Springfield Dive, London IG2 6QS, UK
e-mail: info@tjacupuncture.co.uk

K. Dandridge
Muthill, Perthshire, Scotland

© The Author(s), under exclusive license to Springer Nature Switzerland AG 2024
T. Wang and W. Wang (eds.), *Acupuncture Techniques*,
https://doi.org/10.1007/978-3-031-59272-0_11

associated characteristics. There are six channels directly connected with the head and which enter the Brain; Du, Ren, Stomach, Gallbladder, Bladder and the San Jiao [2].

In the Huangdi Neijing, there are 25 points on the head, It has been calculated in current texts that there are 38 channel points located on the head and indications of many of the points include neurological and psychological disorders [2].

It is common clinical practice to choose points mainly on the channels to treat related conditions, including proximal or distal to local area symptoms. Where the points are located on the head; these are commonly used to treating head and brain related conditions, some according to the channels and some for local area symptoms.

Ancient Chinese doctors have already known about the importance of the channels and acupoints on the head. There were many theories and statements about needling on the head over three millenia.

2 Development of Scalp Acupuncture

Unlike other TCM theory developments, the TCM Brain theory and the related needling therapy was not thoroughly developed. The most rapid development of acupuncture on the head and related to the brain occurred from the 1950s after "new China" was founded and Chairman Mao standardised further the TCM medical system. Inspired by some of the micro-acupuncture systems, such as ear acupuncture, nose acupuncture and eye acupuncture, some acupuncture experts began to practice needling on the head to treat diseases on other parts of the body.

In the early 1970s, influenced by neurological knowledge, head acupuncture was separated from the traditional acupuncture system, i.e., not only via the procedures of channels, acupoints and classical TCM theory. In 1971, this modern acupuncture technique was first published [1], which was combined with traditional acupuncture needling and the knowledge of modern physiology and anatomy of the nervous system and in 1972, it was systematically summarised and named "Tou Zhen" (head acupuncture or in translation in English 'scalp acupuncture: SA'). Later, the other styles of scalp acupuncture were published. Each of them proposed different diagrams and groupings of scalp acupuncture points [3].

3 Brief Introduction of the Anatomy of the Scalp and Brain

The scalp consists of 5 layers: the skin, connective tissue, epicranial aponeurosis, loose areolar tissue, and pericranium. The first 3 layers are bound together as a single unit. This single unit can move along the loose areolar tissue over the pericranium, which is adherent to the calvaria.

A skull consists of the cranium, facial bones and mandible. The brain includes the forebrain, midbrain, and hindbrain. The forebrain consists of the cerebrum, thalamus, and hypothalamus (part of the limbic system). The midbrain consists of the tectum and tegmentum. The hindbrain is made of the cerebellum, pons and medulla. Often, the midbrain, pons, and medulla are referred to together as the brainstem.

The cerebral cortex is the largest part of the human brain and is associated with higher brain functions such as thought and action. The cerebral cortex is divided into four sections, called "lobes": the frontal lobe, parietal lobe, occipital lobe, and temporal lobe. Frontal lobe-associated with reasoning, planning, parts of speech, movement, emotions, and problem solving. Parietal lobe-associated with movement, orientation, recognition, and perception of stimuli. Occipital Lobe-associated with visual processing. Temporal lobe-associated with perception and recognition of auditory stimuli, memory, and speech [4].

4 Chinese Scalp Acupuncture Stimulation Areas and Indications

If not specified, Chinese scalp acupuncture (CSA) or simply scalp acupuncture (SA) in this book refers to Jiao's style [5]. There are some revisions on their locations and indications based on current clinical experiences and research [2, 4].

Motor Area (MTA)
Location: A line connecting 2 points called the upper and lower points of the motor area. The upper point is situated on the antero-posterior midline, 0.5 cm behind its midpoint. The lower point is the point in the temporal region where the supercilio-occipital line intersects the anterior hairline. The whole area line is divided into five equal parts and grouped into three sections: upper one-fifth, middle two-fifths and lower two-fifths (see Figs. 1 and 2).

Indications: Generally, for motor paralysis of the contralateral side.
Upper one-fifth: paralysis of the contralateral lower limb, trunk, spine and neck.
Middle two-fifths: paralysis of the contralateral upper limb.
Lower two-fifths: Central facial paralysis of the contralateral side, motor aphasia, dripping of saliva, disturbance of phonation, etc. (also called First Speech Area, FSA).

Note:

The antero-posterior midline is the line from DU-29 Yintang, or middle of eyebrows, to the lower board of the apex of the external occipital protuberance.

Easy way to find the midpoint of the antero-posterior midline: When the pupil is straight to the front, a line is directly dug from the two ear apexes, and the intersection point with the midline is the midpoint. It is also the acupoint of DU-20 Baihui.

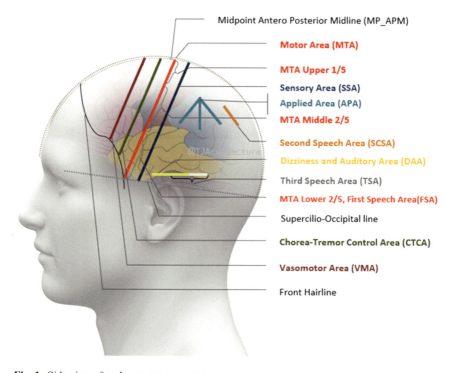

Fig. 1 Side view of scalp acupuncture areas

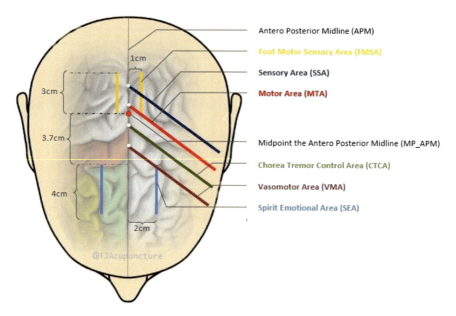

Fig. 2 Top view of scalp acupuncture areas

Sensory Area (SSA)
Location: A line parallel to and 1.5 cm posterior to the motor area. The whole area line is divided into five equal parts and grouped into three sections: upper one-fifth, middle two-fifths and lower two-fifths (see Figs. 1 and 2).

Indications: Generally, for the sensory disorders of the contralateral side.

Upper one-fifth: Pain, numbness and abnormal sensation of the contralateral side in the back, occipital headache, pain of the neck, tinnitus, and phantom low limb pain.

Middle two-fifths: Pain, numbness and abnormal sensation of the contralateral arm, phantom low limb pain.

Lower two-fifths: Numbness and pain of the contralateral side in the head and face, migraine, temporomandibular arthritis, trigeminal neuralgia, etc.

Chorea-Tremor Control Area (CTCA)
Location: Parallel to and 1.5 cm anterior to the motor area (see Figs. 1 and 2).

Indications: Involuntary movement and tremor of the contralateral side head and limbs, Sydenham's chorea, Parkinsonism's disease, tremors, essential tremor and related syndromes.

Vasomotor Area (VMA)
Location: Parallel to and 1.5 cm anterior to the chorea-tremor control area (see Figs. 1 and 2).

Indication: Cortical superficial oedema, essential hypertension, chronic pain, Alzheimer's disease, dementia, brain injuries, etc.

Foot Motor-Sensory Area (FMSA)
Location: Parallel to and 1 cm lateral to the anterior–posterior line. The line is 3 cm long and starts 1 cm posterior to the line representing the sensory area. Or 1 cm lateral to the midpoint of the midline, draw a 3 cm long line to the posterior (see Fig. 2).

Indication: paralysis, pain or numbness of contralateral lower limb, pain of the back and neck, nocturnal enuresis, frequent urination, prolapsed uterus, poor memory, etc.

Dizziness and Auditory Area (DAA)
Location: A horizontal line 4 cm long, midpoint 1.5 cm above the apex of the ear (see Fig. 1).

Indication: Ipsilateral dizziness, deafness, tinnitus, auditory vertigo, Meniere's syndrome, etc.

First Speech Area (FSA)
Location: Lower two-fifths of the motor area (see Fig. 1).

Indications: Motor aphasia, dripping of saliva, disturbance of phonation, etc.

Second Speech Area (SCSA)
Location: A vertical line 3 cm long, parallel to the anterior–posterior midline, its upper end 2 cm posterior-inferior to the parietal tubercle (see Fig. 1).

Indication: Nominal aphasia (cannot express the words who want to say, particularly nouns such as name).

Third Speech Area (TSA)
Location: A horizontal line 4 cm long drawn posteriorly from the midpoint of the auditory area. Or: from the point 1.5 cm above the apex of the ear, draw a horizontal line 4 cm long posteriorly.

Indication: sensory (receptive) aphasia (see Fig. 1).

Application Area (APA)
Location: A 3 cm line from the parietal tuber to the center of the mastoid process and two additional 3 cm lines from the same origin of the first line at the tuber, one in front and another one behind the first line with an angle of 45° between the first line and each of the latter lines (see Fig. 1).

Indication: Apraxia, difficulty with fine movement.

Visual Area (VSA)
Location: A line 4 cm long drawn upwards and parallel to the anterior–posterior midline from the point 1 cm lateral to the external occipital protuberance (see Fig. 3).

Indication: Cortical (central) impairment of vision and cataract.

Balance Area (BLA)
Location: A line 4 cm long drawn downwards and parallel to the anterior–posterior midline from a point at the level of the external occipital protuberance, 3.5 cm lateral to the midline (see Fig. 3).

Indication: Loss of balance due to cerebellar disorders, brain atrophy, etc.

Mania Control Area (MCA)
Location: On the anterior–posterior midline, from the tip of the external occipital protuberance, a line 4 cm long was drawn downwards on the midline (see Fig. 3).

Indication: Mania, anxiety, medulla and brainstem injuries.

Stomach Area (STA)
Stomach area: A line 2 cm long drawn directly backwards and parallel to the anterior–posterior midline from a point on the anterior hairline vertically above the pupil of the eye (see Fig. 4).

Indication: Disorders of the upper abdomen and general malaise, gastritis, stomach pain, poor appetite, oesophageal reflux, and TCM spleen and stomach conditions.

Liver and Gallbladder Area (LGA) or Hepatic Area (HTA)
Location: A line 2 cm long extending anteriorly from the stomach area (see Fig. 4).

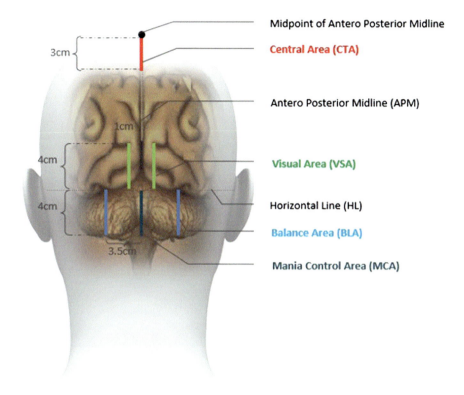

Fig. 3 Back view of scalp acupuncture areas

Indication: Pain or discomfort in the epigastric and right hypochondriac, diseases of the liver and gallbladder system, emotion disorders, general pain, and TCM liver and gallbladder conditions.

Thoracic Cavity Area (TCA) or Chest Area (CHA)
Location: A line 4 cm long, parallel to the anterior–posterior midline, with its midpoint at the anterior hairline, midway between the stomach area and the midline (see Fig. 4).

Indication: Chest pain, palpitation, stable angina, shortness of breath, bronchial asthma, paroxysmal supraventricular tachycardia, and TCM heart and lung conditions.

Reproduction Area (RPA)
Location: A 2 cm long line parallel from the frontal corner upwards. Alternatively, a line 2 cm long, parallel to the anterior–posterior midline, was drawn directly backwards from the anterior extremity of the stomach area at the same distance that separated the stomach area from the thoracic cavity area (see Fig. 4).

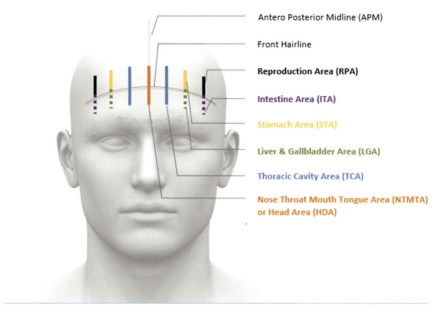

Fig. 4 Front view of scalp acupuncture areas

Indication: Impotence, ejaculation praecox, functional uterine bleeding, frequent urination, cystitis, prolapsed uterus, and TCM kidney conditions.

Intestine Area (ITA)
Location: A 2 cm long line, extending from the reproduction area downwards (see Fig. 4).
Indication: Large intestine and small intestine conditions, IBS, diarrhea, constipation, urinary tract infection (UTI), and TCM small intestine and large intestine conditions.

Nose Throat Mouth Tongue Area (NTMTA) or Head Area (HDA)
Location: From the meeting point of the anterior–posterior midline with the front hairline, draw a line 4 cm long, 2 cm upwards and 2 cm downwards (see Fig. 4).
Indications: Centre of face problems, nose-, throat-, month-, tongue-related conditions, and emotional conditions.

Note: Nose Throat Mouth Tongue Area (NTMTA) and Head Area (HDA) are in the same area. The latter was published in the book "Chinese Scalp Acupuncture" in 2011.

Spirit-Emotion Area (SEA)
Location: 2 cm side of the antero-posterior midline, a 4 cm line from the vasomotor area to the front (refer to Figure T). Or: 2 cm lateral to the point of 3.7 cm front of the middle point of midline, draw a 4 cm line to front parallel to midline (see Fig. 2).

Indication: Emotional disorders, such as depression, stress, anxiety, bipolar disorder, epilepsy, posttraumatic stress disorder (PTSD), insomnia and substance abuse.

Central Area (CTA)
Location: On the anterior–posterior midline, a 3 cm line from the midpoint back ward (see Fig. 3).

Indication: Poor memory, emotion disorders, children stunting, frequency urination, infertility, prolapsed uterus, etc.

Note: This is the only area that is not listed in Jiao's books. It is major based on the ISSA-MS5 and personal clinical experiences [6].

5 Scalp Acupuncture Needling Techniques

Needle Size
The commonly used needle sizes are 0.25×25 mm and 0.30×40 mm. The first three layers of the scalp, skin, sensed connective tissue and epicranial aponeurosis are tightly bound together as a single unit. The stronger material of the needle body is more suitable for scalp insertion, as the scalp skin is thicker than general body skin.

Angle and Depth of Needling
The angle for inserting the needle is $20°–30°$, according to the area of the skull, i.e., flat area lower angle (see Fig. 5). After rapid needle insertion, the angle was lowered slightly to $10°–20°$, and the needle was pushed to a suitable depth according to the length of the stimulation area and the response of the patient. As a sample of foot motor-sensory area, which is 3 cm in length, then the needle depth should be better in 3 cm as well.

Needling Manipulation
After the needle is inserted in the scalp, if the patient has already gained considerable sensation, it does not need more manipulation. If there is not much sensation and the condition requests it, such as in severe cases or if there is not so much of a response for just needling, then further manipulation is needed. Different styles of scalp acupuncture suggest different manipulations. ISSA and Jiao's style require rapid rotation needling. The ideal frequency of rotation is 200 movements per minute.

Needle Removal
When SA needles are removed, the insertion point should be pressed with a cotton ball or cotton stick after the needle is removed, and the pinhole should be pressed for several seconds to reduce pain and avoid bleeding or subcutaneous hematoma. If bleeding occurs, the patient should press for longer than 10–30 s. Occasionally, there are 1–2 areas sore with tension after the needle is removed. We can ask the patient to slightly press or massage the area and warm the area after 12 h, if needed.

Fig. 5 Scalp acupuncture needling angle

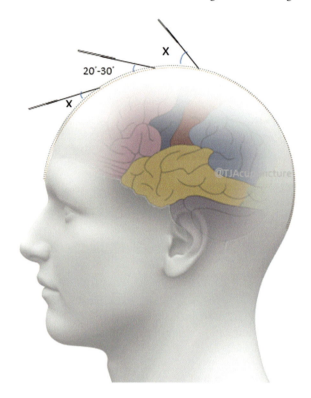

Combination with Electricity
Electrio acupuncture can generate continuous stimulation through needles to points or areas and may stimulate the neuro-humoral regulation system to enhance clinical effectiveness.

Stimulation needle selection: Two needles were chosen on the same line or areas, such as the upper 1/5 and the lower 2/5 of the motor area. You may choose the two different SA lines or areas, such as foot motor-sensory area plus same side of spirit-emotion area.

Regarding the nature or pattern of the electropulses, the frequency, timing, etc., please refer to Chap. 18 Electrio Acupuncture of this book.

Scalp Acupuncture for Children
Compared with body acupuncture, scalp acupuncture is more suitable for children, as it is not visible, and mobility is possible during needling, playing games while needling, and so on.

Combination with Other Techniques
Scalp acupuncture, regardless of the style, can be combined with other acupuncture techniques in addition to electroacupuncture. The most common combination is SA in general body acupuncture, etc.

6 Precautions and Contraindications of Scalp Acupuncture

Scalp Layers

The scalp is the soft tissue envelope of the cranial vault. The scalp has five layers: the skin, connective tissue, epicranial aponeurosis, loose areolar tissue, and pericranium. The first 3 layers are bound together as a single unit. This single unit can move along the loose areolar tissue over the pericranium, which is adherent to the calvaria. Scalp acupuncture needling should pass through this single unit, and the needle tip and main body should reach the layer of loose areolar tissue, which is approximately 4–6 mm underneath the surface of the scalp.

Precautions

- For stroke patients, it is essential to wait until the vital life factors are stable, including blood pressure, heartbeat and breathing, before scalp acupuncture is applied.
- Not suitable for patents with a high temperature without known reason, or heart failure, etc.
- Ensure that the needling does not cause the patient to faint due to strong stimulation.
- Compared with body acupuncture, scalp acupuncture has a greater possibility of bleeding after removing the needle due to the countless arteries and veins on the scalp. Careful attention is required for patients with hemophilia or those prescribed bleed thinning medication. When removing the needles, the needled points should be pressed with cotton balls or swabs for several seconds. If bleeding continues, more pressure should be applied.
- It is inadvisable to apply scalp acupuncture on any scalp area where there is a wound, infection, ulcer, tumour, large scar, or postoperative skull defect and to avoid inserting a needle directly into the shunt.
- If the scalp skin is not clean enough or sweating, the needling point area should be cleaned.

Scalp Acupuncture for Children and Women

- It is inadvisable to treat an infant whose fontanel has not yet closed, similar to other brain delayed developments, with exceptional care. If treatment is necessary, the fontanel should be carefully avoided.
- More attention is required for pregnant women. The general principle is to avoid applying scalp acupuncture for the first three months and last two months of pregnancy if they have a history of miscarriages or risks of miscarriage.

7 Scalp Acupuncture Sample Clinical Treatments

This section lists some commonly seen conditions or symptoms and relevant scalp acupuncture areas for the reference of clinical treatments. They might be combined with general body acupuncture or other acupuncture points and techniques [2, 4].

Stroke

- Hemiplegia: the contralateral motor area is dominantand, the foot motor sensory area can be added
- Coma: Head area, thoracic area, central area
- Aphasia: First speech area, head area
- Central facial paralysis: head area, first speech area
- Double vision or other vision problems: vision area
- Depression: Spirit-emotion area.

Alzheimer's Disease and Other Forms of Dementia
Motor area, sensory area, spirit-emotion area, foot motor-sensory area, balance area, vertigo-auditory area, tremor area.

Parkinson's Disease (Paralysis Tremor) and Chorea
Limb tremor or shaking, back stiffness, limb cramps: chorea-tremor control area.
    Dizziness + Vertigo and auditory area.
    Ataxia or walking instability + Balance area.
    Constipation + Intestine area, Foot motor-sensory area.
    Frequent urination + Foot motor-sensory area.

Multiple Sclerosis (MS)
Motor area, sensory area, foot motor-sensory area, balance area, vertigo-auditory area, tremor area, spirit-emotional area.

Epilepsy
Emotion area, foot motor sensory area, manic control area, central area, head area, central area, liver area, visual area, application area.

Migraine and Tension-Type Headache
Vasomotor area, foot-motor sensory area, sensory area, spirit-emotion area, central area.

Depression
Spirit-emotion area, foot motor-sensory area, head area, central area, manic control area.

Anxiety
Spirit-emotion area, manic control area, central area, head area,

Insomnia
Spirit-emotion area, foot-motor sensory area, head area, central area,

Pain
Sensory area, foot-motor sensory area, vasomotor area, spirit-emotion area.

Hypertension
Central area and vasomotor area.
  Headache + Head area; tinnitus + hearing dizziness area; irritability + spirit-emotion area and liver area; palpitations + thoracic area.

Pseudobulbar Palsy
Head area, central area, lower 2/5 of motor area, and madness control area.

Trigeminal Neuralgia
Lower 2/5 of contralateral sensory area, contralateral vasomotor area; ipsilateral reproductive area.

Peripheral Facial Paralysis
Head area, lower 2/5 of the ipsilateral motor area.

Hemifacial Spasm
Head area, liver area, and reproductive area (all on the same side). Both sides: chorea-tremor control area, vasomotor area, spirit-emotion area.

Vertigo
Head area, central area, dizziness and auditory area.
  Nausea and vomiting + stomach area and liver area.

Neurasthenia/Neurosis
Spirit-emotion area, central area, thoracic area.

Cerebellar Ataxia
Balance area, madness control area.

Autism (ASD)
Foot motor-sensory area, motor area, sensory area, speech area, balance area, chorea tremor area, head area, vertigo dizziness area.

Cerebral Palsy (CP)
Central area, motor area, sensory area, foot motor-sensory area, balance area, vision area, speech area, head area, application area, etc.

Attention Deficit Hyperactivity Disorder (ADHD)
Head area, central area, motor area, madness area, thoracic area, liver area, stomach area.

Tourette's Syndrome, or Tics
Head area, foot motor-sensory area, motor area, chorea-tremor control area, thoracic area, spirit-emotion area, liver area.

Restless Legs Syndrome

Upper motor area and sensory area, foot-motor sensory area, stomach area, and intestine area.

Motor Neuron Disease (MND)

Speech area, foot motor-sensory area, motor area, sensory area, balance area, chorea tremor area, head area, spirit-emotion area, etc.

Skin Problems

Sensory area, foot motor-sensory area, spirit-emotion area, stomach area, liver area, intestine area, etc.

8 Clinical Evidence

Many studies have been conducted on the potential mechanisms of SA in treating brain diseases, especially stroke. Stimulating specific scalp areas in a reflex somatotopic system may result in restoring neurological dysfunction, corresponding to the functional zones of the cerebral cortex, thereby altering the excitability of the cerebral cortex. Applying scalp acupuncture on the scalp areas directly above the cortical motor area could induce collateral circulation, raise cerebral blood flow, lower the risks of infarction, and improve motor function for ischemic stroke patients [3].

Functional magnetic resonance imaging (fMRI) has been widely used to study brain functions related to acupuncture, including scalp acupuncture. Through fMRI, it was observed that the contralateral somatosensory association cortex, the postcentral gyrus, and the parietal lobe were triggered when SA needles were inserted. Among acute ischemic stroke patients, SA was shown to be capable of enhancing functional connectivity, particularly between visual, cognitive, motor control, and planning-related brain regions, or strengthening the functional activities related to sensory integration, language processing, and motor coordination of the dominant cerebral hemisphere and the motor control bilateral frontal lobe [7].

Many studies have shown that scalp acupuncture has remarkable treatment efficacy for motor dysfunction in stroke patients, mostly in China and some in Western countries. Scalp acupuncture intervention combined with rehabilitation training can effectively improve the neurotrophy state and reduce nerve injury in patients with a convalescent period of cerebral haemorrhage [8].

The motor area of Jiao's scalp acupuncture or the anterior oblique line of the vertex-tempora of the international standardised scalp partition is usually selected as the scalp acupuncture stimulatory region to treat motor dysfunction in stroke patients. The motor area specifically used for the treatment of motor dysfunction after stroke is equivalent to the structure of the precentral gyrus of the cerebral cortex on the scalp projection [3].

A number of RCTs on scalp acupuncture for vascular dementia have been reported in the last 10 years. Most of the reports were published in China by Chinese researchers [9].

Complex regional pain syndrome (CRPS) can result from trauma or after surgery. It is often difficult to manage effectively. If not recognised early, it can result in significant debilitation. Scalp acupuncture resulted in improvement in the pain scales. Additionally, decreased sensory changes and improved function were noted on examination and therapy assessments. Notably, the pain reduction, functional improvement, and normalisation of sensation were fully maintained between treatments. Scalp acupuncture provided lasting pain reduction and improved function and sensation in this group of combatants with upper extremity CRPS [10].

9 Summary

Scalp acupuncture, as an independent acupuncture system, started in the early 1970's. The location of scalp acupuncture areas, indications and needling techniques are mostly according to Jiao's style with some revisions which are based on clinical experiences and additional research. The colourful illustrations of scalp acupuncture areas highlight the stimulation zones with measurements which are easy to follow and practice.

All clinical treatments follow the general principle of pattern identification for application of acupuncture and there is an additional benefit to applying scalp acupuncture for many disorders and neurological diseases. This newly developing area of acupuncture is showing promise to add further improvement to very difficult and chronic diseases as well as being useful for acute brain injury and trauma. There will be further clinical evidence emerge in the future for combined treatments of acupuncture plus scalp acupuncture as well as alongside or instead of pharmaceutical intervention.

Comprehension/Review Questions

(1) What are the basic TCM and western medicine theories of scalp acupuncture?
(2) How to locate the Motor Area? How to find the lower point if the front hairline is not clear?
(3) What are the indications of the foot motor-sensory Area?
(4) What is the angle of insertion of a SA needle on spirit-emotion Area?
(5) When is it appropriate for stroke patients to receive SA treatment?
(6) Explain how to treat multiple sclerosis with scalp acupuncture?
(7) What is the mechanism of SA?

References

1. Jiao SF. Scalp acupuncture and clinical cases. Beijing: Foreign Languages Press; 1997.
2. Wang TJ. Acupuncture for brain: treatment for neurological and psychologic disorders. Switzerland: Springer; 2021.
3. Liu Z, Guan L, Wang Y, et al. History and mechanism for treatment of intracerebral haemorrhage with scalp acupuncture. Evid-Based Complement Altern Med. 2012. Article ID 895032. 9 p.
4. Hao JJ, Hao LL. Chinese scalp acupuncture. Boulder, USA: Blue Poppy Press; 2011.
5. Jiao SF. Scalp acupuncture (Chinese). 2nd ed. Beijing: People's Health Press; 2009.
6. WHO Scientific Group on International Acupuncture Nomenclature. A proposed standard international acupuncture nomenclature: report of a WHO scientific group, World Health Organization, Geneva, Switzerland; 1991.
7. Park SU, Shin AS, Jahng GH, et al. Effects of scalp acupuncture versus upper and lower limb acupuncture on signal activation of blood oxygen level dependent fMRI of the brain and somatosensory cortex. J Altern Compl Med. 2009;5:1193–200. https://doi.org/10.1089/acm.2008.0602.
8. Liu H, Jiang Y, Wang N, et al. Scalp acupuncture enhances local brain regions functional activities and functional connections between cerebral hemispheres in acute ischemic stroke patients. Anat Rec. 2021;304:2538–51. https://doi.org/10.1002/ar.247461.
9. Sun L, Fan Y, Fan W, et al. Efficacy and safety of scalp acupuncture in improving neurological dysfunction after ischemic stroke: a protocol for systematic review and meta-analysis. Medicine. 2020;99: e21783. https://doi.org/10.1097/MD.000000000002178.
10. Hommer DH. Chinese scalp acupuncture relieves pain and restores function in complex regional pain syndrome. Mil Med. 2012;177(10):1231–4. https://doi.org/10.7205/milmed-d-12-00193. PMID: 23113454.

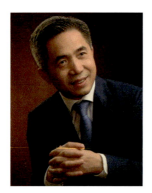

Prof. Dr. Tianjun Wang (王天俊) graduated from Nanjing University of Chinese Medicine (NUCM) in 1989. He completed his Ph.D. of Acupuncture at NUCM. Tianjun moved to the UK and joined the University of East London UK as a Senior Lecturer and the Director of Acupuncture Clinic 2007–2014. He is a Guest Professor of NUCM.

Current Prof. Wang is the Principal of the London Academy of Chinese Acupuncture (LACA). He is also the Vice President of the Scalp Acupuncture Committee of World Federation of Chinese Medicine Societies (WFCMS) and the president of the Academy of Scalp Acupuncture UK (ASA). He owns TJ Acupuncture Clinic and Brain Care Centre in London.

Prof. Wang has authored and co-authored more than 50 academic papers as well as peer reviewers to many international journals. His authored book "Acupuncture for Brain: Treatment for Neurological and Psychologic Disorders" published by Springer 2021.

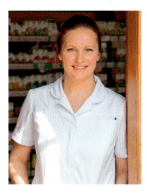

Katherine Dandridge BSc TCM, BMed (Beijing), Dip CHM (Obs/Gyn) runs a busy general acupuncture and Chinese herbal medicine practice in Perthshire, Scotland. She began her complementary medicine career in Hong Kong in 1999 training in holistic aromatherapy and allied therapies, then went on to study the five year TCM degree at Middlesex University twinned with the Beijing University of Chinese Medicine. She has over the last 20 years developed her practice including obstetric, fertility, health coaching and gynaecological studies, five palms qi gong, scalp acupuncture and cosmetic acupuncture and functional medicine training; getting good, consistent results for the community that she serves. She is a member of the UK practitioner groups; British Acupuncture Council, Register of Chinese Herbal Medicine, Institute of Scalp Acupuncture UK, British Acupuncture Federation, Royal Society of Medicine Associate Member and The International Federation of Professional Aromatherapists.

Auricular Acupuncture

Jun She

Learning Objectives
- To impart theoretical knowledge of auricular acupuncture general history and development.
- To produce the learner's ability to locate auricular points accurately.
- To help the learners achieve skills of applying acupuncture needle or pellet to auricular points.
- To develop a critical evaluation of which auricular points are appropriate in commonly seen clinical issues.
- To understand the current auricular acupuncture research evidence.

1 General Introductions of the Technique

1.1 Definition

Auricular acupuncture is one of the microsystems in acupuncture, it can reflect the conditions of the whole body on the outer ears. Acupuncture needles can be inserted into auricular points, producing a gentle stimulation and creating a response in a certain part of the body to promote a natural self-recovery.

J. She (✉)
London Confucius Institute for Traditional Chinese Medicine, London, UK
e-mail: shexiaojun01@gmail.com

1.2 General History and Development of Auricular Acupuncture

Stimulating outer ears were used in ancient India, Ancient Greece, Persian, etc. *Huangdi Neijing* describes the examination of the ears for disease prognosis. In *Zhengzhi Zhunsheng*, it says that a brighter and lustrous helix is a sign of good vitality. In contrast, if the helix is extremely dry, the patient's health condition will be very worrisome. In prescriptions, emergencies, jaundice, and cataracts are treated by stimulating outer ears. French physician Paul Nogier, considered the father of modern auriculotherapy, developed the inverted foetus image on the outer ear. Chinese people further carry on the Nogier's theory and integrated it into one of the microsystems in Chinese medicine.

2 Features

2.1 The Physiology and Pathology of Auricular Acupuncture

Most parts of the outer ear are supported by elastic cartilage and covered by skin. The subcutaneous tissue is less compact and rich in blood vessels and nerves. The pendulous part at the lower end of the ear, without cartilage, is only made up of skin, connective tissue and fat, called the earlobe. The auricular ligaments, auricular muscles, cartilage and skin are attached to both sides of the skull.

When something goes wrong with a certain part of the body, there will be some changes in colour, shape, pain threshold and electric resistance of the outer ear.

Pathological changes in the outer ear include changes in colour, shape, pimpling, vessels and desquamation at the corresponding location.

The ear is regarded as a hologram of the body, and there are 93 auricular points in total [GBT13734-2008]. The auricular points on the ear are for both internal organs and the muscular skeleton. Some of them have multi-functions, for example, Shenmen, Endocrine, Subcortex, etc.

2.2 The Relationship Between Internal Organs, Meridians and Ears

The heart, kidney and ear:

Both the heart and kidney systems are open to the ears in Chinese medicine. The kidney system, a very important system, is called the origin of congenital consititution, and it opens its orifice to the ear. In *Zhenjiu Jiayijing (Acupuncture ABC)*, it says that all five Zang organs have their own orifices; but the tongue is not a real orifice actually, so the heart opens its orifice to ears as well.

The small intestine and ear:

> ...then travels posteriorly towards the ear, where it intersects the Gall Bladder channel at Touqiaoyin GB-11 and the Sanjiao channel at Jiaosun SJ-20 and Erheliao SJ-22 and enters the ear at Tinggong SI-19...

The Sanjiao meridian and the ear:

> ...Another branch: Separates behind the ear and enters the ear, emerges in front of the ear to intersect the small intestine and gallbladder channels at Tinggong SI-19 and Shangguan GB-3...

The Bladder meridian and the ear:

> ... from the vertex, a branch descends to the temples in the region above the ear, intersecting the Gall Bladder channel at points from the vertex, another branch enters the brain, meets the Governing channel at Naohu DU-17.

Gall Bladder meridian and the ear:

> ...crosses to the anterior portion of the ear at Tinghui GB-2 then...descends via points Xuanlu GB-5, Xuanli GB-6 and Qubin GB-7 to the region above the ear where it meets with Erheliao SJ-22, curves posteriorly behind the ear to the mastoid process ...

The stomach meridian and the ear:

> ...ascends anterior to the ear passing via Xiaguan ST-7 to Shangguan GB-3...

The large intestine's luo-connecting channel and the ear: ...divides on the cheek, one branch entering the ear and another branch connecting with teeth...

2.3 *The Names and Distribution of Auricular Points*

There are 93 points in total on the auricle, the ear points are named after the nomination of body's anatomy, the meridians and Zangfu, the nerve, the diseases or symptoms, functions of the auricular point, the locations, the image of auricular point on the out ear and the arranging order of auricular points (Fig. 1 and 3).

See Figs. 2 and 1. The auricular points are distributed on different parts of the outer ear, such as an inverted fetus with the head down, the hips and lower limbs up and the waist and torso in the middle. The earlobe corresponds to the head and face; the tragus is equivalent to the throat, inner nose, adrenal gland; the supra-tragic notch corresponds to the outer ear; the antihelix corresponds to the body trunk; the inferior crus of the antihelix corresponds to the hip; the superior crus of the

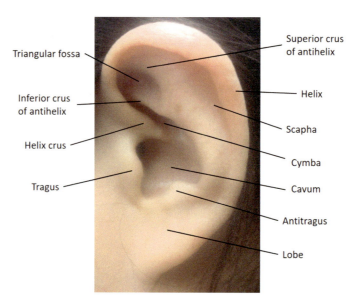

Fig. 1 Structure of auricular area

antihelix corresponds to the lower limb; the scapha is equivalent to the upper limb; the triangular fossa is equivalent to the pelvic cavity and internal genitalia; the helix crus corresponds to the diaphragm; the area around the helix crus is equivalent to the digestive tract; the concha cavum corresponds to the abdominal cavity; and the concha cymba is equivalent to the chest.

Intertragic Notch corresponds to the endocrine gland system. However, some auricular points are not completely located on the corresponding parts of the auricular anatomy, such as the adrenal point.

The Function of Auricular Points (see Fig. 3).

1. Middle ear (diaphragm) HX_1

Location: helix crus, helix area 1.
Application: blood deficiency, skin problems due to blood stagnation or blood heat, ostinate itchiness or urticaria on the skin.

2. Rectum HX_2

Location: at the beginning of the helix crus, anterior to the middle ear (HX1), corresponding to the same level as the large intestine.
Application: constipation.

3. Ear Apex $HX_{6,7}$

Location: at the highest point when the auricle is folded forward.

Fig. 2 Theory of auricular acupuncture

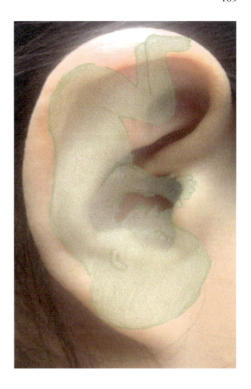

Application: all kinds of acute inflammation of five sense organs on the head, for example hordeolum (Sty), conjunctivitis, sore throat, Bell's palsy, urticaria, eczema, acne, itchy ski, etc.

4. Wind Stream SF_1 and SF_2

Location: anterior to the helix tubercle between the finger and wrist, the place where SF_1 meets SF_2.
Application: allergic skin, itchy skin, urticaria, eczema, Palmer keratosis, acne.

5. Sympathetic AH_6 and HX_4

Location: the area where the end of the inferior crus of the antihelix meets the inner border of the helix.
Application: functional disturbance of vegetative nerves, sleeping disorders, hydrosis, etc.

6. Uterus (Internal Genitals) TF_2

Location: In the lower part of the anterior 1/3 of the triangular fossa.
Application: Irregular period, dysmenorrhea, amenorrhea, metrorrhagia and metrostaxis, increased leucorrhoea, pelvic inflammation, chloasma, acne, and overweight.

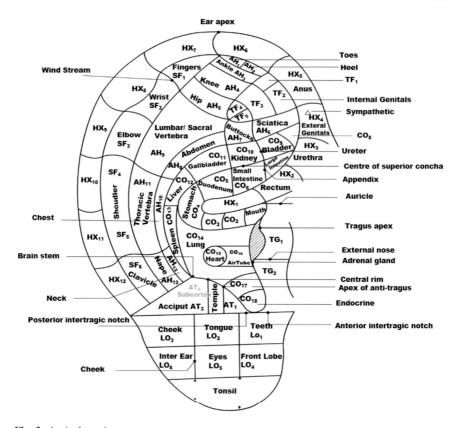

Fig. 3 Auricular points map

7. Shen Men (Spirit Gate) TF_4

Location: In the triangular fossa, the slightly upper part of the bifurcation between the superior and inferior cruses of the antihelix.
Application: Sleeping disorder, dreaminess, irritation, tiredness, headache, facial pain, toothache, urticaria, itchiness and withdrawal syndrome.

8. Pelvic cavity TF_5

Location: the lower part of the posterior 1/3 of the triangular fossa.
Application: leukorrheal disease, pelvic inflammation, and annexitis.

9. Adrenal gland TG_2

Location: the tip of the lower part of the free end of the tragus.
Application: low blood pressure, pale complexion, dizziness, allergic skin.

10. Subcortex AT_4

Location: inside part of the antitragus.
Application: insomnia, dreaminess, memory deterioration, and neuropathic headache.

11. Apex of antitragus AT_1, AT_2, and AT_4

Location: the tip of the free end of the antitragic notch.
Application: allergic skin, itchiness on the skin.

12. Mouth CO_1

Location: anterior 1/3 of the place inferior to the helix crus.
Application: facial paralysis, stomatitis, angular stomatitis, acne around the mouth.

13. Stomach CO_4

Location: the point where the helix crus ends, between the Cymba and Concha Cavity
Application: indigestion, bloating, insomnia, fetid breath, acne, bottle nose, and overweight.

14. Large Intestine CO_7

Location: anterior 1/3 of the upper part of the helix crus.
Application: constipation, overweight, acne.

15. Kidney CO_{10}

Location: inferior to the base of the inferior crus of the antihelix.
Application: premature senility, hair loss, sleeping disorder, irregular period.

16. Liver CO_{12}

Location: inferior and posterior to the cymba.
Application: irregular period, dysmenorrhea, climacteric syndrome, chloasma, acne.

17. Spleen CO_{13}

Location: posterior and inferior to the Concha Cavity.
Application: deficiency of the spleen and stomach, constipation, diarrhea, poor appetite, leukorrhagia, metrorrhagia and metrostaxis.

18. Heart CO_{15}

Location: the depression in the centre of the Concha Cavity.
Application: neurasthenia, oral ulcer and tongue sores, hoarse voice.

19. Lung CO_{14}

Location: the place around the centre of the concha cavity.
Application: hoarseness, laryngolaryngitis, itchy skin, urticaria, acne, flat wart, constipation.

20. Air Tube CO_{16}

Location: anterior to the CO_{15}.
Application: Cough, asthma, breathless, Pharyngitis, tracheitis, Bronchial Asthma, acute and chronic bronchitis.

21. Sanjiao CO_{17}

Location: at the bottom of the concha cavity, superior to the endocrine (CO18), between the Lung (CO14) and endocrine (CO18).
Application: constipation, bloating, simple obesity.

22. Endocrine CO_{18}

Location: medial to the intertragic notch, at the bottom of the concha cavity.
Application: irregular period, dysmenorrhea, climacteric syndrome, overweight, chloasma, acne.

23. Cheek

Location: the place where the LO5 meets LO6 at the lobe.
Application: Facial paralysis, facial pain, acne, chloasma, flat wart.

3 Detailed Techniques of Auricular Acupuncture

Auricular acupuncture can be used in addition to body acupuncture or as a stand-alone therapy to treat a wide range of conditions. Common uses include quitting addictions, pain reduction, anti-stress, fertility support, and weight loss etc.

Advantages of auricular acupuncture:

Points are more easily accessed than body acupuncture; quick to apply; can be performed easily with patient in any position—commonly used for quitting addictions (patients seated) and even in 'battlefield' situations; ear seeds used to continue treatment after auricular acupuncture session ends.

Fig. 4 Probing auricular points

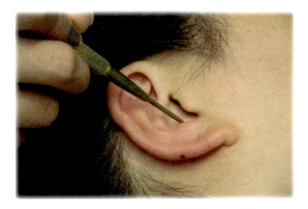

3.1 Health and Safety When Applying Auricular Acupuncture is Similar to Body Acupuncture

Little concern of additional risk of infection when used as part of standard acupuncture treatment. Follow Codes of Practice as the standard acupuncture for cleaning needle technique, disposal of needles, clean field, etc.

Potential for bleeding—have cotton wool ready.

Needles can fall out during the treatment. Make sure they are counted in and out. Fill in an incident report if any are not found.

3.2 Needling the Ear

Make sure the outer ear is clean, swab the auricle with 70% isopropyl alcohol wipes if necessary, allow the skin to dry fully before needling, and wash your hands before needling as normal. use an ear probe to determine the most tender area at the chosen auricular points, gradually apply stronger pressure—the dent is marked at the point for needle insertion, use 13 mm × 0.16 mm needles, obleak tapping insertion and no manipulation.

Inserting a needle with quick 'flick' action, the needling angle is important if needling multiple ear acupoints, the depth of the needle can be approximately 1–2 mm, and caution will be taken not to pierce through to the other side of the auricle. Make sure you make a note of all auricular points used. The auricular treatment duration should be approximately 10–30 min.

3.3 Auricular Plaster with Seeds (See Fig. 4)

After normal auricular acupuncture treatment, for long-lasting effectiveness, the auricular plaster with seeds can be stuck to the chosen points with tweezers, and the tweezers can be gently removed and pressed around the seed with fingers or probes to secure the plaster stuck to the right point. Ask patients to press each seed to make sure they know where the seeds have been exactly placed. Observe them doing this. When removing, normally one week later, tweezers were used to gently peel off the plaster.

4 Clinical Applications

For all kinds of pain symptoms, weight loss, quitting smoking, anti-hypertension, and many other diseases or problems are suitable for acupuncture.

4.1 How to Use Auricular Acupoints

Normally, 4–5 auricular points are chosen, and appropriate anatomical and/or organ auricular points are chosen according to Chinese medicine theory. Some auricular points have more general indications than others, e.g., auricular Shen Men to help calm the Shen.

Host points:

The host points can be explained as the most commonly used and useful points on the outer ear. For example, Shen Men (Spirit Gate) can be used for most problems or diseases; Sympathetic auricular point can balance sympathetic and para-sympathetic nervous systems; and Subcortex point affects the thalamus region, autonomic nerves and endocrine glands and can be used for pain and analgesia issues. Endocrine auricular point can bring endocrine hormones to appropriate homeostatic levels and activate the pituitary gland to regulate glandular secretions.

Guest points:

The guest points can be used based on the pattern differentiation in Chinese medicine.

4.2 Here Are Some Commonly Seen Diseases Clinically as Examples

Sleeping disorder, these auricular points are suggested:

Host points:

Shen Men [TF_4], Subcortex [AT_4].

Guest points:

Kidney [CO_{10}]—tonifying the kidney to calm the Shen;

Heart [CO_{15}]—clearing the heart fire to calm the Shen;

Gallbladder [CO_{11}]—reducing the gallbladder fire to calm the Shen*

Stomach [CO_4]—decreasing the stomach fire to link the heart and kidney*

Spleen [CO_{13}]—tonifying the spleen and pacifying the heart to calm the Shen*

*According to the pattern differentiation clinically to choose the points.

Quitting Smoking
These auricular points are suggested for quitting smoking:

Host points:

Endocrine [CO_{18}], Shen Men [TF_4], Subcortex [AT_4].

Guest points:

Kidney point [CO_{10}]—Tonifying the kidney system to calm the fear [4].

Liver point [CO_{12}]—promoting qi stagnation and regulating emotions (stress, anxiety) [5].

Lung point [CO_{14}]—Regulate the Qi of the lung to promote aeration and help patients let go of sadness [6].

Frozen Shoulder
These auricular points are suggested:

Host points:

Shen Men [TF_4], Endocrine [CO_{18}], Adrenal Gland [TG_2].

Guest points:

Shoulder [4], shoulder joint [5], clavicle [6]: local selection;

Stomach [CO_4] and large intestine [CO_7]: dispelling the phlegm and expelling the dampness from the Yangming meridians.

Osteoarthritis
These auricular points are suggested:

Host points:

Shen Men [TF_4], Endocrine [CO_{18}], Adrenal Gland [TG_2], Subcortex [AT_4].

Guest points:

Knee point: local selection;

Kidney point [CO_{10}]: tonifying the kidney system to strengthen the bone;

Liver [CO_{12}]: tonifying the liver system to strengthen the ligaments.

Constipation
These auricular points are suggested:

Host points:

Subcortex [AT_4], Sympathetic [HX_4].

Guest point:

Large Intestine (CO_7): Promote large intestine's motility;

Spleen [CO_{13}]: Promote small intestine's motility;

Rectum [HX_2]: Promote rectum's motility.

Indigestion
These auricular points are suggested:

Host points:

Subcortex [AT_4], Endocrine [CO_{18}].

Guest point:

Large Intestine (CO_7): Promote the absorptive function of the large intestine;

Small Intestine [CO_6]: Promote the transportation function of the small intestine;

Spleen [CO_{13}]: Promote the absorptive function of the small intestine;

Stomach [CO_4]: Promote gastric motility;

Gallbladder [CO_{11}]: Promote the secretion of bile to aid digestion.

Diarhhea
These auricular points are suggested:

Host points:

Endocrine [CO_{18}], Sympathetic [HX_4], Adrenal Gland [TG_2].

Guest point:

Large Intestine (CO_7), Small Intestine [CO_6], Spleen [CO_{13}], Lung [CO_{14}].

Chest Pain
These auricular points are suggested:

Host points:

Endocrine [CO_{18}], Sympathetic [HX_4], Adrenal Gland [TG_2], Subcortex [AT_4], Shenmen [TF_4], Occiput (AT_3).

Guest point:

Chest.

Asthma

These auricular points are suggested:

Host points:

Endocrine [CO_{18}], Sympathetic [HX_4], Adrenal Gland [TG_2], Shenmen [TF_4], Occiput (AT_3).

Guest point:

Lung [CO_{14}]: local selection.

Bronchopneumonia

These auricular points are suggested:

Host points:

Endocrine [CO_{18}], Subcortex [AT_4], Adrenal Gland [TG_2] and Shenmen [TF_4].

Guest point:

Lung [CO_{14}]: Descending the qi of hand taiyin to dispel the phlegm;

Spleen [CO_{13}]: tonifying qi of foot shaoyin to dispel the phlegm;

Large Intestine [CO_7]: Clearing the large intestine organ to lower qi;

Bronchus: local selection.

Low Blood Pressure

These auricular points are suggested:

Host points:

Sympathetic, Subcortex [AT_4], Adrenal Gland [TG_2], Shenmen [TF_4], Occiput [AT_3].

Guest point:

Heart [CO_{10}], Small Intestine [CO_6], and Stomach [CO_4].

Tachyrhythmia

These auricular points are suggested:

Host points:

Sympathetic [HX_4], Subcortex [AT_4], Shenmen [TF_4], Occiput [AT_3].

Guest point:

Heart [CO_{10}], Small Intestine [CO_6]: clearing the heart to reduce the fire.

Coronary Heart Disease
These auricular points are suggested:

Host points:

Shenmen [TF_4], Sympathetic [HX_4], Adrenal Gland [TG_2], Subcortex [AT_4].

Guest point:

Heart [CO_{10}], Small Intestine [CO_6]: tonifying the heart yang;

Liver [CO_{12}]: regulating the liver and releasing liver qi stagnation;

Spleen [CO_{13}]: Strengthening the spleen and resolving phlegm;

Kidney [CO_{10}]: tonifying the vital qi.

Heart [CO_{10}], Sympathetic [HX_4], Subcortex [AT_4] are the key points.

Irrhythmia
These auricular points are suggested:

Host points:

Shenmen [TF_4], Sympathetic [HX_4], Subcortex [AT_4], Occiput [AT_3].

Guest point:

Heart [CO_{10}] and mall Intestine [CO_6]: tonifying the heart yang.

Liver [CO_{12}]: regulating the liver and releasing liver qi stagnation;

Heart [CO_{10}], Subcortex [AT_4] and Sympathetic [HX_4] are the key points.

Migraine
These auricular points are suggested:

Host points:

Shenmen [TF_4], Endocrine [CO_{18}], Occiput [AT_3].

Guest point:

Liver [CO_{12}]: regulating the liver and releasing liver qi stagnation;

Kidney [CO_{10}]: Tonifying kidney to stop the pain;

Temple (AT_2): local selection.

Liver [CO_{12}] and Temple [AT_2] are key points.

Dreaminess

These auricular points are suggested:

Host points:

Shenmen [TF_4], Subcortex [AT_4], Occiput [AT_3].

Guest point:

Kidney [CO_{10}], Stomach [CO_4], Heart [CO_{10}], Spleen [CO_{13}], Sanjiao (CO_{17}).

Heart [CO_{10}], Spleen [CO_{13}] and Kidney [CO_{10}] are key points.

Intercostal Neuralgia

These auricular points are suggested:

Host points:

Subcortex [AT_4], Adrenal Gland [TG_2], Endocrine [CO_{18}], Shenmen [TF_4], Occiput [AT_3].

Guest point:

Liver [CO_{12}]: regulating the liver and releasing liver qi stagnation;

Spleen [CO_{13}]: tonifying the spleen and nourishing the blood;

Chest: Danzhong Ren17 on the chest is the sea of qi.

Chest and Shenmen are key points.

Hyperhidrosis

These auricular points are suggested:

Host points:

Adrenal Gland [TG_2], Endocrine [CO_{18}], Sympathetic [HX_4] and Occiput [AT_3].

Guest point:

Kidney [CO_{10}]: tonifying the kidney and strengthening the yuan qi;

Lung [CO_{14}]: tonifying taiyin to strengthen defensive qi.

Lung [CO_{14}] and Kidney [CO_{10}] are key points.

Frequent Micturition

These auricular points are suggested:

Host points:

Shenmen [TF_4], Endocrine [CO_{18}], Sympathetic [HX_4].

Guest point:

Bladder and Kidney [CO_{10}]: tonifying kidney to dispel the deficient cold from bladder;

Urethra: local selection.

Kidney [CO_{10}] and Bladder are key points.

Urinary Retention
These auricular points are suggested:

Host points:

Endocrine [CO_{18}], Sympathetic [HX_4] and Subcortex [AT_4].

Guest point:

Bladder and Kidney [CO_{10}]: tonifying kidney to promote diuretic.

Kidney and Bladder are key points.

Leakage of Urine
These auricular points are suggested:

Host points:

Shenmen [TF_4] and Subcortex [AT_4].

Guest point:

Liver [CO_{12}]: regulating the liver to release the liver qi stagnation;

Spleen [CO_{13}]: tonifying the spleen to strengthen the smooth muscle.

Bladder and External Genitals: local selection.

Bladder is the key point.

Dysmenorrhea
These auricular points are suggested:

Host points:

Shenmen [TF_4], Endocrine [CO_{18}], Sympathetic [HX_4], Subcortex [AT_4].

Guest point:

Kidney [CO_{10}]: tonifying the kidney to stop the pain;

Liver [CO_{12}]: regulating the liver to stop the pain;

Spleen [$CO13$]: tonifying the spleen and blood to stop the pain;

Uterus: local selection.

Uterus and Kidney [CO_{10}] are the key points.

Pruritus Vulvae

These auricular points are suggested:

Host points:

Shenmen [TF_4], Adrenal Gland [TG_2], Endocrine [CO_{18}], Occiput [AT_3].

Guest point:

Lung [CO_{14}]: dispersing the lung and relieving itchiness;

External Genitals [HX_4]: local selection.

Lung [CO_{14}] and External Genitals [HX_4] are the key points.

Hyperthyroid

These auricular points are suggested:

Host points:

Shenmen [TF_4], Sympathetic [HX_4], Adrenal Gland [TG_2], Endocrine [CO_{18}].

Guest point:

Cervical Vertebrae [SF6]: corresponding place to the thyroid;

Thyroid [AH_{13}]: local selection.

Cervical vertebrae and thyroid are key points.

Chronic Tonsillitis

These auricular points are suggested:

Host points:

Shenmen [TF_4], Adrenal Gland [TG_2], Endocrine [CO_{18}] and Occiput [AT_3].

Guest point:

Throat [TG_1]: local selection.

Sanjiao [CO_{17}]: clearing shaoyang fire to release the symptom.

Throat [TG_1] is the key point.

Eczema

These auricular points are suggested:

Host points:

Adrenal Gland [TG_2], and Occiput [AT_3].

Guest point:

Large Intestine [CO_7]: clearing the heat from hand yangming large intestine.

Lung [CO_{14}]: dispersing the lung to stop itchiness.

Lung point [CO_{14}] is the key one.

Gonarthritis

These auricular points are suggested:

Host points:

Shenmen [TF_4], Adrenal Gland [TG_2], Endocrine [CO_{18}], Subcortex [AT_4] and Occiput [AT_3].

Guest point:

Knee [AH_4]: local selection;

Liver [CO_{12}] and Kidney [CO_{10}]: Strengthening tendons and bones.

Kidney [CO_{10}] and Knee [AH_4] points are key ones.

5 Clinical Notice and Caution

Sterilize the outer ear strictly to avoid infection. The outer ear is exposed outside, its structure is quite special, and the blood flow is not sufficient to make it easy to become infected. Furthermore, cartilage can be affected easily after infection. For severe cases, this infection can cause the local area to undergo necrosis, atrophy and distortion. Therefore, prevention is quite important;

It is not suggested to take auricular acupuncture if there is eczema, ulcer or broken frostbite;

Do not offer auricular acupuncture treatment for pregnant women who have habitual abortion;

Make sure to have appropriate rest for the old, the weak or the patient who has high blood pressure or other serious diseases, make sure that the hand techniques are gentle instead of strong manipulation;

Be aware of needle faint when taking auricular acupuncture, and do prevention for it;

As with standard acupuncture, care is needed with patients who are hungry, overfull, overtired, too weak or under the influence of alcohol or drugs.

Combined with appropriate movement when the needle in or ear seed plaster on for the patients who has a sprain to get better effectiveness.

Ear seed plaster is very commonly used for patients clinically; it consists of small plasters with seeds, traditionally Vaccaria seeds or metal seeds. Patients can press seeds 2–3 times per day for appropriate stimulation to achieve better effects.

The seeds can be left on for 3–7 days. Patients should be advised to remove seeds after this period of time or when the seeds begin to irritate the skin. Be careful to take shower or wash hair when the seeds are on. Do not press the pellets too hard;

if it is painful without pressing, the local skin might be broken; ask the practitioner for advice.

Ear Seed is useful for continuing treatment after the needling session, it consists of small plaster or film with seed—traditionally vaccaria seed or metal, the metal one can be magnetic, or gold/silver-plated; it is suggested that the practitioner should avoid using overneedled points due to risk of infection.

6 Clinical Research on Auricular Acupuncture

Lan Y mentioned that a total of 1381 records were identified, with 15 studies deemed eligible for the present review. Meta-analyses were conducted in two comparisons separately: participants who received auricular acupuncture were more likely to make an improvement in clinical effective rate, sleep duration, sleep efficiency, number of awakenings and sleep onset latency when compared to sham auricular acupuncture or placebo. Statistical analyses of the outcomes revealed a positive effect of auricular acupuncture for primary insomnia.

Moura et al. [2] suggested that auricular acupuncture is a promising practice for the treatment of chronic back pain in adults. Lan [1] mentioned that statistical analyses of the outcomes revealed a positive effect of auricular acupuncture for primary insomnia.

Ruela LO et al. [3] enrolled 31 cancer patients in the study. After the eight auricular acupuncture sessions, there was a significant difference between the groups regarding the reduction in pain intensity ($p < 0.001$) and the use of medications ($p < 0.05$). Based on the research above, he concluded that auricular acupuncture was effective in reducing the pain of patients receiving chemotherapy.

Comprehensive/Review Questions

(1) Why can pressing auricular points treat holistic health condition?
(2) How many auricular point in auricular acupuncture?
(3) What relationship are between auricular theory and TCM theory?
(4) Is there any other material that can stimulate the auricular points apart from the acupuncture needle?

References

1. Lan Y, Wu X, Tan HJ, Wu N, Xing JJ, Wu FS, Zhang LX, Liang FR. Auricular acupuncture with seed or pellet attachments for primary insomnia: a systematic review and meta-analysis. BMC Complement Altern Med. 2015;2(15):103. https://doi.org/10.1186/s12906-015-0606-7.PMID: 25886561;PMCID:PMC4425871.

2. Moura CC, Chaves ECL, Cardoso ACLR, Nogueira DA, Azevedo C, Chianca TCM. Auricular acupuncture for chronic back pain in adults: a systematic review and metanalysis. Rev Esc Enferm USP.2019;53:e03461. https://doi.org/10.1590/S1980-220X2018021703461
3. Ruela LO, Iunes DH, Nogueira DA, Stefanello J, Gradim CVC. Effectiveness of auricular acupuncture in the treatment of cancer pain: randomized clinical trial. Rev Esc Enferm USP. 2018;52:e03402. Portuguese, English, Spanish. https://doi.org/10.1590/S1980-220X2017040503402. PMID: 30570087

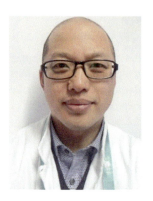

Jun She(佘军) Graduated from Heilongjiang University of Chinese Medicine in China and got his Ph.D. degree in 2007. He came to the UK in 2008 to work as a Chinese herbal practitioner, Senior lecturer, Acupuncturist, Tai Chi instructor in London South Bank University, and he also is a senior lecturer and clinic director in London Academy of Chinese Acupuncture.

Based on his knowledge and academic background, his main areas of interest are delivering Chinese medicine knowledge, practice six meridian method and Wu's acupuncture train clinically for the people and help them keep healthy in Chinese medicine way.

Cheek Acupuncture

Yongzhou Wang and Yongzheng Wu

Learning Objectives
- To learn the acupoints of cheek acupuncture and indications of this technique.
- To understand the principle of cheek acupuncture and the procedures for manipulation.
- To know the safety precautions of cheek acupuncture.
- To demonstrate the common diseases that can be treated by cheek acupuncture and the acupoints that were used for the corresponding disease.
- To show the application of cheek acupuncture in the clinic and to understand the potential mechanism of action of this technique.

1 Introduction

The microneedling system, characterized by performing acupuncture only on the local surface of a special organ or the limited location of the body to treat diseases originally occurring in another part of the body, has been widely applied in the clinic. It includes scalp acupuncture, ear acupuncture, wrist-ankle acupuncture, and cheek acupuncture. Cheek acupuncture, also referred to as buccal acupuncture, is introduced in this chapter. All other techniques of microacupuncture are described in the other chapters of this book.

Y. Wang (✉)
International Cheeks Acupuncture Therapy Institute, 30 Bd de Picpus, 75012 Paris, France
e-mail: wyongzhou@yahoo.fr

Y. Wu
CNRS UMR3691, Cellular Biology and Microbial Infection Unit, Institut Pasteur, Université Paris Cité, Paris, France
e-mail: wuyzh@pasteur.fr

© The Author(s), under exclusive license to Springer Nature Switzerland AG 2024
T. Wang and W. Wang (eds.), *Acupuncture Techniques*,
https://doi.org/10.1007/978-3-031-59272-0_13

The idea of cheek acupuncture originated in 1991 when the author observed by chance that an acupoint on the cheek could be used to relieve pain in the back and legs by acupuncture. This discovery encouraged the author to explore this technique further. In 2000, our group published the first paper on cheek acupuncture, identifying the acupoints on the cheek used to relieve corresponding pain [1]. With subsequent efforts to enrich and standardize the acupoints, and to develop supporting theories, the book 'Cheek Acupuncture Therapy' was published in 2017 by People's Health Publishing House Co. Ltd. [2], the best and largest medical press in China. This publication marked a milestone in the establishment of the cheek acupuncture system. The standardised acupoints on the cheek, the specific and holographic targeting of the body reflected on the cheek, the application in treating a wide range of diseases, the simple operating procedures, and the painless and safe nature of the technique are its distinctive features.

Three major theoretical systems, including holography, Da San Jiao, and physical and mental integration, have been developed as the guiding principles and practical system of cheek acupuncture, with Da San Jiao being the core. Based on the basic concepts of traditional Chinese medicine, such as zang-fu viscera and meridian theories, we combine the Da San Jiao theory of traditional Chinese medicine with the physical-mental theory of Western medicine and the biological holographic theory. This integration establishes a coherent holographic-San Jiao-physical-mental theoretical system that provides a multidimensional understanding of life development and the pathogenesis, prevention, and treatment of diseases.

In detail, several theories and systems contribute to the system of cheek acupuncture. First is the theory of the Qi pathway, which recognises the head as an important location where the Qi of the meridians gathers, circulates, and penetrates to connect the whole body. Hence, the cheek area of the head is chosen for the cheek acupuncture system to treat body diseases. The second is holographic theory, which is based on the author's observations in clinical practice and refinement of a holographic system of the entire body, including the zang-fu organs on the buccal area, through acupuncture. This theory provides guidance for performing cheek acupuncture. Third is the traditional meridian-collateral theory, which recognizes that the yangming and shaoyang meridian of the hand/foot travel and cover the cheek area. The yangming meridian has an excess of Qi and blood, while the shaoyang meridian acts as a modulating hub. In addition, the conception and governor vessels pass through the head and connect the ying and yang meridians in the body. Fourth is the system of nerves, with the trigeminal and facial nerves, two cranial nerves responsible for sensation and movement, also being distributed in the cheek needling area. Fifth is the Da San Jiao theory, which is based on the action of the Qi transformation of San Jiao from the "Zhongzang Classic". The author proposes that vitality is the key element during the process of the Qi transformation of San Jiao, and the theory emphasizes the importance of traditional Chinese medicine in understanding the nature of life. Indeed, when travelling in the body along meridian-collaterals, the vitality descends in the right (wood) of the body and ascends in the left (mental), maintains balance between up (fire) and down (water) and is adjusted by the earth located in the centre of the 5-element model. Therefore, vitality can eventually modulate and control its distribution and travel in the body, including the viscera, all limbs and bones, 5 sense organs and orifices, and 5 minds and 7 emotions. Finally, psychosomatic theory recognizes the unity of the body and spirit as the principle for cheek acupuncture. The five Zang organs are considered the generators of the five spirits, and Qi serves as the natural link between the physical body and spirit, allowing for intervention on both the physical body and the spirit by modulating the Qi flow. In particular, cheek acupuncture combines modern brain/neuron science with the theories of traditional Chinese medicine to optimize physiological functions and psychological states of the human body. Therefore, cheek acupuncture not only preserves one's health and prevents and treats diseases but also modulates spirit and psychology at the same time.

In summary, cheek acupuncture is a unique technique within the microacupuncture system. It has its own set of theoretical systems, including holography, Da San Jiao, and physical and mental integration, which guide its practice. The cheek acupuncture system is based on the concepts of the Qi pathway, holographic theory, meridian-collateral theory, nerve distribution, Da San Jiao theory, and psychosomatic theory. This technique not only promotes health and prevents and treats diseases but also modulates the spirit and psychology of individuals.

2 The Acupoints and Indications

The Acupoints

The cheek acupuncture system contains 16 standard acupoints (Fig. 1), which can be divided into 4 groups. ① The acupoints for the head and San Jiao include the head point, the point of the upper energizer, the point of the middle energizer, and the point of the lower energizer; ② The cervical point, back point, lumbar point, and sacral point belong to spine-associated acupoints; ③ There are 4 acupoints for the upper extremities, including the shoulder point, the elbow point, the wrist point, and the hand point; ④ The acupoints for the lower limbs are the hip point, the knee point, the ankle point, and the foot point. The detailed position of the standard acupoints is described in Table 1, and the acupoint diagram of the cheek acupuncture (from "Cheek Acupuncture Therapy" written by Wang Yongzhou [2]) is shown in Fig. 1.

Indications for Cheek Acupuncture

As described in the introduction, holography, Da San Jiao, and physical and mental integration are the major architectural theories of cheek acupuncture. Therefore, the treatment indications of this technique mainly work at these three levels. At the holographic level, cheek acupuncture therapy predominantly relieves acute and chronic pain in the limbs and spine. Indeed, acute and chronic pain in the neck, shoulder, lumbar spine, and legs caused by soft tissue injuries are very common in the clinic. Certain types of pain induced by complicated disorders, such as cervical spondylosis, herniated disc, and spinal stenosis, can also be relieved by cheek acupuncture.

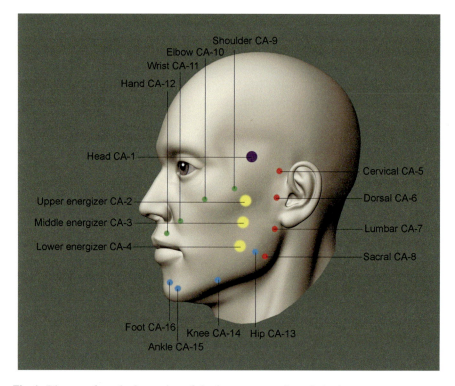

Fig. 1 Diagram of standard acupoints of cheek acupuncture (lateral view)

At the level of Da San Jiao, cheek acupuncture is effective in treating diseases occurring in the chest and abdomen. These symptoms include chest tightness, palpitation, coughing and wheezing, phlegm, breast distension, stomachache, esophageal reflux, heartburn, abdominal distension, diarrhoea, constipation, frequent urination, urgent urination, dysmenorrhea, and neck, back, lumbar, and sacral pain associated with respiratory and digestive diseases.

The third part of the indications of cheek acupuncture is at the physical and mental level, including irritability, stress, anxiety, depression, and moody allergic diseases, rheumatoid disease, endocrine diseases, persistent skin diseases, chronic allergic asthma, persistent insomnia, Alzheimer's disease, headache, migraine, etc. However, these three levels are usually integrated and intermingled, and the disease may be dominated at one of the levels, the interaction of two levels, or even touch all three levels in certain chronic diseases. Thus, it is very important to adjust the treatment in the clinic according to the diagnosis, target selection, and immediate effectiveness of the acupuncture.

Table 1 Anatomical orientation of the acupoints and their main applications

Name	Orientation	Applications
Head point (CA-1)	1 inch above the upper edge of middle point of zygomatic arch	Headache, dizziness, toothache, insomnia, stress, anxiety, depression, stroke, etc.
Upper energizer point (CA-2)	The cross of posterior coronoid of mandible and lower edge of zygomatic arch	Headache, cervical pain, chest pain, chest tightness, breast swelling and pain, tachycardia, arrhythmia, asthma, etc.
Middle energizer point (CA-3)	The middle point of connecting line between upper and lower energizer acupoints	Stomach cramp, acute/chronic gastritis, heartburn with acidity, hiccups, vomiting, digestive diseases, etc.
Lower energizer point (CA-4)	Anterior oblique line of mandible	Abdominal bloating and pain, colitis, dysmenorrhea, pelvic inflammatory disease, menstrual irregularities, leukorrhea, gynecological disease
Cervical point (CA-5)	Top edge of the root of zygomatic arch	Neck pain, stiff neck after sleeping, cervical spondylosis, sore throat, dizziness, stress, scalene spasm, tinnitus, etc.
Dorsal point (CA-6)	The cross of lower edge of zygomatic arch and inferior capsule of temporomandibular joint	Back pain, rhomboid muscle strain, chest tightness, shortness of breath, stomachache, heart palpitations, etc.
Lumbar point (CA-7)	The middle of connecting line between dorsal and sacral points	Lower back pain, lumbar muscle strain, acute lumbar sprains, sciatica pain, herniated disc, etc.
Sacral point (CA-8)	0.5 inch to anterior & superior angle of mandible	Sacrospinous muscle strain, lower back pain in women, injuries of sacroiliac ligament, bedwetting, prostatitis, etc.
Shoulder point (CA-9)	The middle point of temporozygomatic sature	Shoulder pain, frozen shoulder, tendonitis of biceps brachii, synovitis of infra-acromion of scapula, tendonitis of supraspinatus muscle, etc.
Elbow point (CA-10)	The middle point of connecting line between lateral canthus and bottom of zygomatic bone	Elbow pain, tennis elbow, golf elbow, wrist extensor tendonitis, wrist flexor tendonitis, etc.

(continued)

Table 1 (continued)

Name	Orientation	Applications
Wrist point (CA-11)	The point of nasolabial folds at the horizon level of lower edge of nostrils	Wrist pain, injuries of wrist joint, carpal tunnel syndrome, finger pain
Hand point (CA-12)	The middle of connecting line between the middle point of lower edge of nostril and vermilions border	Finger arthritis, tenosynovitis, finger numbness, hand numbness
Hip point (CA-13)	1 inch of anterior & superior of angle of mandible on the masseteric tuberosity	Sciatica pain, wound-induced hip osteoarthritis, injury of piriform muscle, groin pain
Knee point (CA-14)	The middle point of connecting line between angle of mandible and chengjiang point	Knee pain, superficial fibular nerve pain, arthritis of knee joint, hamstring muscle injury, gastrocnemius muscle spasm, etc.
Ankle point (CA-15)	1/3 proximity of connecting line between knee and Chengjiang points	Ankle joint sprain, ankle joint swelling and pain, ankle arthritis, Achilles tendinitis, heel pain
Foot point (CA-16)	0.5 inch lateral to Chengjiang point	Gout, metatarsals fascia sprain, plantar fasciitis, heel pain, toe pain

3 The Manipulation of the Check Acupuncture

The Principle of Cheek Acupuncture Treatment

The fundamental principle of cheek acupuncture treatment is to regulate Qi flow and the spirit by acupuncturing specific points on the cheek, thereby achieving the harmonization of the body's yin and yang and maintaining homeostasis and stability.

Qi can be divided into Wei Qi, Ying Qi, and Yuan Qi. In general, regulating the Qi by acupuncture not only adjusts the Ying and Wei Qi of internal and external meridians but also, more importantly, adjusts the Yuan Qi. Indeed, a better circulation and balance of Yuan Qi in the body assure the transportation and transformation of Zang-Fu to function well. Thus, fine-tuning the ascension-descension, going-out, and coming-in of Qi is an important rule of clinical treatment for cheek acupuncture, which should be considered by the practitioner. Needling should also follow the movement of Qi, e.g., ascending on the left and descending on the right part of the body, in treating the patient.

Tuning the spirit is another key issue for cheek acupuncture, which contains three aspects. First, the practitioner performing acupuncture should carefully conduct a physical examination for the patient to make the diagnosis and concentrate on the treatment. Second, we must be aware that the spirit treatment is not only to tune the mental activity of the patients but, to speak broadly, to adjust the five-zang spirits, including the ethereal soul, vitality, ideation, corporeal soul, and will of the patient.

This is because Zang-Fu viscera disease is the consequence of emotional disorders in patients. In other words, the disorder of the spirit results in the problem of the physical body, which is also the sequential order of the treatment by which the spirit disorder needs to be cured first. Therefore, the treatment of the patient's spirit is the principal rule throughout the entire process of acupuncture treatment. Once the soul and spirit become smooth, the activities of five-zang work well, and the disease is resolved. Finally, the highest level of treatment by acupuncture is to follow the natural way of maintaining health and preventing and treating diseases together with the body's internal stability and self-adaptation.

Physical Examination and Acupoint(s) Selection
According to the basic theories of cheek acupuncture, precise diagnosis is critical for selecting corresponding acupoint(s), which is the premise for efficient treatment by acupuncture. Thus, a physical examination is essential for the correct diagnosis and subsequent acupuncture. Based on the patient's complaints, the local muscles, tendons, bones, their movement, and nerve sensation should be checked carefully. For the spine and surrounding tissues, the pathological reaction points in the joints, bones, muscles, and nerves associated with the spine should be examined. The practitioner can also identify abdominal diseases by directly touching the patient's abdomen and even diagnose various signs and diseases of internal medicine due to Qi reversal in the internal organs and meridians by pressing, feeling, touching, probing, and leaning on the abdomen. A detailed physical examination can help the practitioner make decisions on the diagnosis, followed by choosing the standard acupoint corresponding to the target organ, tissue, or disease for cheek acupuncture.

Cheek Acupuncture Commonly Used Method
Generally, a single needling is performed at the acupoint on the cheek that corresponds to the target, such as a muscle or organ in the body. However, we must note that cheek acupuncture considers the acupoint as a point area that is determined according to the size and involvement of the target disorder/injury, although the acupoint is positioned precisely. Therefore, sometimes the same point area will be enhanced by using multiple needles to achieve the maximum effective treatment, including double needles, triangular pricks, diamond-shaped pricks, plum blossom pricks, single-row pricks, and double-row pricks. These special methods are mainly applied to patients with more severe, longer duration, and larger size of the lesion/pain.

Sensation of Cheek Acupuncture
Compared to classical acupuncture, which can cause sensations of soreness, numbness, swelling, and pain at the site of needling, cheek acupuncture typically produces only slight or even no special sensation. Once the needle tip reaches the appropriate depth, it provides the right amount of stimulation to promote the flow of Qi, blood, and meridians. The practitioner then needs to verify whether the symptoms or pain of the patient's target organ/tissue have improved or been relieved, either by communicating with the patient or by checking and comparing the abdomen situation before and after acupuncture.

4 The Depth of Needling and the Sequential Order of Cheek Acupuncture

In general, the depth of acupuncture is determined by the patient's condition and the location of the target area, as well as the abdominal diagnosis. For instance, shallow needling is used for mild diseases, while deep needling is used for severe diseases. Regarding the sequential order of needling, resolving chest and abdominal disorders takes priority over treating extremities. For localized diseases, needling is performed on the same side of the cheek, while bilateral Sanjiao points are needled for systemic diseases. Under certain circumstances, enhanced needling in the Sanjiao acupoint area may be necessary, according to the problem of the corresponding target organ and abdominal diagnosis.

5 Maintaining Time of Acupuncture

The needling of acupuncture can be maintained for 20–60 min, depending on the patient's situation. During this period, the needling can be adjusted or replenished based on the patient's response. For patients with chronic or persistent pain and mental relaxation, needling can be maintained for a longer time, while a shorter time is recommended for other diseases.

Frequency and Duration of Treatment
Generally, cheek acupuncture is performed once a week for 3 weeks depending on the situation of the patient. Five acupuncture sessions were considered one cycle of treatment.

The Error Correction System for Cheek Acupuncture
One of the features of cheek acupuncture is its precision, and the establishment of a reliable correction system is at the core of this accurate acupuncture in the clinic. To achieve this, the physical body and Qi of Zang-fu and body-mind must be correctly determined based on the diagnosis of local tissue and abdomen, followed by needling the corresponding point on the cheek. If the clinical efficacy is unsatisfactory, it is essential to check whether the location of selected acupoints is precise, whether the target was missed during the physical examination, whether the integrity of the body was considered, and whether the depth or direction of needling is correct, among other factors. To verify this, another physical examination is necessary, and the practitioner needs to reconsider the patient's main symptoms, followed by the adjustment or replenishment of needling to achieve the maximal efficacy of on-site treatment.

Safety Precautions
There are only 16 basic acupoints for cheek acupuncture, including four for each of the upper and lower extremities, four for the spine, and the Sanjiao and head

Cheek Acupuncture 213

points. These acupoints on the cheek correspond to the organ, muscle, or tissue target on the body. If the patient's problem is relatively simple, it is usually easier to control by needling the corresponding acupoint. However, in certain situations, needling should be performed around the area of the individual acupoint's anatomical location, according to the influenced target of the injury and the area involved, even though the acupoints of cheek acupuncture are relatively accurate. Particularly, it is not recommended to follow the diagram of typical cases in the chapter entirely. Instead, needling should be modified according to the individual's condition and disease.

Attention

1. Acupuncture can cause dizziness, retained needles, bent needles, broken needles, hematoma, pneumothorax, internal organ damage, and other abnormalities, which should be avoided.
2. If one side of the cheek has a dermatological problem, the acupoint on the other side of the cheek is usually used for treatment.
3. Eating and talking are generally prohibited during acupuncture to prevent retained or broken needles caused by excessive chewing or facial muscle movement.
4. The situation of pregnant women, especially those with a history of miscarriage or artificial insemination, should be carefully evaluated before acupuncture. In particular, beginners of acupuncture should avoid treating these patients.

Cheek Acupuncture is not Recommended in the Clinic Under the Following Conditions

1. The patient has a dermatological lesion or local infection on the face.
2. The patient has a fever with high temperature, convulsions, lung or heart failure, or other emergent health conditions.
3. The patient's physiological parameters and laboratory examinations showed severe abnormalities. Patients with thrombocytopenia or bleeding tendencies should not receive acupuncture.
4. No acupuncture should be performed near the periocular tissue.
5. The patient is too hungry, fatigued, or overly nervous. For patients who are thin and deficient in Qi and blood, the lying position should be used for acupuncture.
6. For patients who have had plastic surgery, face slimming injections, or anti-wrinkle injections, the details should be asked and evaluated for risk before performing cheek acupuncture.
7. Cheek acupuncture should be used with caution in patients with trigeminal neuralgia and facial muscle spasms.

6 Acupoints Selection for Common Diseases

Dysautonomia

A patient had symptoms of dry mouth and sweating accompanied by tension throughout the body. The physical examination showed pressing pain of the scalene muscles on both sides. The patient was considered to have sympathetic nerve excitation. The acupoints of the head and enhanced positions were selected for needling. After acupuncture, the patient felt completely relaxed, and the symptoms of dry mouth and sweating disappeared.

Tennis Elbow

A patient had been experiencing elbow pain in his left arm for 10 days. The physical examination showed pressing pain on the lateral epicondyle of the left arm and the scalene muscle on the left side. The diagnosis of tennis elbow was determined. The acupoints of the elbow and neck were selected for acupuncture. Pain relief was achieved immediately after needling.

Uterine Fibroid

A patient had excessive bleeding during her period and was diagnosed with uterine fibroids by ultrasonography. The physical examination revealed pressing pain in the lower abdomen. The lower energizer point, sacral point, and corresponding enhanced positions were needled. The abdominal pain disappeared after needling. Acupuncture was conducted every two weeks for a total of four times. Menstrual bleeding recovered to a normal volume without pain in the belly.

Nerve Entrapment Syndrome

A patient presented with symptoms of numbness in the thumb, index finger, and middle finger and difficulty raising her right arm. The physical examination revealed pressing pain in the back of the neck, scalene, pronator teres muscle, and wrist. The diagnosis of nerve entrapment syndrome with multiple sites was given. The acupoints of the upper neck, shoulder, elbow and wrist were chosen for needling. After needle insertion, the symptoms of numbness in the fingers improved immediately.

Sport Injury

A male had left leg pain for a couple of days when raising his leg or during sports activities. Physical examination showed pressing pain in the upper hip on the left side. The symptoms improved after inserting needles into the sacral acupoint. Based on holographic theory, subsequent treatment was given on the neck point, and the symptoms completely disappeared.

Post Surgery Pain

A female was diagnosed with breast cancer and underwent mastectomy and axillary lymph node dissection on the right side three weeks prior. She then could not raise her right arm and was experiencing insomnia. During physical examination, it was found that the pain limited the range of motion of her right arm to only 70 degrees. Pressing pain was detected at the trapezius, coracoid process, and lower back on the right side of her body. Acupuncture was performed on the acupoints of the shoulder and head, as well as the corresponding enhanced points. The pain was alleviated, and she was able to raise her right arm overhead.

Cancer Pain

A male with lymphoma complained of a sore throat and inability to raise his left arm after undergoing chemotherapy and radiotherapy. The arm could be raised passively but not by himself. The patient also reported experiencing pressing pain around his throat. The acupoints on the shoulder, enhancement sites, and upper energizer were selected for needling. After needle insertion, the patient reported no more sore throat when swallowing and was able to raise his arm to approximately 160°.

Insomnia

A male patient complained of poor quality sleep and difficulty falling back asleep after waking up at 5 AM in the morning. During the physical examination, mild pressing pain was detected in the abdomen. The acupoints of the head and corresponding enhanced points, as well as the upper and lower energizer points for both cheeks, were selected for acupuncture treatment. Abdominal pain was relieved after needle insertion.

Sciatica Pain

A female patient had been suffering from long-term sciatica pain and knee pain for 2 weeks. Physical examination revealed pressing pain in the vertebrae from the chest to the lumbar area, as well as in the knee and gastrocnemius muscle. The holographic points of the back, lumbar spine, sacrum, knee, and corresponding enhancement points were selected for acupuncture. The pressing pains were immediately alleviated.

Gastroenteritis

A male had acute gastroenteritis with vomiting and severe diarrhoea after consuming contaminated food. Acupuncture was performed on the acupoints of the upper, middle, and lower energizer on both cheeks. After acupuncture, there was no more diarrhoea, and the feeling of nausea significantly improved.

Excessive Tension of Erector Spinae Muscles

A woman complains of lumbar pain and pain in the upper side of her left leg without a history of injury or falling down. Physical examination shows diffusing pain upon compression. The problem of erector spinae muscles is considered. Acupuncture points at the cervical, chest, dorsal, and sacral regions are used. After needle insertion, the compression pain was immediately alleviated.

7 Current Cheek Acupuncture Application and Latest Research

The Use of Cheek Acupuncture Has Become Widespread in Clinical Practice

In the past few decades, acupuncture departments have been established as independent departments in hospitals nationwide. This has led to a large number of patients who would be suitable for acupuncture treatment being treated by other clinical departments. Consequently, the range of diseases treated in acupuncture departments has decreased, and the therapeutic efficacy of acupuncture has gradually weakened. However, with the progressive development of cheek acupuncture in China, an increasing number of specialists have learned and applied this technique in their clinical practice. Currently, cheek acupuncture is widely used in many specialties, including internal medicine (gastroenterology, endocrinology, cardiology, neurology, etc.), otolaryngology, breast, dermatology, gynaecology, paediatrics, anaesthesia, orthopedic injuries, etc. It has achieved fantastic efficacy and immediate effects in treating certain diseases that are difficult to be treated by conventional therapy.

Interestingly, with the application of buccal acupuncture in different specialties, the efficacy of cheek acupuncture against specialized diseases has been widely explored and confirmed. This has also promoted the generalization of this new technique.

The Theoretical System of Cheek Acupuncture Has Been Further Enriched and Improved

As described in the introduction section, the three theoretical systems of cheek acupuncture (holographic, Da San Jiao, and mind and body) have been established and further enriched and improved in the process of inheritance and standardization of cheek acupuncture therapy. For instance, Liang et al. (2018) [3] reported that the holographic theory could serve as a principal guide for cheek acupuncture in treating tendon and bone diseases. Combining traditional Chinese medicine theory, abdominal diagnosis, and holographic theory, they used our specialized Da San Jiao theory specifically for Zang-Fu disease. Sun et al. (2019) also applied the doctrine of spine-related diseases to the diagnosis and treatment of cheek acupuncture, which has achieved excellent clinical efficacy in treating spine-related extremity pain, spine-originated pain, spine-related head and face diseases, and spine-related visceral diseases [4].

Preliminary Exploration of the Potential Molecular Mechanism of Action of Cheek Acupuncture Therapy

Based on the clinical and animal experimental data obtained in recent years, the potential molecular mechanisms of action of cheek acupuncture have been explored. For example, in patients with cardiac X syndrome, cheek acupuncture significantly increases the level of nitric oxide (NO) and decreases the concentration of plasma endothelin (ET-1) and serum high-sensitivity C-reactive protein (hs-CRP) in the blood, thus reducing the inflammatory response in patients [5]. The cheek acupuncture therapy of patients with postoperative visceral pain after gynaecological laparoscopic surgery may achieve analgesia by reducing the levels of neutrophil elastase (NE) and 5-hydroxytryptamine (5-HT) [6]. A rabbit animal model of rheumatoid arthritis [7] has been used to determine the clinical retention time and reasonable regimen development for cheek acupuncture therapy. A significant difference in the quantitative efficacy curve of the analgesic effect by acupuncture is observed between the 1st and the 7th acupuncture, but no further difference is detected at the 10th acupuncture compared to the 7th, indicating that the analgesic effect induced by acupuncture gradually strengthens with the increase in the number of buccal acupuncture treatments but does not increase after a certain number of treatments. This study verifies the rationality of the 7-day regimen of treatment in the clinical practice of cheek acupuncture therapy.

8 Summary

Since the author's initial idea in 1991, cheek acupuncture has been clinically applied to more than 200,000 patients, achieving local and systemic therapeutic effects through this technique. In particular, cheek acupuncture has demonstrated reliable efficacy and immediate therapeutic effects on common diseases such as pain (neck, shoulder, waist, leg, etc.) and stress syndrome (a representative of physical and mental diseases and subhealth states). Due to its safety, painlessness, standardization, accuracy, and generalization, check acupuncture has been rapidly and widely applied in various specialties in China. Importantly, cheek acupuncture is applicable not only to Asian populations but also to other populations (European, African, American, etc.) with similar effects, based on the author's practical experience in China and abroad. However, there is still a lack of accumulation of a large quantity of populations with repeated efficacy. Furthermore, the exploitation and improvement of cheek acupuncture for more diseases need to be further investigated. Finally, the mechanism of this acupuncture therapy remains unclear, and further laboratory research is required to elucidate its mechanism of action, which will promote the wide application of cheek acupuncture therapy.

Comprehension/Review Questions

(1) What are the differences between traditional acupuncture and cheek acupuncture?
(2) What are the characteristics of cheek acupuncture?
(3) What are the major theories of cheek acupuncture?
(4) What's the name of acupoints of cheek acupuncture and how to determine those acupoints?
(5) What is the application of cheek acupuncture, and how can this technique be manipulated?
(6) Which kind of diseases can be efficiently treated by cheek acupuncture?
(7) What is the potential mechanism of action of cheek acupuncture?

References

1. Wang YZ, Wang. HD, Fang XL, et al. Application of buccal acupuncture in clinical pain relief. Chinese Acupuncture & Moxibustion **S1**, 2 (2000).

2. Wang YZ. *Cheeks Acupuncture Therapy*. 287 (People's Health Publishing House Co. Ltd. 2017).
3. Liang LY, Zhou Y, Zhong Z, et al. Discussion on the clinical application of cheek acupuncture points. Guangming Journal of Chinese Medicine. 2018;23:4.
4. Sun JF, Li. HJ., Liao JF, et al. Clinical overview of buccal needle for spine-related diseases. *Journal of New Chinese Medicine* **53**, 4 (2021).
5. Wu CJ. The holographic therapy of cheek acupuncture in patients with cardiac X syndrome and its effect on the vascular endothelium. *Shanxi Medical Journal* **51** (2022).
6. Sun Y, Zhao. Q, Xiao JY, et al. The effect of buccal acupuncture on the postoperative visceral pain in patients undergone gynecological laparoscopic surgery and its action mechanism. *Jiangxi Medical Journal* **57**, 584–586, https://doi.org/10.3969/j.issn.1006-2238.2022.06.009 (2022).
7. Pu RS, Fang XL, Jie WJ, et al. Characterizing analgesic effect of cheek acupuncture in rabbit model with rheumatoid arthritis. Chinese General Practice. 2017;20:5. https://doi.org/10.3969/j.issn.1007-9572.2017.00.142.

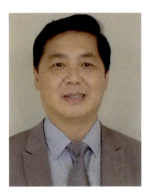

Dr. Yongzhou Wang(王永洲) a chief physician and the founder of cheek acupuncture therapy, serves as the president of the French Association of Traditional Chinese Medicine. Additionally, he is the dean of the French International College of Cheek Acupuncture, the chairman of the Acupuncture Committee of the All-European Federation of Traditional Chinese Medicine Experts. Dr. Wang also holds the position of vice president of the Appropriate Technology Promotion Committee of the World Federation of Traditional Chinese Medicine and is the executive director of the Naturopathic and Orthopedic Research Association.

Simultaneously, he is among the first batch of distinguished clinical experts at Beijing University of Chinese Medicine and an expert at Wang Yongzhou's Academic Experience Inheritance Studio at Guangdong Provincial Hospital of Traditional Chinese Medicine. The "Cheek Acupuncture Therapy" founded by Dr Wang is one of the first ten finalists in the "Hundred Talents and Hundred Projects" program of overseas Chinese medicine. It is also the ninth traditional Chinese medicine technology promotion program, "Xinglin Treasure Hunt", at Guangdong Provincial Hospital of Traditional Chinese Medicine.

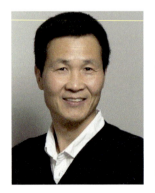

Dr. Yongzheng Wu(毋永正) graduated from Xi'an Medical University and obtained a clinical master's degree from Second Military Medical University. He joined Institut Pasteur at the beginning of 2000 and earned a Ph.D. from the University of Paris VI in 2003. He had his post-doc training at the University of Pennsylvania (USA). Since 2007, Dr. Wu has worked as tenured researcher at Institut Pasteur in Paris.

He worked as pediatrician for 7 years and have 20 years of experiences in scientific research. Currently, his main research interest is to understand the pathogenesis of infectious diseases, especially the interaction between the host and bacteria in the respiratory and reproductive systems. More than 35 papers have been published in peer-reviewed international scientific journals. In recent years, he has also developed an interested in cheek acupuncture.

Wrist-Ankle Acupuncture

Yu Sun and Katherine Dandridge

Learning Objectives

- To help students understand wrist-ankle acupuncture completely.
- To increase student clinical ability.
- To raise and amplify clinical effects.
- To broaden students' knowledge.

1 General Introduction

Wrist-ankle acupuncture (for short: WAA) is considered a newly formed 'microsystem' acupuncture technique, alongside other microsystem acupuncture techniques, such as ear acupuncture and scalp acupuncture. In wrist-ankle acupuncture, the doctor (张心曙) had been enlightened by electric shock therapy, combined with the traditional Chinese medicine meridian, points and needling technic theory, and study and practice repeatedly for approximately ten years [1].

It was shared with the public in 1976, and then many doctors learned and used it in the clinic, and the evidence continued to grow and develop, leading to further understanding and features:

1. It is a simple acupuncture technique: It has a total of only 24 points divided into 12 pairs.

Y. Sun (✉)
Sunny International (UK) Ltd., 39 Leahurst Court Road, Brighton BN1 6UL, UK
e-mail: doctorsun88@yahoo.co.uk

K. Dandridge
Muthill, Perthshire, Scotland
e-mail: info@katherinedandridge.com

2. It elicits a quick reaction: If the physician restricts themselves to the basic needling technique, the patient can feel that the symptom improves immediately.
3. Highly effective: Many symptoms can improve with wrist-ankle acupuncture, they will certainly be a good effect.
4. Wide range of treatment care: It can be used for many disorders.
5. Comfort for the patient: When the needle is effectively applied, the patient should not feel any discomfort around the needle, even if the patient moves the arm or leg.
6. Convenient: the patient does not need undress, just expose the lower arm or lower leg.

2 Area with Organs and Tissues

The important principle of wrist-ankle acupuncture is to divide the body surface into six areas in the longitudinal direction, from head to toe, and in symmetry from left to right. In addition, the areas of the upper part and lower part are divided in the transverse by diaphragmatic line, the arm belonging to the upper part (herein 'UPPER'), and the leg belonging to the lower part (herein 'LOWER').

Each of the six areas are organized by the following acronyms to differentiate the areas clearly and correspond with the areas to effect treatment on the arm points and leg points. See the diagram and match the following.

Six Areas and Two Parts

Six Areas by Longitudinal Direction
The body surface is divided into six areas in the longitudinal direction: torso (including head) areas, arm areas and leg areas.

The Torso (Including Head) Six Areas
Area 1: Each side of the anterior median line in every direction 1.5 individual cun. The left side area and right side area are symmetrical and identical. They are called left area 1 and right area 1 respectively (see Fig. 1a).

Area 2: Area 2 is located between the anterior axillary line to the outside left edge of area 1 or to the outside right edge of area 1. The left side area and right side area are symmetrical and identical. They are called left area 2 and right area 2 respectively (see Fig. 1a).

Area 3: Area 3 is located between the anterior axillary line and the mid-axillary line. The left side area and right side area are symmetrical and identical. They are called left area 3 and right area 3 respectively (see Fig. 1a).

Area 4: Area 4 is located between the mid-axillary line and the posterior axillary line. The left side area and right side area are symmetrical and identical. They are called left area 4 and right area 4 respectively (see Fig. 1b).

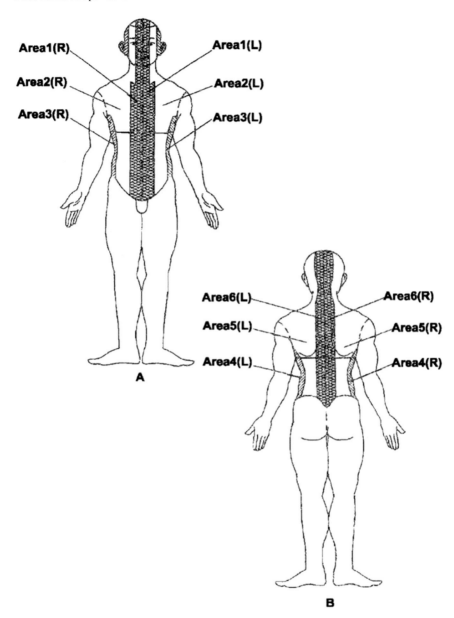

Fig. 1 The torso six areas

Area 5: Area 5 is located between the posterior axillary line to the outside left of the edge of area 6 or to the outside right of the edge of area 6. The left side and right side areas are symmetrical and identical. They are called left area 5 and right area 5 respectively (see Fig. 1b).

Area 6: Area 6 is similar to Area 1, but from the posterior median line in every direction 1.5 individual cun. The left side area and right side area are symmetrical and identical. They are called left area 6 and right area 6 respectively (see Fig. 1b).

The Arm Six Areas
The arm surface is divided into six equal areas along the longitudinal direction.

For the Left Arm: Start from the anterior margin of the ulna, keep moving clockwise through point P6 (Nei Guan), and continue to the anterior margin of the radius. continues again towards the posterior margin of the radius, and then through to point SJ-5 (Wai Guan), until you reach the posterior margin of the ulna. They leave each other in the following order: left arm area 1, left arm area 2, left arm area 3, left arm area 4, left arm area 5, and left arm area 6 (see Fig. 2a, b).

For the Right Arm: The right arm is the same as the left arm, but moves anticlockwise to divide the areas. They leave each other in the following order: right arm area 1, right arm area 2, right arm area 3, right arm area 4, right arm area 5, and right arm area 6 (see Fig. 2a, b).

The Leg Six Areas
It divided the leg surface into six equal areas along the longitudinal direction.

For the Left Leg: Start the medial edge of the Achilles tendon, keep moving clockwise through point SP-6 (San Yin Jiao), extend to the medial edge of the tibia crest, continue toward the lateral edge of the tibia crest, and then extend through point GB-39 (Xuan Zhong) up to the lateral edge of the Achilles tendon. They leave each other in the following order: left leg area 1, left leg area 2, left leg area 3, left leg area 4, left leg area 5, and left leg area 6 (see Fig. 3a, b).

For the Right Leg: Same as the left leg, but move anticlockwise to divide the areas. It leaves each other in the following order: right leg area 1, right leg area 2, right leg area 3, right leg area 4, right leg area 5, and right leg area 6 (see Fig. 3a, b).

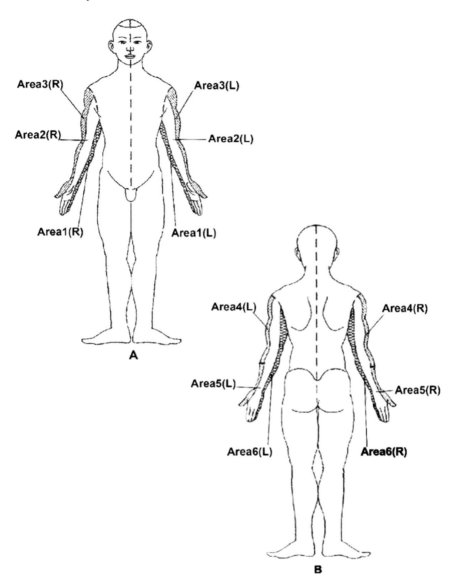

Fig. 2 The arm six areas

Upper-Part and Lower-Part by Transvers

Another important principle of wrist-ankle acupuncture is to divide the body surface into two parts: the transvers by diaphragmatic line, the arm belonging to the upper part, and the leg belonging to the lower part.

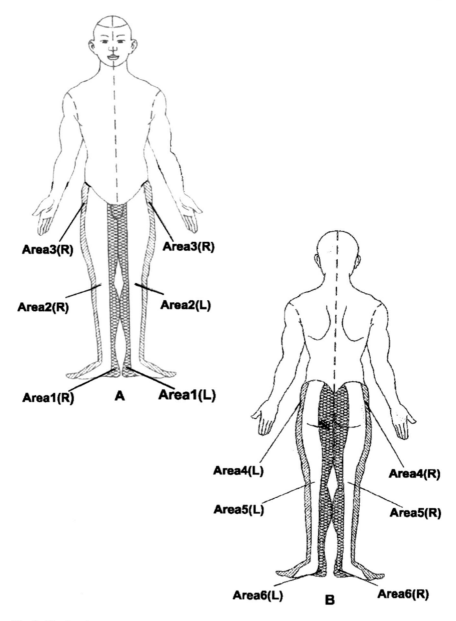

Fig. 3 The leg six areas

Upper-Part Six Areas

The head and torso upper part area plus the corresponding arm area. It leaves each other in the following order: Upper-Area 1, Upper-Area 2, Upper-Area 3, Upper-Area 4, Upper-Area 5, and Upper-Area 6, and in symmetry from left to right. It leaves each other in the following order:

Left-Upper-Area 1, Left-Upper-Area 2, Left-Upper-Area 3, Left-Upper-Area 4, Left-Upper-Area 5, Left-Upper-Area 6. And **Right-Upper-Area 1, Right-Upper-Area 2, Right-Upper-Area 3, Right-Upper-Area 4, Right-Upper-Area 5, Right-Upper-Area 6** (see Fig. 4a, b).

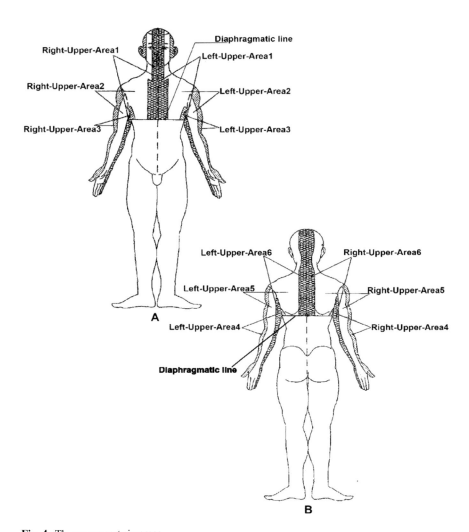

Fig. 4 The upper-part six areas

Lower-Part Six Areas

The torso lower part plus the corresponding leg area are called in order: Lower-Area 1, Lower-Area 2, Lower-Area 3, Lower-Area 4, Lower-Area 5, and Lower-Area 6 and in symmetry from left to right. It leaves each other in the following order:

Left-Lower-Area 1, Left-Lower-Area 2, Left-Lower-Area 3, Left-Lower-Area 4, Left-Lower-Area 5, Left-Lower-Area 6. And **Right-Lower-Area 1, Right-Lower-Area 2, Right-Lower-Area 3, Right-Lower-Area 4, Right-Lower-Area 5, Right-Lower-Area 6** (see Fig. 5a, b).

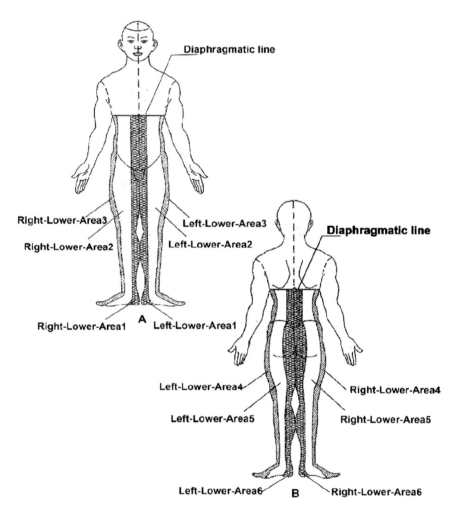

Fig. 5 The lower-part six areas

The Area with Main Organs and Main Tissues
Our body has many organs and tissues. According to the body surface area, it will stay in different areas, and some organs or tissues could be in one or two, even staying in more than that. Here, if you can refer to basic anatomy knowledge, you will determine more details. Here dose nothing more than give you some reference.

The Upper Area with Main Organs and Main Tissues
Upper-Area 1: Inner canthus portion of the eyes, nose, incisors, tongue, pharynx, tonsils, throat, trachea, breastbone, weasand, anything along this area as well as the muscles and tendons in arm area.

Upper-Area 2: Frontal portion of the eyes, cheekbone, molar, lunge. heart (left-upper-area 2), anything along this area as well as the muscles and tendons in arm area 2.

Upper-Area 3: Frontal angle, cheek, side neck, frontal side chest, anything along this area as well as the muscles and tendons in arm area 3.

Upper-Area 4: Temporal bone, ear, backside chest, anything along this area as well as the muscles and tendons in arm area 4.

Upper-Area 5: Backside head, backside next, back chest, back heart (left-upper-area 5), upper back, anything along this area as well as the muscles and tendons in arm area 5.

Upper-Area 6: Back head, back neck, cervical spinal column, spinal column of chest, anything along this area as well as the muscles and tendons in the arm area 6.

The Lower Area with Main Organs and Main Tissues
Lower-Area 1: Stomach, bladder, uterus (female), vagina (female), prostate (male), penis (male), anything along this area as well as the muscles and tendons in leg area 1.

Lower-Area 2: Stomach, spleen (Left-Lower-Area 2), liver (Right-Lower-Area 2), gallbladder (Right-Lower-Area 2), large intestine, small intestine, anything along this area as well as the muscles and tendons in the leg area 2.

Lower-Area 3: Spleen (Left-Lower-Area 3), liver (Right-Lower-Area 3), gallbladder (Right-Lower-Area 3), colon ascendens (Right-Lower-Area 3), colon descendens (Left-Lower-Area 3), frontal flank, anything along this area as well as the muscles and tendons in leg area 3.

Lower-Area 4: Spleen (Left-Lower-Area 4), liver (Right-Lower-Area 4), colon ascendens (Right-Lower-Area 4), colon descendens (Left-Lower-Area 4), back flank, anything along this area as well as the muscles and tendons in the leg area 4.

Lower-Area 5: The kidney, lower back, anything along this area as well as the muscles and tendons in leg area 5.

Lower-Area 6: Spine (lumbar), anus, anything along this area as well as the muscles and tendons in the leg area 6.

3 The Points and Applications

The Points
Wrist-ankle acupuncture has just 24 points in total, which are divided into 12 pairs of points. There are 6 pairs on the arm near the wrist (12 in total, 6 on each side left and right) and 6 pairs on the leg near the ankle (12 in total, 6 on each side left and right).

The Arm Points
Simply circle the arm surface, make a circle line through the point P-6 (Nei Guan) and the point SJ5 (Wai Guan). The circle line is divided into six equal parts, and the central point of each part is the acupuncture point. According to the point in which the area of the arm will be named, for example, if the point stays in left arm area 1, the point will be called Left-Upper-Point 1, and the like be called Left-Upper-Point 2, Left-Upper-Point 3, Left-Upper-Point 4, Left-Upper-Point 5, Left-Upper-Point 6.

In addition, symmetry is observed from the left arm to the right arm. It is leaving each other called in order: Right-Upper-Point 1, Right-Upper-Point 2, Right-Upper-Point 3, Right-Upper-Point 4, Right-Upper-Point 5, Right-Upper-Point 6.

All of the points could be called for short-hand: LUP1, LUP2, LUP3, LUP4, LUP5 LUP6 and RUP1, RUP2, RUP3, RUP4, RUP5, RUP6 (see Fig. 6a, b).

The Leg Points
Simply circle the leg surface, make a circle line through point SP-6 (San Yin Jiao) and point GB-39 (Xuan Zhong).

The circle line is divided into six equal parts, and the central point of each part is the acupuncture point. According to the point in which the area of the leg will be named, for example, if the point stays in left leg area 1, the point will be called Left-Lower-Point 1, and the like will be called Left-Lower-Point 2, Left-Lower-Point 3, Left-Lower-Point 4, Left-Lower-Point 5, and Left-Lower-Point 6.

In addition, symmetry is observed from the left leg to the right leg. It is leaving each other called in order Right-Lower-Point 1, Right-Lower-Point 2, Right-Lower-Point 3, Right-Lower-Point 4, Right-Lower-Point 5, and Right-Lower-Point 6.

All of the points could be called for short-hand: LLP1, LLP2, LLP3, LLP4, LLP5, LLP6 and RLP1, RLP2, RLP3, RLP4, RLP5, RLP6 (see Fig. 6a, b).

Using the Points for Symptom and Disease Care
Wrist-ankle acupuncture can be used to treat many problems, any problems associated with the corresponding organ or tissues, and any problems associated with the area.

'The problem' is nothing more than reference. Actually, 'the problem' has many symptoms; for example, eye problems could be eye try, eye itching, eye dropping, eye pain and so on.

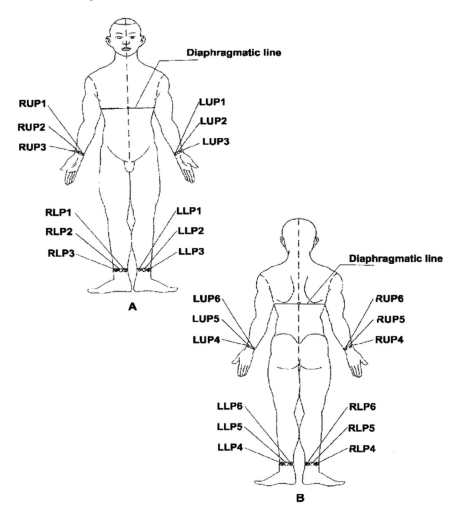

Fig. 6 The arm points and the leg points

Arm Points with Common Problems as Treatment

Upper-Point 1: Forehead problem, eye problem, noise problem, mouth problem, throat problem, tongue problem, front tooth problem, cough, and bronchitis, chest pain, high blood pressure, hives, insomnia and all of the symptoms as reactions in upper area 1. Left-Upper-Point 1 is the same as the right one.

Upper-Point 2: Forehead problem, eye problem, sinus problem, mouth problem (on side), throat problem (throat wall), tongue problem (on side), tooth problem (canine tooth), front neck problem, chest pain, breast problem, heart problem (left-upper-area 2), and all of the symptoms as reactions in upper area 2. Left-Upper-Point 2 is symmetric with the right one.

Upper-Point 3: Frontal angle problem, frontal side head problem, face pain, canthus (outwards) problem, side neck problem, side chest problem, and all of the symptoms as reactions in upper area 3. Left-Upper-Point 3 is symmetric with the right one.

Upper-Point 4: Side head problem, ear problem (front), side neck problem, side chest problem, and all of the symptoms as reactions in upper area 4, and so on. Left-Upper-Point 4 is symmetric with the right one.

Upper-Point 5: Backside head problem, ear problem (back side), side neck problem, back side chest problem, heart problem (left-upper-area 5), and all of the symptoms as reactions in upper area 5. Left-Upper-Point 5 is symmetric with the right one.

Upper-Point 6: Back head problem, back neck problem, up central back problem, and all of the symptoms as reactions in upper area 6, and so on. Left-Upper-Point 6 is the same as the right point.

Leg Points with Common Problems as Treatment
Lower-Point 1: Stomach problem, navel or around it pain, bladder problem, uterus problem, vaginal problem, prostate problem, genitalia problem and all of the symptoms as reactions in lower area 1, and so on. Left-Lower-Point 1 is the same as the right one.

Lower-Point 2: Stomach problem, liver problem (right-lower-area 2), gallbladder problem (right-lower-area 2), spleen problem (left-lower-area 2), annexed uterus problem, intestine problem, genitalia problem and all of the symptoms as reactions in lower area 2. Left-Lower-Point 2 is symmetrical with the right one.

Lower-Point 3: Frontwards side belly problem and all of the symptoms as reactions in lower area 3, and so on. Left-Lower-Point 3 is symmetrical with the right one.

Lower-Point 4: Backwards side belly problem and all of the symptoms as reactions in lower area 4, and so on. Left-Lower-Point 4 is symmetric with the right one.

Lower-Point 5: Kidney problem, lower-back problem and all of the symptoms as reactions in lower area 5, and so on. Left-Lower-Point 5 is symmetrical with the right one.

Lower-Point 6: Central lower-back problem and all of the symptoms as reactions in lower area 6, and so on. Left-Lower-Point 6 is the same as the right point.

According to the Area of the Corresponding Point Prescription Guidance
For successful application of wrist-ankle acupuncture, two considerations are important to include:

1. Choose according to the anatomical area that the symptom is presenting and reacting on the surface of the body:
   - Be guided by the main symptom and to which area it is associated and then choose the right point for that area.

- Normally, the area would correspond with the point, e.g., cervical spine pain towards the left of the spine would correspond with upper-left-area 6, the point is LUP6. And so on.

2. Choose according to the anatomical site of area of the root of the symptom:
   - If we know in clinical practice what is the reason or root cause of the problem, e.g., a neck problem is causing the forehead pain, we would be best to choose the point for the forehead and another point for the neck.

Basic Principles

- For issues in the upper area, choose the upper point. For issues in the lower area, choose the lower point.
- If the main symptom is in the left area, choose the left side point, in contrast, choose the right side point prescription.
- If the symptom cannot be confirmed as left or right or upper or lower, it is sometimes hard to define the cause as being rooted in any area. In this case, for the blood pressure problem, insomnia, hives, and so on, choose LUP1 and RUP1.

Extraordinary Principles Can Be Followed in Some Circumstances

- The upper points can work with the lower points together, and vice versa. For example, if the symptom is around the diaphragmatic line, either up or lower. it would be best to use upper and lower points together.
- The left points can work with the right points together, which are especially useful if the problem is around the anterior or posterior median line. A better result may be achieved if using both the left and right corresponding points together.
- The front points can work together with the back points. A better result may, for example, for belly pain using LLP2 and RLP2 plus LLP5 and RLP5. Usually, area 1 corresponds to area 6, area 2 corresponds to area 5, and area 3 corresponds to area 4; vice versa, if we need to add on, can according to this do it.
- Three adjacent points can work well together when the pain or problem area is extensive. You can choose a point for the main symptom and then a point neighbouring both side points for a more powerful result.

Using the Point Guide for Common Symptoms

Symptom	Main Points	Adjunct Points
1. Forehead Pain	RUP 1 and LUP 1, RUP 2 and LUP 2	If it is caused from the neck, add on RUP 6 and LUP 6, even add on RUP 5 and LUP 5
2. Stiff or painful neck	RUP 6 and LUP 6, RUP 5 and LUP 5	
3. Blocked, runny or bleeding nose	RUP 1 and LUP 1	
4. Red eye, myopic eye, presbyopia, dry or itching or painful eyes	RUP 2 and LUP 2	RUP 1 and LUP 1, RUP 3 and LUP 3
5. Ptosis, droopy eye	RUP2 and LUP2	If the drooping is from inner-canthus, add on RUP 1 and LUP 1. If the drooping is from external-canthus, add on RUP 3 and LUP 3
6. Toothache	RUP 2 and LUP 2	If it is incisor pain, add on RUP 1 and LUP 1. If it is molar pain, add on RUP 3 and LUP 3
7. Cough	RUP 1 and LUP 1	If the lung has a problem, add on RUP 2 and LUP 2, even add on RUP 5 and LUP 5. If the bottom of the lung has a problem, add on LLP 2 and RLP 2, LLP 1 and RLP 1, LLP 3 and RLP 3
8. Stomach-ache	LLP 1 and RLP 1, and LLP 2 and RLP 2	If the top of the stomach has the problem, add RUP 1 and LUP 1 and RUP 2 and LRP 2, sometimes add RLP 5 and LLP 5
9. Whole abdomen pain	LLP 2 and RLP 2, LLP 1 and RLP 1	RLP 3 and LLP 3 sometimes need to be added to RLP 5 and LLP 5, RLP 6 and LLP 6
10. Dysmenorrhea	LLP 1 and RLP 1, LLP 2 and RLP 2	RLP 6 and LLP 6, RLP 5 and LLP 5
11. Abnormal leukorrhea	LLP 1 and RLP 1	RLP 6 and LLP 6, RLP 5 and LLP 5
12. Urinary infection	LLP 1 and RLP 1	LLP 2 and RLP 2, even add on RLP 6 and LLP 6
13. Hay-fever	RUP 1 and LUP 1	RUP 2 and LUP 2
14. Hypertension or hypotension	RUP 1 and LUP 1	
15. Hives	RUP 1 and LUP 1	

(continued)

(continued)

Symptom	Main Points	Adjunct Points
16. Insomnia	RUP 1 and LUP 1	
17. Emotional Issues	RUP 1 and LUP 1	
18. Lumbago	RLP 6 and LLP 6	RLP 5 and LLP 5
19. Lumbar muscular degeneration	RLP 5 and LLP 5	RLP 6 and LLP 6, or RLP 4 and LLP 4
20. Myofascial pain syndrome (MPS)	RLP 5 and LLP 5	RLP 4 and LLP 4, or RLP 6 and LLP 6. If the pain area is on the upper back. add RUP 5 and LUP 5, RUP 4 and LUP 4, RUP 6 and LUP 6

4 WAA Needling Technique

Basic Needling Technique

If you are already a proficient acupuncturist, this will be simple for you. You can use your normal needle insertion technique. It is suggested that you use the needle tube technique for ease.

- The needle tip with the tube slightly touches the patient's skin, one hand holds the tube at an angle of 15°–30° and then uses the index or other finger of another hand to click the bottom of the needle quickly to ensure that the needle tip passes through the initial layer of the skin quickly to the subcutaneous fat level.
- Then, lay down the body of the needle parallel to the skin surface and push the needle slowly to enter the subcutaneous level further until just 3–5 mm left of the body of the needle.
- The needle gauge and length are usually 0.25–0.35* with a length of 25–40 mm.
- The needle tip is applied to the point towards the main symptom you are treating.

Needling Aspects to Pay Attention to

In wrist-ankle acupuncture, to achieve a better result, along with the basic techniques above, it is important to pay attention to further needling parameters:

The Right Depth: In clinical practice, it is important that the needle is not too shallow where the patient will feel discomfort or even pain, and it should also not be too deep where the patient will feel similar needling sensations as per traditional acupuncture. When the patient takes wrist-ankle acupuncture for treatment, it should not feel any sensation or discomfort.

One appearance could help us to ensure the right depth. When you push the needle enter, if you could see a stealth line in the skin surface when the pinpoint is moving on, it will be the right depth.

The Right Direction: To support the efficacy of wrist-ankle acupuncture, it is important to point the needle tip direction towards the main symptom. For example, if the main symptom is on the head or hands or feet, the needle tip must point towards the head or hand or feet.

The Adjusting: If you have applied all the guidance and the patient is still not feeling a positive effect of the treatment. Now, we must perform the adjustment. The needle is withdrawn until the needle tip was still inserted approximately 3–5 mm. and adjust the needle direction in another angle and then again push in the needle to the side of the original direction, either left or right a small way.

Try this until the main symptom has been feeling better, even subsided a little.

Course of Treatment

The course of treatment is same as the traditional acupuncture, refer to it should be fine.

Other Needle Technique

Wrist-ankle acupuncture is same as traditional acupuncture. Like electric connect, and so on. Refer to it you will be understand.

Abnormality Precaution

In clinical practice, wrist-ankle acupuncture is similar to traditional acupuncture and could have some abnormalities, such as the following: fainting spell during acupuncture. Bend the needle. Broke the needle. Stagnating the needle. Local pain (or local discomfort). Local hematoma or local bleeding. For all of this, refer to traditional acupuncture should be fine.

5 Modern Study Summary

From 1976 to now, many doctors have practiced and studied the use of wrist-ankle acupuncture. They have proven that wrist-ankle acupuncture can be used for any problem or symptom by living example, such as headache, vertigo, neck problem, occipital neuralgia, insomnia, hives, herpes, hypotension, hypertension, addiction to smoke or drugs, emotional problems, Tourette syndrome, posttraumatic stress disorder, vegetative system dysfunction, myopia, hyperopia, cough, frozen shoulder, arthritis, gout, tennis elbow, MPS, soft tissue disorder, facial paralysis, acne, facial spasm, ear rings, toothache, chest pain, functional premature ventricular contractions, acute mastitis, hypochondriac pain, hiccup, stomach pain, belly pain, IBS, bed-wetting, dysmenorrhea, premenopausal syndrome and postmenopausal syndrome, FUTS, renal colic, ankylosing spondylitis, lumbar disc herniation, piriformis syndrome, Bernhardt-Roth Syndrome, peripheral polyneuritis, chronic fatigue syndrome, and so on [1–4].

Some doctors have used wrist-ankle acupuncture combined with herbal medicine or western medicine to treat the pain after operation or the pain brought about by cancer, not only enhancing the clinical effect but also reducing some western medicine leading to side effects [5, 6].

Some doctors have been trying to determine what, how or where the working material basis of wrist-ankle acupuncture is. Some researchers found that the local electrolyte near the wrist-ankle acupuncture point changed slightly before the needle was inserted and after the needle was inserted [7]. One study found that wrist-ankle acupuncture could affect some local areas of the network of the brain as the brain is in a resting state [8].

Author Comments

Wrist-ankle acupuncture works immediately. You must use the basic technique, needle in the right direction and at the correct depth. "**if the patient feels the needle sensation as per traditional acupuncture or any discomfort around the needle, could be too shallow or too deep**". Either too shallow or too deep, it is not **right**.

Follow the above guidelines, practice repeatedly to make yourself an experienced wrist-ankle acupuncture practitioner.

As you get more experienced you should be able to get good effects straight away, especially for the problems where the main symptom is pain.

Note: Individual Cun (拇指同身寸-Mu Zhi Tong Shen Cun): The width of the thumb knuckle is one individual cun.

Comprehension/Review Questions

1. How long has the history of wrist-ankle acupuncture been?
2. How many area of the body surface dose the Wrist-Ankle Acupuncture has by longitudinal direction?
3. How many parts of the body surface dose the wrist-ankle acupuncture has by transverse?
4. How many points dose the Wrist-Ankle Acupuncture has?
5. How many things do you do to choose the point?
6. Is the wrist-ankle acupuncture technique same as traditional acupuncture?
7. What is the right depth of the needle in wrist-ankle acupuncture?
8. What is the right direction of the needle in wrist-ankle acupuncture?

References

1. Sun Y, Gao BX. Chinese wrist-ankle acupuncture therapy. Press of Shanghai University of Traditional Chinese Medicine 1999:1–8.
2. Sun G, Zhou ZHL, Zhao L. Clinic curative effect analysis for wrist-ankle acupuncture to treat the disease with the pain. Hebei Tradit Chin Med. 2011;33(11):1715–9.
3. Zeng K, Zhou QH. Evolving of the clinic applying and studying for wrist-ankle acupuncture to treat the disease with the pain. J. Clin. Acupunct. Moxibustion 2012;28(09):69–72.

4. Lu FF, Qian XL. Evolving of the studying for wrist-ankle acupuncture to treat the disease without the pain. J Liaoning Univ Tradit Chin Med. 2018;20(01):117–9.
5. Chen XY. Evolving of the clinic applying and studying for wrist-ankle acupuncture to relieve the patient's pain leaded by operation after. Gen Care. 2020;18(27):3615–8.
6. Yu YM, Liu Y, Xie J, et al. Evolving of the clinic applying for wrist-ankle acupuncture to treat the cancerous pain. Chin. Med. Combine W. Med. Care 2019;5(10):77-81
7. Chen MH, Yu SX, Xie YY, et al. Studying the transformation of the electrolyte by wrist-ankle acupuncture was inserted and after. Med Diagn. 2022;12(01):38–42.
8. Qi C, Xiang AF, Chen MY. A study of multi-frequency band and resting-state FMRI for analgesia effect of wrist-ankle acupuncture. In: The symposium of annual conference of China Association of Acupuncture-Moxibustion 2022:6.

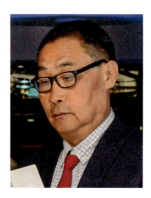

Yu Sun (孙瑜) born 1963 in Shaanxi, China. Studied Chinese Medicine at Shaanxi University of Traditional Chinese Medicine, graduating in 1988. He is a distinguished expert in Chinese Medicine and Acupuncture.

He has been deeply immersed in the study of wrist-ankle acupuncture since 1985 and has continually practiced it ever since. has made significant contributions to this field, notably authoring the seminal book 'Chinese Wrist-Ankle Acupuncture Therapy' and twelve other publications. He has also disseminated his extensive knowledge through thirteen theses and an instructional video on the subject. A notable milestone in his career was receiving personal tutelage from Professor Xinshu Zhang (张心曙) in 1997.

He spent fourteen years taught acupuncture at Ningxia Medical University in China and was an associate professor in 1999.

His ongoing dedication to studying and practicing Chinese Medicine and Acupuncture has established him as a respected figure.

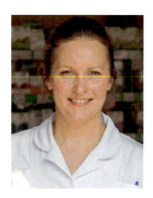

Katherine Dandridge BSc TCM, BMed (Beijing), Dip CHM (Obs/Gyn) runs a busy general acupuncture and Chinese herbal medicine practice in Perthshire, Scotland. She began her complementary medicine career in Hong Kong in 1999 training in holistic aromatherapy and allied therapies, then went on to study the five year TCM degree at Middlesex University twinned with the Beijing University of Chinese Medicine. She has over the last 20 years developed her practice including obstetric, fertility, health coaching and gynaecological studies, five palms qi gong, scalp acupuncture and cosmetic acupuncture and functional medicine training; getting good, consistent results for the community that she serves. She is a member of the UK practitioner groups; British Acupuncture Council, Register of Chinese Herbal Medicine, Institute of Scalp Acupuncture UK, British Acupuncture Federation, Royal Society of Medicine Associate Member and The International Federation of Professional Aromatherapists.

Acupuncture Techniques with Special Needles

Yuan Li Needling

Songyan Chen

Learning Objectives

- To impart basic knowledge about the history and development of Yuan Li needling therapy.
- To enhance students' ability to accurately identify pathological knots and acupoints along the sinew meridian.
- To equip students with Yuan Li needling manipulation techniques, including Guan needling, Hui needling, Hegu needling, and Turtle probing needling.
- To help students understand the primary clinical indications for Yuan Li needling therapy.

1 Introduction

1.1 History of Yuan Li Needling Therapy

Ancient Yuan Li needling is the sixth of the ancient "Nine Needles". It is documented in "The Yellow Emperor's Classic of Internal Medicine", written over 2000 years ago. According to the "Spiritual Axis. Nine Needles Theory", the Yuan Li needle has a short, slender body and a large tail with a rounded tip that comes to a sharp point. It was traditionally used to treat carbuncle disease and Bi syndrome. The design of the Yuan Li needle is derived from another ancient needle, the Mao needle, which resembles the tail of a horse (see Fig. 15.1). The needle is slightly larger at the end and smaller at the body, allowing for deep penetration [1]. Although it was historically used for the treatment of carbuncle disease, this application is no longer prevalent today.

S. Chen (✉)
London Academy of Chinese Acupuncture, London, UK
e-mail: 514438926@qq.com

Fig. 15.1 Ancient Yuan Li needle illustration

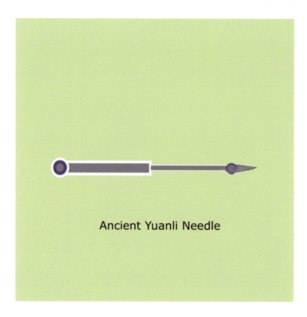

The ancient Yuan Li needling technique had several shortcomings: its large tip made insertion and operation difficult, and patients often experienced severe pain during the procedure. As a result, ancient acupuncturists rarely used this technique.

1.2 Modernisation of Yuan Li Needling

Since the 1970s, some Chinese acupuncturists have made improvements to the ancient Yuan Li needling method. Compared to the ancient version, the tip of the modern Yuan Li needle is specially and repeatedly polished, making it more acceptable to patients. Furthermore, the modern needle retains the advantages of its ancient counterpart, specifically its thick and sturdy body.

From a visual standpoint, the modern Yuan Li needle looks similar to the filiform needle, except that its body is thicker. This raises the question: if the appearance is so similar, why are there two different names? To answer this question, one must first understand the Traditional Chinese Medicine theory underlying Yuan Li needling.

1.3 Traditional Chinese Medicine Treatment Mechanism of Yuan Li Needling

Yuan Li needling is commonly employed to treat Bi syndrome, which falls under the category of meridian sinew diseases in Traditional Chinese Medicine (TCM).

Meridian sinews primarily refer to the muscles, sinews, and ligaments located along the pathways of the primary meridians and their associated connecting vessels. These pathways typically start at the extremities and separate from the primary meridians at the fingertips and toes. They then extend toward the trunk or even further, reaching the head and face [1].

The ancients likened the operation of meridians to rivers—starting small and becoming mighty, moving from shallow to deep. If the regular meridians are considered rivers, then the meridian sinews can be thought of as riverbeds. These sinews rely on the nourishment and regulation provided by the twelve regular meridians. The circulation routes of the meridian sinews are described in detail in the "Spiritual Axis. Meridian Sinews".

To illustrate, let's compare the circulation routes of the Hand Taiyin Lung Meridian and the Hand Taiyin Meridian Sinew. The "Spiritual Axis. Meridian" describes the Hand Taiyin Lung Meridian as follows: "The meridian starts at the stomach of the middle burner and connects with the large intestine. It moves back along the upper entrance of the stomach, passes through the diaphragm, and links to the lung and lung system. It then runs horizontally from the upper part of the chest wall toward the armpit, continuing along the outer side of the upper arm's front. It moves down to the middle of the elbow, proceeding along the radial side of the forearm to Cunkou, and exits at the radial end of the thumb, following the outer edge of the greater thenar." (see Fig. 15.2) [1].

For the Hand Taiyin Meridian Sinew, the "Spiritual Axis. Meridian Sinews" states: "The sinew starts above the big finger, travels up along the big finger, and gathers behind the thenar. From the outside of the Cunkou pulse, it ascends along the forearm and converges in the middle of the elbow. It then passes up through the inner side of the arm, enters the armpit, exits at ST-12 Quepen, and gathers in front of the acromion. It moves inward and downward, knots in the chest, scatters through the diaphragm, converges under the diaphragm, and reaches the hypochondriac region." (see Fig. 15.3) [1].

Comparing the Hand Taiyin Lung Meridian with the Hand Taiyin Meridian Sinew reveals that their circulating distributions are largely similar. However, the circulation of the meridian sinews is not strictly confined to that of the main meridians, their scope of circulation can also vary to some extent.

As shown in Figs. 15.2 and 15.3, the main meridian line is narrower than the meridian sinew. The depth of the primary meridians usually does not exceed 2 cm, while the meridian sinews cover a much larger area. They often form a band and create spindle-shaped bindings (Jie) at the joints and other areas of the body. According to the original text of "The Yellow Emperor's Classic of Internal Medicine", the twelve meridian sinews should be considered independent of the twelve main meridians. However, this point is rarely emphasized in current acupuncture and moxibustion textbooks.

Regarding the treatment principles of meridian sinew diseases, "Spiritual Axis. Cijiezhenxie" states: "When acupuncturists use needles, they must first determine whether the meridians are in a state of deficiency or excess. If the upper part of a meridian is overflowing with Qi and Blood while the lower part is deficient, this

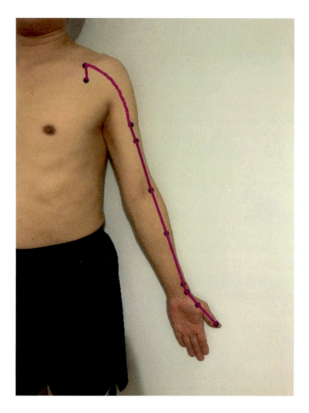

Fig. 15.2 The Lung Meridian of Hand Taiyin

indicates that transverse collaterals (pathological nodes) are compressing the main meridian, causing blockage. In such cases, the reducing method, or 'Untie Knots Therapy' should be employed." The term "transverse collaterals" refers to pathological knots formed by repeated damage to the meridian sinews. These knots block the meridians, hindering the normal circulation of Qi and Blood. This leads to an excess above the point of compression and a deficiency below it. This concept aligns with what is stated in "Spiritual Axis. Meridians": "Meridians determine life and death, treat most types of diseases, regulate deficiency and excess, and must not be blocked" [1]. Transverse collaterals can manifest as bands, masses, or cord-like tissue on the meridian sinews, blocking the flow and causing obstruction. From the perspective of modern anatomy, these obstructions can be located in muscles, fasciae, tendons, sheaths, bursae, and ligaments.

As illustrated in Fig. 15.4, if the twelve main meridians are likened to rivers and the twelve meridian sinews to riverbeds, then the transverse collaterals can be thought of as silt in the riverbeds, obstructing the flow. The most common cause of meridian sinew diseases is that these pathological knots (transverse collaterals) block the main meridians. The treatment process is akin to clearing silt from a blocked river. First, remove the silt (pathological knots), then increase water flow (activate Qi and Blood), and the problem will be resolved. The same principle applies to treating diseases:

Fig. 15.3 The Hand Taiyin Meridian Sinew

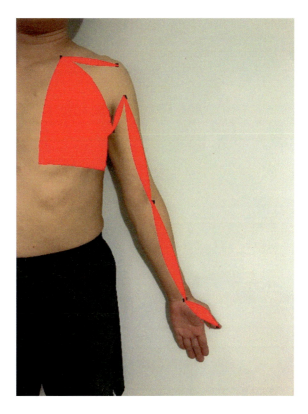

first untie the pathological knots (transverse collaterals), then regulate the meridians and activate Qi and Blood to ultimately achieve the treatment's purpose.

The "Untie Knots Therapy" serves to dredge meridians, strengthen the body's resistance to eliminate pathogenic factors, and regulate yin and yang. This therapy functions both as a guiding ideology and as a method of diagnosis and treatment in acupuncture clinics. Practitioners who understand "Untie Knots Therapy" can better guide and improve clinical outcomes. Generally speaking, if there are no transverse collaterals pressing on the meridians, patients are unlikely to fall ill. Even if they do, the condition is typically mild and can be remedied through self-healing or minor medical intervention. Conversely, if transverse collaterals block the meridians, the resulting disease can be difficult to treat. Treatment involves locating the transverse collaterals and then dredging these blockages while activating Qi and Blood flow, leading to a cure. "Untie Knots Therapy" was also an important therapeutic principle in ancient times, well understood and commonly practiced by ancient acupuncturists. Therefore, it should be the first consideration in treatment planning.

Filiform needle therapy is primarily used for treating diseases related to the twelve main meridians, while meridian sinew therapy is applied for diseases of the twelve meridian sinews. Yuan Li needling therapy is a subset of meridian sinew therapy and serves as an important representative of "Untie Knots Therapy".

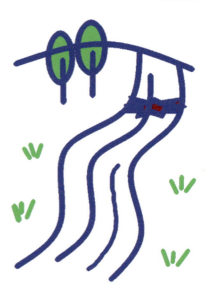

Fig. 15.4 The diagram figuratively shows the relationship among main meridians, meridian sinew, and transverse collaterals

2 Yuan Li Needling Manipulation Techniques

2.1 Preparation Before Treatment

Before delving into the manipulation techniques, it is essential to understand the preparatory steps involved in the therapy.

2.2 Selection of Needles

The choice of needles plays a crucial role in the success of Yuan Li needling therapy. Several factors influence the selection of the appropriate needle, including the patient's sex, age, physique, medical condition, and the location of the ailment. Commonly used needle specifications include 0.5 × 75 mm, 0.5 × 60 mm, 0.5 × 50 mm, and 0.4 × 50 mm, among others. Acupuncturists carefully consider these factors to ensure the chosen needle is suitable for the specific treatment [2].

2.3 Selection of Patient's Body Position

The patient's body position during treatment is another critical consideration. Different body positions are suitable for specific ailments and acupoints. Common positions include the supine position, lateral position, prone position, and sitting position. The choice of position is tailored to the patient's comfort and the nature of the condition being treated.

2.4 Hand Disinfection for the Acupuncturist

Hygiene is paramount in acupuncture practice. Acupuncturists thoroughly disinfect their hands with sanitizers before commencing treatment. This precaution helps prevent the introduction of infection or contaminants during needle insertion.

2.5 Principles of Acupoints Selection

The selection of appropriate acupoints is a fundamental aspect of successful acupuncture therapy. During the needle operation, acupuncturists use both hands in tandem—one for diagnosis and the other for manipulation. The diagnostic hand tightens the pathological tissue, guiding the needle through it until resistance ceases, signaling that the needle has navigated through the pathological knots [3].

The technique primarily employs palpation, utilizing the sense of touch to identify pathological tissues along the twelve meridian sinews. Yuan Li needling therapy follows specific principles for acupoint selection, which are essential to its effectiveness. These principles include:

Select Pain points as Acupoints: This principle, recorded in "Spiritual Axis. Meridian Sinews". Shangshan Yang elaborated on it in his book, "The Yellow Emperor's Classic of Internal Medicine. Taisu". He suggests that acupuncturists should identify acupoints based on the presence of pain. According to the theory, the meridians are nourished by the flow of Yin and Yang Qi, which circulates continuously along the meridian pathways. When a pathogenic influence enters the striae (meridian sinews) and disrupts the flow of Yin and Yang Qi, the affected acupoint becomes immobile, causing pain. Thus, pain points are considered acupoints in Yuan Li needling therapy [1].

Select Pathological Knots Along the Meridian Sinews as Acupoints: Pathological knots often form along meridian sinews due to repeated soft tissue strain. These knots can manifest as subcutaneous knots or cord-like structures. Granular nodules are typically found at the beginning and end of tendons, tendon sheaths, and around joints. They vary in shape and size, are firm to the touch, and can be tender. Cord-like knots, on the other hand, are commonly observed within muscles, such as those in the neck, shoulder, waist, hip, and leg. They feel hard to the touch and may elicit pain when pressed, resembling the texture of a rope when palpated. In treating conditions associated with these knots, "Spiritual Axis. Cijiezhenxie" introduces the "Untie knots therapy", considering the knots as acupoints [1].

Principle of Meridian Acupoint Selection: In Yuan Li needling therapy, acupoints with the same name as the meridian sinew are often chosen. Meridian sinews are distributed alongside their corresponding primary meridians, relying on the Qi and Blood from these meridians for nourishment. Targeting these acupoints helps clear meridians and guide the Qi of the meridian sinews.

Treatment Example: Piriformis Syndrome: Piriformis syndrome is a common condition where the piriformis muscle, after injury, forms a hematoma and eventually develops pathological scar tissue. This compresses the sciatic nerve, causing pain. Yuan Li needling directly targets the affected muscle, reopening the scar tissue, softening the muscle, and alleviating pain. Anatomically, the piriformis muscle and the sciatic nerve are closely related; in some cases, the sciatic nerve even passes directly through the piriformis muscle. Therefore, it's crucial to restore the rigidity of the affected muscle to a soft and normal state. The treatment method offers immediate effects, supported by convincing therapeutic mechanisms.

3 Yuan Li Needling Method Techniques

Guan Needling Method

The Guan needling method originates from "Spirit Pivot". In this context, the Guan Needle is described as follows: "Puncture the ends of tendons on both the body's left and right sides to treat muscle Bi syndrome; be careful not to cause bleeding" [1]. The treatment points, or pathological knots, are generally located near the tendons around the joints of the extremities. Due to the deep penetration directly around the tendon, caution is advised to avoid bleeding during acupuncture.

Hui Needling Method

The Hui needling method also comes from "Spirit Pivot", where it's noted: "For Hui needling, place the needle directly beside the tight tendons and muscles, lift and insert the needle forwards and backwards, thus relaxing the tight tendons and muscles to cure the Bi syndrome" [1]. This technique treats conditions like muscle contractures, acute arthralgia, and pain. The method involves stabbing the needle directly beside the tendons and muscles, then lifting and inserting it to alleviate tension. This approach is multifaceted and resembles the modern multidirectional penetration method.

Hegu Needling Method

The Hegu needling method is detailed in "Spirit Pivot. Guan Needle" as follows: "Obliquely insert the needle into the lesion, retract it to a subcutaneous level, then insert it left and right, resembling a chicken claw, towards the skin and muscles. This method is mainly used to treat muscular Bi syndrome" [1] (see Fig. 15.5)

Turtle Probing Cave Needling Method

Originating from Xu Feng's book "Jinzhenfu" from the Ming Dynasty, the turtle probing cave needling method instructs: "Insert the needle into tightened muscle

Fig. 15.5 Hegu needling manipulation

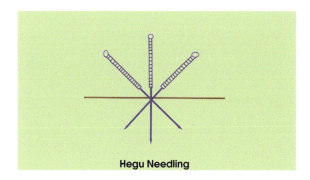

areas, then retract it to the subcutaneous layer. Change direction for multidirectional penetration: up, down, left, and right, similar to how a tortoise seeks a hole".

4 Matters Needing Attention

Personal Notice

- Needling should not be performed immediately if patients are overly hungry, tired, or nervous. For those with a frail constitution or deficiencies in qi and blood, lighter manipulation should be employed, preferably while the patient is in a recumbent position.
- Women within their first three months of pregnancy should avoid needling. Beyond that period, abdominal and lumbosacral acupoints are contraindicated. Specific points like SP-6 Sanyinjiao, LI-4 Hegu, BL-60 Kunlun, and BL-66 Zhiyin, which activate meridians and blood circulation, are also contraindicated.
- Needling should be avoided on the top of the head for children whose fontanels have not yet closed, as well as in patients with spontaneous or continuous bleeding, and those with skin infections, ulcers, scars, or tumours.

Area Notice

- Special care must be taken when needling areas such as GV-16 Fengfu and GV-15 Yamen, particularly in the eye and neck regions, as well as spinal acupoints. The angle and depth of the needle should be carefully controlled to prevent damage to vital tissues and organs.
- This is especially true for patients with urinary retention when needling lower abdominal acupoints to avoid injuring the bladder and other organs.

- Comprehensive knowledge of human anatomy is crucial for acupuncturists. When treating areas like the chest, back, waist, and abdomen—where the five viscera reside—the depth of needle insertion must be strictly regulated. Extra attention should be given to patients with conditions like hepatosplenomegaly and emphysema to prevent medical mishaps, such as liver or spleen puncture and pneumothorax.

Needling Notice

- If a patient experiences severe pain and distension during needle insertion, it's likely that the periosteum has been punctured. In such cases, the needle should be lifted or retracted by 1–2 mm. Some pain or subcutaneous ecchymosis may occur one- or two-days post-treatment, though this is rare. Such bruising will generally fade within a few days, but patients should be advised beforehand.

In summary, acupuncturists must remain highly focused during needling, ensure patients are in appropriate positions, and strictly control the needle's depth and angle to prevent accidents. Moreover, it's important to avoid inserting the entire needle body into the acupoints during treatment.

5 Subcutaneous Acupuncture Technique

The Yuan Li needle insertion technique is straightforward. The needle is slowly inserted through the skin, but there is less emphasis on lifting, inserting, twisting, and rotating the needle. Only the needle's tip is required to pass through pathological knots. Unlike traditional filiform needles, this method does not aim to promote Qi during treatment. Yuan Li needling typically involves selecting only a few specific acupoints, making the technique more precise.

Do not Require "Deqi": Traditional acupuncture considers the appearance of a needling reaction (Deqi) crucial for clinical effectiveness. Various techniques are used to promote and maintain Deqi during treatment. However, Yuan Li needling does not emphasize the importance of Deqi, indicating that its presence or absence has no impact on therapeutic outcomes. This approach eliminates the need for manual needle manipulation, reducing pain and increasing patient comfort [3].

Needle Retention: The standard for needle retention in Yuan Li needling varies. If the patient feels no needle sensation, the needle can be immediately removed upon insertion. If there is a sensation, the needle is generally left in place for a few minutes until the sensation disappears [3]. By contrast, traditional acupuncture requires the needle to be retained for over 30 min or even longer to achieve Deqi.

6 Needle Insertion Methods

Yuan Li needles can be inserted using either cannula or non-cannula methods. The non-cannula method includes both single-hand and two-hand needle insertions:

Single-Handed Needling

Mostly used for short-needle operations.

Two-Handed Needling

Includes aiding with finger pressure, gripping needle, stretching needle, and pinching needle techniques.

Aiding with finger pressure: The thumb or index finger presses beside the acupoint while the other hand inserts the needle.

Gripping needle: Ideal for long needles, this involves holding a sterilized, dry cotton ball and inserting the needle while twisting the handle.

Stretching and pinching: Both methods involve stretching the skin with the fingers during needle insertion.

Currently, the cannula method is widely used internationally. In this approach, a Yuan Li needle with a tube is employed. The needle is removed from its packaging, and the tube is positioned on the skin over the selected acupoint. The needle is then quickly tapped into the subcutaneous tissue before removing the tube.

7 Indications

7.1 The Primary Indications

The primary application of Yuan Li needling therapy is to address pain syndrome. It is prevalent in clinical practice, can be categorized into early, middle, and late stages. In the early stage, the short duration of the illness results in milder pain without noticeable pathological knots upon physical examination. Traditional treatments like filiform needling therapy, massage, cupping, and oral Chinese herbs usually yield positive outcomes.

However, the middle and late stages, characterized by prolonged illness and recurring episodes, can lead to the formation of rigid pathological knots. Due to these knots, treatments often become challenging. For instance, massage therapy struggles to alleviate hardened knots, especially when they're situated in deeper tissue layers. Similarly, the slim nature of the filiform needle makes it difficult to untangle these knots.

Concerning the middle and late stages of pain syndrome, questions arise. Why are the outcomes of traditional filiform needle therapy and massage so inconsistent? Why is pain relief fleeting and prone to recurrence? Why do patients consistently experience residual pain? These challenges were pondered upon by ancient Chinese acupuncturists.

Lingtai Xu, a renowned Chinese medicine expert from the Qing Dynasty, elaborated in his book, "On Acupuncture Not Inherited to the Next Generation." He noted, "Historically, there were 9 types of needles and 21 acupuncture techniques. The needle type and method must be tailored to the disease and not chosen indiscriminately. A wrong selection means the ailment remains untreated. Contemporary acupuncturists predominantly employ the filiform needle and the direct needling technique. With such limited tools, how can they effectively treat challenging diseases?" Xu's insights not only highlighted the pitfalls of his contemporaries but remain relevant for today's practitioners.

Drawing from "The Medical Classic of the Yellow Emperor," the text emphasizes the importance of selecting the appropriate needle from the nine available types. Using a large needle for a minor ailment could harm the vital energy, while a small needle for a grave illness might not dispel the pathogenic Qi. If the disease is superficial, deep acupuncture can damage healthy muscles, and vice versa, failing to disperse the pathogenic Qi [1].

The discourse underscores that ancient acupuncturist believed in tailoring needling techniques to the specific depth of the pathological factors. Precise diagnosis and treatment of the lesion's location are crucial. The pathological acupoints, often multi-layered and three-dimensional in the late stage of pain syndrome, are essential for effective treatment.

In conclusion, Yuan Li needling stands out as a potent technique for addressing the challenges of middle and late-stage pain syndrome.

7.2 More Clinical Indications

The twelve meridians and tendons form the extensive tissue foundation of the human body. While they don't directly connect to the viscera, pathological changes in these tissues inevitably affect both the meridians and the internal organs, manifesting in various diseases. Yuan Li needling therapy is particularly effective in treating tendon-related ailments, visceral disorders, and other complex conditions by untying sinew knots. Let's delve into the specific indications and applications of Yuan Li needling therapy.

Cervical spondylosis and neck pain: Cervical spondylosis, stiff neck, and other cervical spine-related conditions can benefit from Yuan Li needling. By targeting specific acupoints along the affected meridian sinews, this therapy can relieve pain and improve neck mobility.

Shoulder and elbow joint disorders: Conditions such as periarthritis, tennis elbow, and golf elbow often involve musculoskeletal issues in the shoulder and elbow joints. Yuan Li needling can alleviate pain, reduce inflammation, and enhance joint function.

Thoracic spine disorders: Disorders of small joints and hyperostosis in the thoracic spine can cause significant discomfort. Yuan Li needling therapy can address these issues by targeting the meridian sinews in the thoracic region.

Lumbar and leg disorders: Yuan Li needling is effective for conditions like lumbar intervertebral protrusion, lumbar hyperostosis, lumbar spinal stenosis, and other lumbar and leg-related issues. It can improve mobility, reduce pain, and enhance overall function.

Knee disorders: Conditions such as knee osteoarthritis and rheumatoid arthritis can lead to knee pain and reduced joint mobility. Yuan Li needling therapy can target acupoints associated with knee function, providing relief and improving joint health.

Nervous system disorders: Neurological conditions like headache, migraine, facial paralysis, trigeminal neuralgia, intercostal neuralgia, sciatica, stroke sequelae, and peripheral neuritis can benefit from Yuan Li needling therapy.

Cardiovascular disorders: Conditions such as cervical hypertension and cervical heart disease, which have musculoskeletal components, can be managed with Yuan Li needling therapy.

Urinary system disorders: Yuan Li needling therapy can help address urinary incontinence and urinary retention by targeting acupoints related to the urinary system.

Digestive system disorders: Gastrointestinal conditions like acute and chronic gastritis, gastroduodenal ulcers, irritable bowel syndrome, functional dyspepsia, chronic colitis, and constipation can be managed with Yuan Li needling.

Reproductive system disorders: Both male and female infertility, as well as menopausal syndrome, can benefit from Yuan Li needling therapy.

Gynaecological disorders: Gynaecological conditions like breast hyperplasia, pelvic inflammation, irregular menstruation, dysmenorrhea, and pelvic inflammatory disease can be addressed using this technique.

Endocrine system disorders: Yuan Li needling can help manage conditions such as diabetes neuropathy and simple obesity related to the endocrine system.

Dermatological disorders: Skin conditions like eczema, skin pruritus, psoriasis, urticaria, and herpes zoster may show improvement with Yuan Li needling therapy.

Disorders of the five senses: Visual and auditory conditions like myopia, tinnitus, deafness, inner ear vertigo, and sinusitis can be managed using this technique.

Respiratory system disorders: Conditions such as chronic cough, bronchial asthma, chronic bronchitis, and allergic rhinitis with musculoskeletal components can benefit from Yuan Li needling therapy.

8 Modern Research

Modern research has shed light on the effectiveness of Yuan Li needling therapy. Studies have explored its mechanisms of action, clinical outcomes, and potential applications in various medical fields. Here are some notable findings:

Pain Management: Yuan Li needling has shown promise in pain management, especially for conditions like myofascial pain syndrome and fibromyalgia. Research suggests that the therapy can help relieve pain by releasing endorphins and modulating pain pathways [2].

Neuromuscular Disorders: Some studies have investigated the use of Yuan Li needling in neuromuscular disorders such as muscular dystrophy and multiple sclerosis. While further research is needed, preliminary results indicate potential benefits in improving muscle function and reducing spasticity.

Sports Medicine: Athletes and sports enthusiasts have increasingly turned to Yuan Li needling for injury prevention and rehabilitation. It is believed to enhance muscle flexibility, reduce the risk of injury, and expedite recovery [2].

Stress Reduction: Yuan Li needling has been linked to reduced stress and anxiety levels. Acupuncture, in general, is thought to influence the autonomic nervous system, promoting relaxation and reducing stress hormones.

Complementary Therapy: Yuan Li needling is often used as a complementary therapy alongside conventional treatments for a wide range of conditions. Its non-invasive nature and minimal side effects make it an attractive option for many patients.

Studies by acupuncturists have provided experimental evidence that Yuan Li needling has a lasting effect on muscle and ligament disorders. Specifically, upon needle insertion into pathological points, disordered muscle cells rearrange and spasms in muscles are immediately alleviated. This suggests that the treatment goes beyond merely providing temporary anaesthetic relief, thereby establishing Yuan Li needling therapy on a foundation of modern science [3].

Some critics argue that acupuncture is mere pseudoscience or a placebo effect. However, scientific research on Yuan Li needling therapy confirms that the technique leads to significant cellular and muscular changes in the targeted areas.

9 Summary

The clinical efficacy of Yuan Li needling hinges on precise point selection. During the needle operation, acupuncturists use both hands in tandem—one for diagnosis and the other for manipulation. The diagnostic hand tightens the pathological tissue, guiding the needle through it until resistance ceases, signalling that the needle has navigated through the pathological knots.

The technique primarily employs palpation, utilizing the sense of touch to identify pathological tissues along the twelve meridian sinews.

Advantages: Yuan Li needling therapy offers several benefits, including fewer required acupoints, rapid effects, and ease of operation. The technique is particularly effective for treating later stages of pain syndrome. The sturdiness of the Yuan Li needle allows it to penetrate intractable knots, a task difficult for filiform needles to accomplish.

Pain Management: Despite having a diameter greater than 0.5 mm, the Yuan Li needle can be inserted painlessly with the proper technique. Speed and precision are key during skin penetration, while slow and steady movements are essential when navigating through pathological knots.

Treatment Principles: When administering Yuan Li needling therapy, acupuncturists must prioritize clinical safety, followed by patient comfort and treatment efficacy. Finding a balanced approach among these three factors is crucial for successful treatment outcomes.

Self-healing: The ultimate goal of Yuan Li needling is to stimulate the body's innate self-healing mechanisms. It can reliably treat myogenic pain arising from acute or chronic muscle strain, provided the needle is accurately inserted into the pathological tissues.

Comprehension/Review Questions

(1) What are the main disadvantages of ancient Yuan Li needles?
(2) What is the basic TCM mechanism of YL needling?
(3) What are transverse collaterals?
(4) Describe the 'untie knots' therapy.
(5) What are the commonly used specifications of modern YL needles?
(6) Describe the Hegu needling technique.
(7) Is "deqi" required when treating diseases by YL needling therapy?
(8) What is the most widespread clinical application of YL needling?

References

1. Organized by Tian D, Liu G. Spiritual axis. People's Medical Publishing House; 2017.
2. Hu C. Yuan Li needling therapy. Hubei Science and Technology Press; 2016.
3. Lu D. Muscle injuries and pain involving back and limbs. TCM Press; 2000.

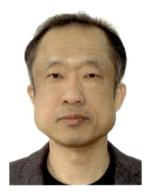

Songyan Chen (陈松岩) an accomplished Traditional Chinese Medicine (TCM) practitioner, brings nearly thirty years of clinical experience to his field. After completing his education at Changchun Traditional Chinese Medicine College, he spent thirteen years working as a TCM doctor in China. Chen's career later took an international turn when he joined a Chinese medical aid team in Kuwait, working as an acupuncturist at a Physical Medicine and Rehabilitation Hospital for three years. In 2008, he was elevated to the role of associate professor, coinciding with his relocation to the UK. Chen is particularly renowned for his expertise in treating Pain Syndrome using the Yuanli needling technique, a method distinct from traditional acupuncture. This innovative approach is known for providing immediate and effective relief, further cementing Chen's status as a skilled and forward-thinking practitioner in the realm of TCM.

Fire Needling

Defeng Wang and Shunchang Wang

Learning Objectives
- Learn theoretical knowledge about the history and development of fire needles.
- Understand fire needles and fire needle operating practices.
- Learn the mechanism and efficacy of fire needles.
- Understand the acupoint selection ideas and clinical application of fire acupuncture.

1 Brief History of Fire Needles

Through the comprehensive collection, systematic analysis, research and arrangement of fire needle literature, the historical development of fire needles can be objectively divided into five stages.

2 "Huang Di Nei Jing" Laid the Theoretical Foundation of Fire Acupuncture Therapy

Fire acupuncture therapy first appeared in the "Huang Di Nei Jing", which is one of the nine needles. The "Nei Jing" made a clear discussion from the fire needle tools to 4 kinds of indications and treatment taboos. This study has laid a solid theoretical foundation for the wide application of fire acupuncture in the clinic. "Huang Di Nei Jing" regards tendon disease as one of the major indications.

D. Wang (✉) · S. Wang
France Académie Wang de MTC, 33 Rue Bayard, 31000 Toulouse, France
e-mail: awmtc@free.fr

3 From the Han Dynasty to the Tang and Song Dynasties, the Fire Needle Developed Widely

(1) In "Shang Han Lun", Zhang Zhongjing used thirteen articles to talk about the taboos of fire acupuncture, wrong treatment, and treatment after wrong treatment.
(2) During the Tang and Song Dynasties, some famous doctors expanded the scope of use of fire needles from tendon diseases and joint diseases to internal diseases and surgical diseases. Sun Simiao proposed fire acupuncture to treat external boils and carbuncles in "Qian Jin Fang", so he pioneered fire acupuncture to treat surgical diseases. In the Song Dynasty, Wang Zhizhong described a case of using fire acupuncture to treat allergic asthma in his "Zi Sheng Jing".

4 The Ming and Qing Dynasties Developed into the Mature Period and Heyday of the Fire Needles

(1) The representative physician is Gao Wu. In his book "Zhen Jiu Ju Ying", he discussed the fire needle in a very comprehensive and systematic way from the operation method, indications, and contraindications of the fire needle, which can be used as a sign of the maturity of the fire needle.
(2) Chen Shigong introduced the method of using fire acupuncture to treat scrofula in "Wai Ke Zheng Zong", which has been verified by many later generations of doctors. This is his great contribution to fire acupuncture.
(3) Yang Jizhou, who collected the achievements of various acupuncture doctors, although he did not make new developments in fire acupuncture, played a great role in the promotion and dissemination of fire acupuncture with his famous book "Zhen Jiu Da Cheng".
(4) The historical facts of Zhou Hanqing using fire acupuncture to treat intestinal ulcers are recorded in the "History of Ming Dynasty. Biography of Zhou Hanqing".
(5) In the Qing Dynasty, Wu Yiluo creatively used fire needles for ophthalmic diseases in his book "Ben Cao Jian Xin".
(6) Wu Qian explored the scope of application of fire acupuncture in his book "Yi Zong Jin Jian" and pointed out that "All kinds of evil energy in the whole body, such as wind or water, overflow the body and stay in the joints, stab it with fire needles."

Through the efforts of the abovementioned doctors in the Ming and Qing dynasties, fire acupuncture therapy was fully developed and matured.

From the end of the Qing dynasty to the period of China's reform and opening up, the development of fire acupuncture lagged seriously, and fire acupuncture therapy was stagnant, even declining, and was on the verge of being lost.

5 The Instrument and Operation of the Fire Needle

5.1 Needles for Fire Needling

(1) The material of the fire needle

It is best to use tungsten-manganese alloy material or stainless steel to make the fire needle. They have the property of being hard and not bent at high temperatures, can be punched into extremely thin needles (diameter = 0.3 mm), and do not leave black marks when entering and exiting the skin.

(2) Regarding the thickness of the fire needle

Ultrafine fire needle: $\Phi = 0.25 \sim 0.30$
Fine fire needle: $\Phi = 0.3 \sim 0.5$
Medium fire needle: $\Phi = 0.5 \sim 0.8$
Coarse fire needle: $\Phi = 0.8 \sim 1.1$

(3) Regarding the choice of fire needles

The principle is that the finer, the better. Never use coarse or medium fire needles when fine or ultrafine fire needles work, especially when acupuncture is performed on normal skin points. (See Fig. 16.1).

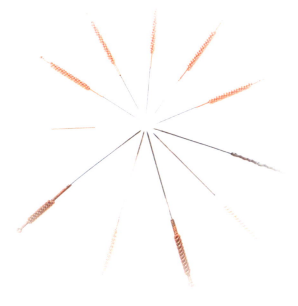

Fig. 16.1 Fire needles commonly used in clinics. Choose a fire needle with the appropriate thickness according to your needs.

6 Operation of Fire Needle Therapy

The operation process of fire needling therapy is very different from general acupuncture methods. Generally, it is divided into seven steps:

(1) Positioning problem before acupuncture

Make a mark before applying the needle and tap the selected point with a fingernail or an alcohol swab. Never use colored pens to mark.

(2) Disinfection

After the acupoints were selected, 70–75% alcohol cotton balls were used to sterilize the acupoints. During the fire needle operation, the procedure of disinfection cannot be omitted or simplified. In fact, fire needle acupuncture itself will not cause infection, but the possibility of postoperative infection exists, so this disinfection is mainly to reduce postoperative infection.

(3) Heat the fire needle

Hold a 90° high-alcohol cotton ball with a hemostat and ignite it 3–4 cm away from the acupuncture point. Then, the tip and front body of the fire needle are moved to the upper end of the flame since the temperature at the upper end of the flame is the highest. It must be burnt to a reddish-white state. (See Fig. 16.2).

The reddish-white state can bring two benefits. One benefit is that the temperature of the needle body is very high. After piercing the human body, it can bring much heat energy to the patient's body to eliminate diseases. Therefore, we say that the

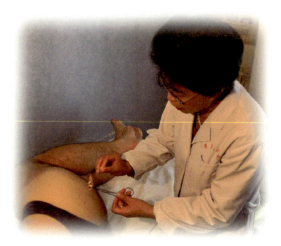

Fig. 16.2 Professor Wang Defeng uses fire acupuncture to treat sciatica

reddish-white state is effective, and the nonreddish-white state is ineffective. The second benefit is that the high-temperature fire needle has strong penetrating power and can quickly penetrate the skin.

(4) Quickly and briefly prick

The fire needle that burns until it turns red and whitish is stabbed into the acupuncture point and then pulled out at a speed of a few hundredths of a second. The faster the action, the shorter the time, the less heat is dissipated, and the faster the needle is inserted, the less pain the patient suffers.

(5) Retaining the needle or not

Fire needle therapy is mainly based on instant acupuncture, most of which does not retain needles. However, for some diseases, it is still necessary to maintain the needle for two to five minutes, such as abscesses, lymphatic tuberculosis, cysts, nodules, and calcifications; that is, when the temperature of the needle body drops to the same temperature as the human body, the needle can be pulled out.

(6) Pull out the needle

The process of needle withdrawal must be stable to reduce the patient's pain and avoid leaving scars.

(7) Treatment after acupuncture

Immediately after the needle is removed, the needle hole must be pressed with a dry cotton ball but must not be rubbed. The patient was asked not to wet the needle hole within 24 h, including not taking a bath, not using any disinfectant or any ointment or oil on or around the needle hole, and not doing strenuous exercise to prevent the patient from sweating, since sweat may flow into the pinhole and bring the chance of infection.

7 Three Key Points of Fire Acupuncture Therapy

The first point is whiteness; that is, when the fire needle is burned, it must be burned until it turns red and then turns white.

The second point is the accuracy, including the accuracy of acupoint selection and needle insertion, which are very important.

The third point is speed; that is, the needle must be inserted quickly.

These three key points are the key to ensuring the success of fire acupuncture and the curative effect.

8 About Frequency of Treatment

According to our clinical experience, when performing fire acupuncture, the best interval between two treatments is approximately five to ten days. Too frequent treatment will not only fail to improve the curative effect but will damage the curative effect.

9 Experimental Study and Preliminary Study on the Mechanism of the Fire Needle

Through the inductive analysis of the indications of fire acupuncture recorded in the literature of the past dynasties, fire acupuncture is not only suitable for cold syndrome but also for heat syndrome; not only for deficiency syndrome but also for excess syndrome; not only for superficial syndrome, it can also be used for internal syndrome. External and internal, cold and heat, deficiency and excess, and various diseases and syndromes can be applied. Therefore, the fire needle has a wide range of applications, which means that the fire needle has multiple functions. Then, is there any internal connection among the multiple functions of fire needles, or in other words, is there any dominant effect of fire needles? What is this leading effect (or basic effect)?

Fire needling burns the needle body until it turns red and white and pierce the acupoints quickly, that is, to pierce the acupoints at a speed of a few hundredths of a second. Instant fire needling therapy inputs two powerful energies into the patient's body: thermal energy and kinetic energy. The heat source comes from the high temperature of the needle body, and the kinetic energy comes from the high speed at which the instant fire needle penetrates into the body (because the kinetic energy is proportional to the square of the speed). Therefore, the two powerful energies, thermal energy and kinetic energy, are injected into the human body in such a short period of time, which can effectively promote the circulation of Qi and blood in the human body and promote the local temperature rise of the patient. If explained in terms of traditional Chinese medicine, fire needles have the effect of warming and dredging meridians, promoting Qi and blood circulation. Warming and dredging the meridians, promoting qi and promoting blood circulation are the main effects of fire needles.

To prove this inference, we designed two experimental studies in 1987:

The first experimental study was to observe the changes in nail fold microcirculation in 20 patients before and after fire acupuncture treatment (completed with the help of Mr. Xia from the Beijing Institute of Traditional Chinese Medicine at that time, thanks again) and found that after fire acupuncture treatment, the blood flow velocity of the patient's nail fold microcirculation was significantly faster than before treatment, and the blood flow state was obviously improved. The two results were processed statistically, and there were significant differences. This result indicates that fire needles can improve microcirculation. That is, the experimental results support our inference: the basic or dominant effect of fire acupuncture therapy is to warm and dredge meridians and promote Qi and blood circulation.

The second experimental study was on 23 patients who received fire acupuncture treatment. During the treatment period, that is, 20 min before and after the fire acupuncture treatment, the infrared thermal image was measured (this experiment was conducted by the Institute of Acupuncture, China Academy of Chinese Medical Sciences). Researcher Zhang Dong helped to complete it, thanks again). The research method was to test the average temperature and the maximum temperature of the lesion with an infrared thermal imager before and after the fire acupuncture treatment. The statistical results show that these two temperatures increased significantly after the treatment, and there are significant differences, which shows that fire acupuncture therapy has a positive effect on the lesion. Warming effect, an increase in temperature indicates that local blood circulation increases and local tissue metabolism strengthens. This result also supports our inference that the basic or dominant effect of fire needles is warming the meridians, dredging collaterals, promoting Qi and activating blood.

10 Efficacy of Fire Needle Therapy

The main effect of fire acupuncture therapy is to warm the meridians, dredge the collaterals, promote Qi and activate blood, and it has derived eleven subeffects.

11 Dispelling Cold and Dehumidification

Due to the function of warming the meridians and collaterals, promoting Qi and activating blood, the meridians are ventilated, and the blood flows. Cold pathogens and dampness pathogens blocked in the meridians will also be loosened, and they are easily driven out of the body by the meridians. Therefore, as early as the "Huang Di Nei Jing" period, fire acupuncture was used for the treatment of cold arthromyodynia and bone arthromyodynia. All kinds of rheumatic joint diseases are still the first major indications of fire acupuncture therapy [1].

12 Clear Heat and Detoxify, Remove Putrefaction and Discharge Pus

People habitually think that fire needles belong to the method of warming and can only be used for cold syndrome, not for heat syndrome, and they think this is the theory from "Huang Di Nei Jing". However, the clinical practice of many later generations of physicians has proven that fire acupuncture therapy has miraculous effects on many syndromes caused by fire-heat toxins, such as treating mastitis and waist-wrapped dragons. This is the clinical application of the theories of "using heat to induce heat" and "fire stagnation must be vented". The poisonous heat inside is very strong, and it resists the cold; then, the method of clearing heat and purging fire will not work. Fire acupuncture therapy has the function of warming the meridians, promoting Qi and activating blood, so it can induce the fire pathogen to go out so that the heat can be dissipated, and the poison can be released [3].

13 Eliminate Blood Stasis and Dissipate Stagnation

The blood stasis eliminated by fire acupuncture includes tumors, lumps, nodules, and even some calcified foci formed by the accumulation and coagulation of various pathological products, such as Qi, blood, and phlegm dampness. It can be on the body surface or inside the body, such as ovarian cysts and uterine fibroids in the body, ganglion cysts on the body surface, joint effusion, etc. The reason why fire needle therapy can dissipate the crux is because it has the function of warming and dredging the meridians, promoting Qi and blood circulation. If the crux is caused by the accumulation of phlegm dampness, on the one hand, since the meridians become unobstructed and the meridian Qi can flow well, the stagnant phlegm dampness can be washed away. On the other hand, because fire acupuncture therapy enhances Yang Qi and helps Qi flow, it can promote the circulation of water and liquid and can also eliminate the pathogen of phlegm and dampness. (See Fig. 16.3) [2].

14 Promoting Muscle and Reducing Sores

Fire needles promote muscle and reduce sores. It has a good healing effect on some chronic ulcers that have not healed for a long time, such as chronic lower extremity ulcers caused by varicose veins, ulcerated lymphatic tuberculosis, and anal fistula. Should be based on the size of the wound, choose fine fire needle or medium fire needle. If the sore surface was very large, three to four needles were punctured around the sore and one in the middle. If the sore surface was small, a needle was pricked in the center of the sore surface. The mechanism is that the fire needle has the leading effect of warming the meridians, promoting Qi and activating blood, which

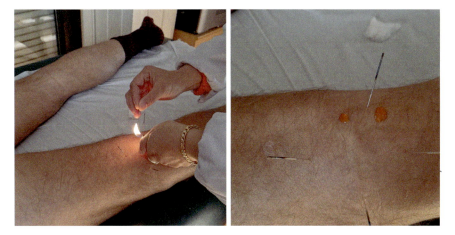

Fig. 16.3 Fire needle removal of joint effusion

increases the blood flow around the sore, thereby increasing the nutrient supply of the surrounding tissue and promoting the metabolism of the tissue, thus enhancing the regeneration ability of the tissue, and the sore easily heals.

15 Tonify Kidney and Strengthen Yang

Applying fire needles to acupoints such as BL-23 Shenshu and DU-4 Mingmen can stimulate the Qi of the kidney meridian, make the Qi and blood of the kidney meridian unobstructed, strengthen the Qi transformation function of the kidney, and thus achieve the effect of tonifying the kidney and strengthening Yang. Clinically, it can be used for patients with low sexual function, chronic kidney deficiency and low back pain.

16 Warm and Unblock the Spleen and Stomach

Applying fire needles to acupoints such as ST-36 Zusanli, REN-12 Zhongwan, BL-21 Weishu, and BL-20 Pishu can warm and unblock the meridians of the spleen and stomach, stimulate the movement of spleen and stomach Qi, invigorate Yang of the spleen and stomach, transport and transform the pathogen of cold and dampness in the middle burner, and restore the digestion of the spleen and stomach. The functions of absorbing, raising clearness and lowering turbidity can be used clinically to treat stomach cramps, chronic gastritis, chronic enteritis, gastroptosis and Crohn's disease and often achieve miraculous effects.

17 Propagating Lung Qi and Calming Asthma

Fire needles can warm and dredge the lung meridian Qi by stimulating BL-13 Feishu, EX-B-1 Dingchuan, DU-14 Dazhui and other points so that the lung Qi can be ventilated and descended, phlegm and fluid retention can be eliminated, and cough and asthma can be relieved. It has special effects on intractable asthma diseases such as allergic asthma and chronic bronchitis.

18 Analgesia

Pain relief is the strong point of fire acupuncture. It warms and dredges the meridians, activates Qi and activates blood circulation to achieve "no pain".

19 Anti-itch

According to the theory of traditional Chinese medicine, all itches belong to deficiency and wind. The warming and dredging of the meridians and the circulation of Qi and blood in fire acupuncture therapy can not only promote the supply of Qi and blood in the itching area but also induce the wind to disperse, and the blood will flow and the wind will extinguish itself, thereby achieving the effect of relieving itching. During treatment, for pruritus caused by skin diseases such as hyperplasia and hypertrophy, such as psoriasis, it is advisable to prick the diseased tissue with a medium or thick fire needle. For pruritus without skin hyperkeratosis, such as senile pruritus, it is advisable to use filiform fire needles and fine fire needles to puncture GB-31 Fengshi, SP-10 Xuehai, BL-17 Geshu and local areas.

20 Antispasmodic

The theory of traditional Chinese medicine believes that convulsions are internally caused by wind pathogens or blood that cannot moisten and nourish tendons. A filiform needle was used to puncture LR-3 Taichong, GB-34 Yanglingquan, SP-10 Xuehai and local areas of convulsions to promote blood circulation. Extinguishing the wind and softening the tendons will stop the twitching on its own. Clinically, we use this method to treat facial muscle spasms, gastrocnemius muscle spasms and other diseases, and we often obtain good results.

21 Denumbing

Numbness is caused by the inability of Qi to direct the blood to nourish the meridians and skin. Therefore, through the fire needle to warm the meridians, activate Qi and blood circulation, the blood can reach the meridians and relieve numbness. Clinically, we use filiform or fine fire needles to perform scattered needling to remove anesthesia, such as in the treatment of lateral femoral neuritis.

22 Acupoint Selection Strategy for Fire Needle Therapy

There are two ways of selecting acupoints for fire needling.

22.1 Acupoint Selection Based on Syndrome Differentiation and Meridian Differentiation

Through syndrome differentiation and meridian differentiation, take meridian points. Generally, filiform or fine fire needles are used on the meridian points to stimulate the movement of meridian Qi, promote Qi and blood circulation, strengthen the body and eliminate pathogens, balance Yin and Yang, and adjust the functions of the viscera. It is mainly used for diseases of the viscera, and deficiency syndrome and cold syndrome are the main ones. For example, fire acupuncture is applied at BL-13 Feishu, EX-B-1 Dingchuan and DU-14 Dazhui points to treat allergic asthma and chronic bronchitis. Another example is to prick BL-13 Feishu and BL-12 Fengmen with fire needles to treat allergic rhinitis. Another example is to apply fire needles on ST-36 Zusanli, RN-12 Zhongwan, BL-21 Weishu, BL-20 Pishu et al. to treat diseases such as chronic gastritis and enteritis of deficiency-cold syndrome. In addition, fire acupuncture was applied to BL-23 Shenshu, DU-4 Mingmen and other acupoints to treat impotence.

22.2 Selecting Acupoints Locally

(1) Select acupoints based on pain points

Filiform or fine fire needles were used at the most obvious tender points, mainly for lesions of muscles, tendons, fascia, joints, and nerves.

(2) Swift pricking

For dry and cracked skin, especially cracked feet and hands in cold seasons, prick fire needles in the cracks quickly.

(3) Intensive acupuncture method

For keratotic diseases of the skin, such as molluscum contagiosum, corns, and psoriasis, thick-fire needles or medium-fire needles should be selected for intensive acupuncture according to the size of the lesion.

(4) Surrounding stab method

For example, patients with surgical carbuncle sores (recurrent, deep abscesses and chronic abscesses that cannot be cured by multiple operations, such as deep breast abscesses and anal fistula) can choose fine, medium or thick fire needles according to the size of the sore surface. Acupuncture was performed around the lesion with a fire needle at a certain depth.

(5) Scattered needling method

For example, for skin pruritus, numbness, or paresthesia diseases, filiform or fine fire needles are used to perform scattered acupuncture on the lesion.

23 Clinical Research on Fire Needle Therapy

Since 1986, Wang Defeng's research team has been persistently conducting uninterrupted, objective and scientific clinical research on fire acupuncture therapy.

On the one hand, we explored and improved the operation technique and acupoint selection method of fire acupuncture therapy to improve the curative effect; on the other hand, we scientifically observed, analyzed, evaluated, and improved the clinical efficacy of fire acupuncture therapy for various diseases.

The following diseases that are most suitable for fire acupuncture therapy have been screened out, and the norms for the application of fire acupuncture have been established: tendinitis, tennis elbow, frozen shoulder, calcific tendinitis, sciatica, facial spasm, degenerative arthritis of the knee joint, deformed knuckles arthritis, cervical spondylosis, lumbar degenerative disease, rheumatoid arthritis, ankylosing spondylitis, joint sprain, ganglion cyst, joint effusion, abscess, anal fistula, mastitis, cleft foot, cleft hand, corn, contagious soft warts, neurodermatitis, chronic gastritis, Crohn's disease, asthma, ovarian cysts, uterine fibroids, gastrointestinal spasms, lower extremity ulcers, hemiplegia, gout, heel pain, etc.

24 Case Study of Recurrent Pain in the Shoulder Joint (Calcific Tendonitis of the Supraspinatus Muscle)

Patient Yves, male, 44 years old, came to our clinic on March 29, 2012, with the main complaint of "repeated pain in the right shoulder joint, limited mobility for two and a half years, and aggravated in the past three months".

Current medical history: Two and a half years ago, his right shoulder joint began to ache without obvious triggers. He was treated by a physical therapy masseuse for several courses and took anti-inflammatory drugs many times, but the pain could not be cured. The pain had been aggravated and not relieved in the past 3 months, and it affected sleep. After steroid injection, the symptoms were still not relieved. Ultrasound examination revealed 2 shadows of calcification in the supraspinatus muscle, which were 13 and 20 mm in size. The rotator cuff was thick, the subacromial bursa was edematous, and the X-ray film also confirmed that the calcification still existed, and it was larger than that two years ago. Introduced by his homeopathic doctor, he came to our clinic to seek acupuncture treatment.

Current symptoms: Severe pain on the outside of the right shoulder, inability to sleep at night, limited movement, especially difficulty in abduction (only 60°), which affects putting on and taking off clothes. There was obvious tenderness in the posterosuperior of the greater tuberosity of the humerus and the subacromial bursa area. The tongue is dark red. The tongue coating is thin and yellow and slightly greasy. There are saliva lines attached to both sides of the tongue, and the pulse is stringy and slippery.

Diagnosis of traditional Chinese medicine: Arthralgia of the shoulder (liver does not nourish tendons, phlegm and blood stasis intertwine, obstruction of tendons);

Western medicine diagnosis: supraspinatus calcific tendonitis.

Therapeutic principles: soothe the liver and soften tendons, resolve phlegm and activate blood circulation, dredge meridians and collaterals to relieve pain, break up stones and absorb calcium.

Treatment method: The mild reinforcing-reducing method was applied on both sides of LR-3 Taichong, SP-9 Yanglingquan, SP-10 Xuehai and ST-40 Fenglong. Warm needles were applied to SJ-14 Jianliao and LI-16 Jugu on the affected side. On the affected side, the mild reinforcing-reducing method was applied to SJ-13 Naohui.

One treatment was administered every 4 days.

After 3 treatments, the shoulder pain was greatly reduced, and he no longer woke up with pain at night. Improved shoulder joint mobility, no pain when putting on and taking off clothes.

At the fourth visit, after the abovementioned acupuncture, the needle on the shoulder was removed, and fire acupuncture was applied on the SJ-14 Jianliao and Ashi points (subacromial induration) once a week.

During the seventh visit, the patient reported no pain in the affected shoulder, sleep well, and fully returned to normal activities. After two consolidation treatments, the tenderness point of the affected shoulder disappeared completely. A review of X-rays on June 20, 2012, showed that the two calcifications had disappeared. (See Fig. 16.4).

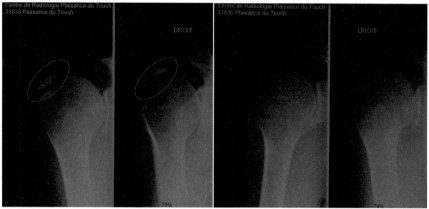

Jan 18, 2012 before treatment   Jun 20, 2012 after treatment

Fig. 16.4 Fire acupuncture removed the calcified foci of supraspinatus calcific tendonitis

25 Clinical Analysis of 30 Cases of Tennis Elbow

We summarize the clinical results of 30 patients with tennis elbow (lateral epicondylitis) treated with fire acupuncture between January 2002 and December 2004 as follows:

(1) Clinical data

Among the 30 patients, there were 18 males and 12 females. The patients were between 27 and 71 years old. The time of illness was within 3 months in 4 cases, 3–6 months in 10 cases, 6 months to 1 year in 11 cases, and more than one year in 5 cases. There were 21 cases of onset on one side and 9 cases on both sides.

(2) Diagnostic criteria
- Localized pain near the lateral epicondyle of the humerus, with obvious pressing pain. Severe cases can radiate to the forearm, wrist, and upper arm.
- Elbow joint movement was normal, but pain was aggravated during movement, especially when flexing and rotating the wrist.
- In severe cases, the lateral condyle of the humerus is thickened and deformed.

(3) Treatment method

Look for tender points (1–3 points) on the lateral epicondyle of the humerus and mark them.

Local disinfection with alcohol cotton balls.

Use a thin fire needle, burn the tip of the needle red, and then puncture the tender point quickly without retention of needle.

Then, LI-12 Zhouliao, LI-10 Shousanli or LI-11 Quchi was added, and the needle was pricked with a fire needle or kept in place for 3 min.

Press gently with a dry cotton ball for 30 s after the needle is removed, and instruct the patient not to immerse the part with water within 24 h.

The cells were treated once every 5–7 days.

(4) The standard to measure the cure of the disease

The patient's elbow pain disappeared, and there was no pain when pressing and moving.

(5) Treatment results

Six cases were cured after 2 treatments, accounting for 20%; 8 cases were cured after 3 treatments, accounting for 26.7%.

Eleven cases were cured after 4 treatments, accounting for 36.7%; 3 cases were cured after 5 treatments, accounting for 10%.

One case was cured after 6 treatments, accounting for 3.3%.

One patient stopped treatment after one treatment.

The cure rate reached 96.7%.

After 6 months of follow-up, 26 cases did not relapse, accounting for 86.7%, and 3 cases relapsed, accounting for 10%, which was related to occupation.

(6) Typical case introduction

ML, 71 years old, has had tennis elbow in both elbows for approximately 1.5 years, and it has worsened in the past 4 weeks.

At that time, she had pain on the outside of both elbows, the right side was worse than the left side, and she could not do housework. She had 20 massages, 1 steroid injection, and 5 acupuncture sessions, all of which were ineffective, so a friend introduced her to the clinic for trial treatment.

After the first fire acupuncture, the elbow pain became worse on the first day, but the pain decreased from the second day.

After the second fire needling session, the pain in the elbow was greatly reduced, with only slight tenderness.

The elbow pain almost disappeared after the third fire acupuncture, but she still felt unwell when doing housework.

After the 4th treatment, I went on a trip for 3 weeks. When I came back, she told me that the first 2 weeks were fine, but there was a slight relapse in the past few days, so the 5th fire acupuncture was performed.

During the one-year follow-up, the elbow pain did not recur.

26 Some Case Studies from Published Papers

Liu Liu, Yi Lu, et al. discussed the efficacy and safety of fire needle therapy for blood stasis syndrome of plaque psoriasis. Their studies have indicated that fire needle treatment for psoriasis provides satisfactory results with few side effects and a low recurrence rate based on a multicenter, randomized, single-blind, placebo-controlled trial.

Jing PANG, Hong-Na YIN, et al. investigated the clinical efficacy of surrounding fire needling combined with electroacupuncture (EA) at Jiājǐ (夹脊EX-B2) on acute herpes zoster and explore the potential mechanism of this combined treatment by measuring the changes of serum inflammatory cytokines and pain mediators. Surrounding fire needling therapy combined with EA at EX-B2 on the base of western medicine obtained better therapeutic effect on acute herpes zoster when compared with western medicine. This combined treatment may effectively relieve pain and depressive emotions, improve sleep quality, and reduce the incidence of post-hepatic neuralgia. The underlying mechanism may relate to regulation of pain mediators and reduction of inflammatory cytokines.

Kai-feng DENG, Liang-huizhi LI, et al. discussed their studies of conducting the meta- analysis and trial sequential analysis (TSA) on clinical trials of fire needling therapy in treatment of gouty arthritis and review systematically the clinical therapeutic effect of fire needling therapy on gouty arthritis to provide the medical evidence of the extensive application of this therapy in treatment of gouty arthritis. A total of 10 trials were included with 775 patients involved. Based on the analytic results, it can be determined that fire needling therapy, as an effective approach to the treatment of gouty arthritis, has a certain advantage as compared with western medication. Given the low overall quality of trials, it still needs high-quality clinical trial to verify the findings of this study results.

Comprehension/Review Questions

(1) What is the origin of fire needle therapy? Who is the physician who made the greatest contribution to fire acupuncture in history?
(2) What are the seven operating steps and three key points of a fire needle?
(3) What is the main function of fire needles? Please list five or six derived effects of fire needles.
(4) What is the idea of acupoint selection for fire acupuncture?
(5) Which diseases are more suitable for fire acupuncture treatment?

References and Key Reading Materials

1. Deng KF, Li LH, Pan TZ, et al. Meta-analysis and trial sequential analysis on blood uric acid and joint function in gouty arthritis treated with fire needling therapy in comparison with western medication. World J Acupuncture—Moxibustion. 2022;32(1):49–60. ISSN 1003–5257, https://doi.org/10.1016/j.wjam.2021.08.010.
2. Liu L, Lu Y, Yan XN, et al. Efficacy and safety of fire needle therapy for blood stasis syndrome of plaque psoriasis: protocol for a randomized, single-blind, multicenter clinical trial. Trials. 2020;21(1):739. https://doi.org/10.1186/s13063-020-04691-7. PMID: 32843084; PMCID: PMC7446129.
3. Pang J, Yin HN, Sun ZR, et al. Acute herpes zoster treated with surrounding fire needling combined with electroacupuncture at Jiājǐ: a randomized controlled trial. World J Acupuncture—Moxibustion. 2023;33(2):111–17. ISSN 1003-5257, https://doi.org/10.1016/j.wjam.2023.02.002.

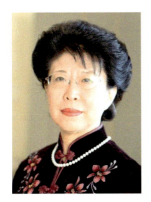

Prof. Dr. Defeng Wang (王德凤) graduated from the Department of Traditional Chinese Medicine at Beijing University of Chinese Medicine in 1985 and continued her postgraduate studies in the same year.

In 1989, she began to engage in clinical and teaching work of traditional Chinese medicine in Toulouse, France. In 1997, she founded the Academy WANG of Traditional Chinese Medicine.

She is currently the dean of the Academy WANG of Traditional Chinese Medicine in France, the vice-president of the Pain Rehabilitation Professional Committee of the World Federation of Chinese Medicine, the vice-president of the European Federation of Traditional Chinese Medicine Experts, the distinguished clinical expert of Beijing University of Chinese Medicine, and the president of the French Association of Traditional Chinese Medicine. She published multiple papers at French, European and international medical seminars and published the book of "Treatment of Pain with Traditional Chinese Medicine (French Edition)".

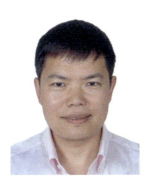

Shunchang Wang (王顺昌) a traditional Chinese medicine practitioner practicing in France, graduated from the French Academy WANG of Traditional Chinese Medicine. The acupuncture technique is inherited from Mr. Yu Jiajian, the 13th generation inheritor of Yu Family Tai Chi Kung Fu Acupuncture. He is currently the assistant to the dean of the French Academy Wang of Traditional Chinese Medicine and the executive chairman of the European Tai Chi Cultural Centre.

Three-Edged Needle, Plum-Blossom Needle and Gua Sha

Bo Sheng

1 Three-Edged Needle

Learning Objectives

To introduce theoretical knowledge of TEN, PBN and GS and development.
To improve the learners' ability to use TEN, PBN and GS correctly.
To help the learners achieve the skills of applying TEN, PBN and GS to the body.
To develop an essential evaluation of which areas are suitable in the clinical environment.
To understand the TEN, PBN and GS evidence from clinical research.

2 General Introductions of the Technique

2.1 Definition

The three-edged needle is a thick needle with a round handle, a trigonous body and a very sharp tip and is used to puncture blood vessels for the purpose of bloodletting. (See Fig. 17.1).

General history and development of three-edged needles

Three-edged needles, an important part of the acupuncture apparatus, have been widely used for 2000 years. The three-edged needle has experienced a number of different development stages to form a modern three-edged needle. The ancient famous Chinese medicine doctor *Hua Tuo* used a three-edged needle to treat serious headache 2000 years ago. Another Chinese medicine doctor, Sun Simiao, used a

B. Sheng (✉)
Confucius Institute for Traditonal Chinese Medicine, London, UK
e-mail: shengbo_hljucm@163.com

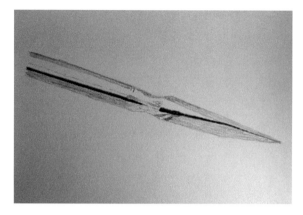

Fig. 17.1 Three-edged needle

three-edged needle to treat serious sore throat by needling the middle part of the little finger in the Tang Dynasty.

Not only used in China but also three edged needles to make bloodletting are still very popular in Western countries. The doctor in ancient Egypt used the blood-letting method, and this treatment method was recorded in papyrus to make the blood out. Furthermore, Avicenna in the Middle Ages mentioned the blood-letting method in detail, and he elaborated how to choose the veins, the sizes and the shapes of the incision, according to the patient's constitution, age, indication and contraindication when taking the blood-letting method. Dr. Broussais in the nineteenth century highly praised bloodletting and mentioned that it is an effective method for inflammation.

3 Features

In comparison with other acupuncture techniques, a three-edged needle is especially designed to draw a few drops of blood on certain acupoints of the body when applied. The three-edged needle technique is also known as superficial blood-letting therapy, but normally, we need to be aware that this treatment method does not need to draw out any more than a tiny amount of blood.

4 Detailed Techniques of Three-Edged Needle

4.1 The Operating Techniques Include

1. Slow needling method

The practitioner uses an elastic band to tighten the upper or lower part of the place needled, and the three-edged needle is held by the thumb, index and middle fingers to slowly puncture the point or the vein targeted 0.5–1 cun deep. Then, the needle is withdrawn slowly to let the blood out until the blood turns from black to red, releasing the elastic band, and the practitioner stops the bleeding by pressing the point with a cotton ball. This treatment method is good for superficial veins on certain acupoints to cause bleeding. For example, Weizhong (BL40) and Chize (LU5).

2. Swift needling method

The acupoint targeted is pinched up by the thumb, middle and ring fingers of the left hand, the three-edged needle is held by the right hand and punctured onto the point 0.5–1 fen (1 cun = 10 fen) deep, and the practitioner presses and squeezes the local area to make it bleed more. For example, Shaoshang (LU11) for sore throat, Shixuan (extraordinary acupoints) for sun stroke or high fever, and 12 spring-well acupoints for stroke.

3. Pricking needling method

This can be applied on the chest, abdomen and back. The skin area is pinched up by the left hand. The practitioner uses a three-edged needle to prick the skin area to make the blood or mucus out and sterilizes the local area after an appropriate amount of blood runs out.

4. Encircling needling

The practitioner uses the three-edged needle to digitally puncture a couple of times or decades of times around the swelling and red area (inflammation) and presses the local area with both hands to make all the extravasated blood out, reducing pain and swelling. This needling method is applied on Bi syndromes and carbuncles.

5. Acu-cupping

Do cupping treatment to let the blood out after three-edged needling. It can be applied on the body trunk or proximal areas of four limbs, which can be sucked by fire cups. The local area was sterilized by an alcohol cotton ball, punctured with a three-edged needle, and then cupped for approximately 10 min. Finally, the cups were taken away after a certain amount of blood was sucked out. This can be applied to some diseases covering more areas. For example, neurodermitis, erysipelas, leukodermia and acnes.

6. Fire needling

This is a fire cupping treatment combined with bloodletting. Heating up the three edged fire needle until it is getting red and puncturing it into a certain place to let the blood out, stop the bleeding and sterilize the local area when the blood colour turns from dark to light. There are advantages of fire needling and bloodletting, which can get better effectiveness. Clinically, it is used for Cold-Bi syndrome, phlebitis of the lower legs, varicose veins of the lower limbs.

5 Clinical Applications of Three-Edged Needles

1. Fever-reducing

There are two kinds of fever: fever due to excess Yang and fever due to Yin deficiency. Fever reduction with a three-edged needle is good for fever due to excess Yang because excess Yang leads to excess blood heat, and bloodletting can eliminate the condition of excess blood to reduce pathogenic heat in the body and decrease fever. It is not suitable for fever due to Yin deficiency.

2. Pain-stopping

If there is blockage, there is pain; if there is no blockage, there is no pain. This means that there must be some blockages if the problem or disease is accompanied by pain. Treatment can allow the blood to drain and dredge Qi stagnation and blood stasis, smooth the meridian and stop pain. For example, three-edged needle treatment is good for sore throat and migraine.

3. Detoxification

The treatment is good for people who suffer from acute lymphangitis (Red Thread Ding) with insufficient Qi and pathogenic toxins accumulating inside, resulting in dysfunction of the body. Bloodletting with a three-edged needle can eliminate toxins; furthermore, it can regulate Qi and blood to turn the body's function back to normal.

4. Fire-reducing

Fire belongs to the heart. Some fire symptoms will occur if Heart-Yang is overactive. For example, irritation, ulcers in the mouth and tongue, and even fever with delirium. The heart dominates blood and vessels; therefore, bloodletting with a three-edged needle can directly reduce the condition of Heart-Yang excess to reduce fire. The liver stores blood, so bloodletting can treat some diseases that are due to excessive yang of the liver and gallbladder, such as severe conjunctivitis and dizziness.

5. Itch-stopping

It is said in Chinese medicine that we have to treat the blood at first when we are going to treat the wind. Therefore, bloodletting with a three-edged needle is to 'regulate blood' because blood is running smoothly and wind will have no place to stay, thus achieving the goal of dispelling wind.

6. Oedema-eliminating

Swelling is mostly due to stagnated Qi, deficient blood and blocked meridians; therefore, bloodletting with a three-edged needle can directly eliminate 'the old' blood and pathogenic factors to smooth meridians and dispel swelling.

7. Numbness treatment

Blood flow cannot reach the extremities because of Qi deficiency, so the three-edged needle can be used to puncture the points of the affected body side to let a small amount of blood out to stop the numbness. Because bloodletting can remove the blood stasis to promote the generation of 'the new' blood, the numbness will be stopped under the good circulation of Qi and blood.

8. Anti-diarrhoea

Heat-diarrhea caused by food in the stomach and intestines or due to the plague can be treated by bloodletting with a three-edged needle, the mechanism of which is to reduce the heat from the small intestine to achieve the function of ascending the clear and descending the turbid. Clinically, Weizhong (BL40) is one of the commonly used acupoints.

9. Emergency use

It is used in treating coma, convulsion, epilepsy and sunstroke. When people get stroke suddenly with unconsciousness, abundant phlegm, and clenched teeth, the 12 Jing-well points can be punctured by a three-edged needle to dispel the extravasated blood.

6 Example of Three-Edged Needle Treatment

6.1 High Fever

High fever can be commonly seen in acute infections, like some acute infectious diseases in Western medicine, summer stroke, rheumatic fever, paediatric respiratory infections, digestive tract infections and other diseases.

The main acupoint is Shixuan acupoints. Dazhui DU-14, Quchi LI-11, and Hegu LI-4.

Operating procedures: Before puncturing Shixuan acupoints, the practitioner first uses his fingers to massage from the base of the patient's fingers to the fingertips to allow more blood to accumulate at the fingertip. Then, clamps the patient's fingers with the thumb and index finger of the practitioner's left hand, holds the needle with his right hand, pricks Shixuan acupoints approximately 0.2–0.5 cm deep, then withdraws quickly, gently squeezes around the needle hole to cause 10 drops of bleeding (one drop per fingertip), and then presses the needle hole with a sterilized dry cotton ball. Three-edged needle pricking was used at Dazhui DU-14, Quchi LI-11 and Hegu LI-4 to cause 3–5 drops of bleeding at each point.

Course of treatment: Once a day, the left and right Shixuan acupoints are used alternately. Two days constitute a course of treatment.

Note: While performing bloodletting treatment with three-edged needle acupuncture, the primary disease should be actively treated.

6.2   Precautions and Contraindications

The three-edged needle method is quite a strong treatment method, and it has very good effectiveness for excess symptoms and heat symptoms. However, there are some very strict contraindications as follows:

Patients: Yin deficiency, hyperhidrosis from over-exertion, over-tired, or the pulse is very weak, patients who bleed easily; or very hungry, thirsty, inebriated by drugs or alcohol or highly emotional and upset.

Hand manipulation: the hand techniques should be gentle otherwise the patient can faint because of the heavy stimulation.

Location: the practitioner should puncture the places very superficially or not needle at all if the location is very close to internal vital organs.

Acupoints: Avoid needling Hegu LI4, Sanyinjiao SP6, Shimen Ren5 and some acupoints on the lower back and sacrum area and other relevant points if the patient is pregnant.

6.3   Clinical Research on Three-Edged Needles

Zhao et al. [6] used a three-edged needle plus bloodletting to treat Bell's palsy of wind-heat syndrome at the acute stage, which has achieved good therapeutic effects. Wang et al. [4] used pricking blood therapy with three-edged needling plus cupping of TCM to treat Bi syndrome of wind-dampness type with obvious therapeutic effects.

Fig. 17.2 Plum-blossom needle

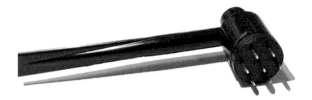

7 PlumBlossom Needle

7.1 Introduction to the Technique

7.1.1 Definition

A plum-blossom needle, also known as a seven-star needle, is an acupuncture technique that uses a small tool with 5 or 7 tiny binding needles to apply a series of light taps on a certain area, puncturing the superficial layer of the skin very slightly to help or treat a variety of problems or diseases. (See Fig. 17.2).

7.1.2 General History and Development of Plum-Blossom Needles

Huangdi Neijng laid the theoretical foundation for the plum-blossom needle, as it summarized medical experiences for acupuncture. It mentioned the detailed treatment methods of bloodletting, such as 'Luo Ci', 'Zan Ci' and 'Baowen Ci'. In another article in *Huangdi Neijing*, the mechanism of bloodletting was mentioned, and the bloodletting method was used to remove blood stasis.

Unfortunately, we could not find treatment methods, treatment tools or any records on treating diseases of plum-blossom until the 1940s. More Chinese medicine practitioners have developed the theory of plum-blossom needles, since then more diseases can be treated by plum-blossom needles.

7.1.3 Features

In comparison with a three-edged needle, a plum-blossom needle is especially designed to apply many times of tapping on a certain skin area with tips of binding small needles when applied. However, we need to be aware that this treatment method only needs to make the local area a very tiny amount of blood or without any blood.

7.1.4 Detailed Techniques of Plum-Blossom Needle

Local tapping is the stroke on the affected area or encircling needling or sparse needling from outside to the centre.

1. **Tapping on the Positive Points**

When tapping the positive points, you must first clearly feel the shape, size, softness, hardness, shallowness, distribution range of the positive points, as well as its starting point, terminal and direction, whether there is any painful reaction when pressing with your fingers, whether there is any adhesion between the base and the surrounding tissue, etc. Then, use heavier techniques to prick the skin area on and around the surface of the positive points. To tap the positive points accurately, the practitioner can fix the positive points with his left thumb or index finger and then tap it. Pay attention to the tapping of the starting and terminal points of the cord-like objects.

2. **Tapping on the Positive Areas**

Positive reaction areas refer to areas of soreness, pain and numbness. During treatment, this skin area should be punctured intensively and the technique should be harder than other areas.

3. **Tapping on the Painful and Sore Areas**

When tapping on this area, you must carefully find the most painful reflecting point, focus on the painful skin area and use auxiliary techniques, that is, use the left index finger or thumb tip to rub the pain point from time to time and spread the rubbing to the surrounding areas.

4. **Tapping on the Numb Areas**

For tapping on numb areas, in addition to intensive puncture on the positive areas where skin sensation is slow or disappearing, dredging tapping should also be performed on the healthy skin surrounding the numb area. That is, the plum-blossom needle taps the normal skin area first and then gradually taps centripetally toward the numbness-positive reflecting area. This method of tapping from the surrounding area of healthy skin to the numb positive reflecting area is called the dredging tapping method. For some affected areas (such as dermatitis, eczema, and hair loss areas), tap from all directions to the centre.

8 Clinical Applications of Plum-Blossom Needling

1. Internal medical diseases and paediatric diseases.
2. Neurological diseases and mental health.
3. Surgical diseases and dermatological diseases.

   Here are some examples.

8.1 Lateral Femoral Cutaneous Neuritis

Clinical symptoms: unilateral or bilateral formication, burning sensation, numbness or pain on the lateral thigh, which can be aggravated by exertion, standing or walking for too long, or exposure to cold.

Use the plum blossom needle to tap from top to bottom along the three Yang meridians of the thigh on the affected side. Stimulate each meridian 3 times until the skin flushes. Then, the local area was tapped. Centrifugally tap from the center outwards until the edges feel normal. Use wrist force and the elasticity of the needle handle to achieve the effect of pricking and tap until there is a tiny bleeding point.

8.2 Alopecia Areata

Alopecia Areata, also known as Patchy Hair Loss, is a condition in which hair is lost from some or all areas of the body. It often results in a few bald spots on the scalp, each about the size of a coin.

Routinely disinfect the plum-blossom needle and tap the affected area with 75% alcohol. Tap the plum-blossom needle slightly on the affected area and its edges. When tapping, the needle tip should be evenly punctured at the tapping area and move sequentially. Tapping was selected flexibly according to the skin colour changes in the hair loss area. If the colour of the scalp on the affected area does not change significantly compared with normal hairy skin, it is appropriate to tap with a moderate amount of stimulation to flush and congest the local scalp.

8.3 Precautions and Contraindications

(1) Check and explain

A detailed examination of the patient was performed before treatment to obtain an accurate diagnosis, clarify treatment principles, produce a treatment plan, and select the correct treatment position. Before the treatment, the patient must relax the muscles of the whole body and the practitioner needs to explain to the patient that it is normal to feel slightly painful during tapping to prevent the patient from being nervous.

(2) Disinfection

The skin at the puncture area (including acupuncture points) must be disinfected before treatment. After a relatively strong puncture, the local skin must be disinfected with alcohol cotton balls or swabs and care should be taken to keep the punctured area clean to prevent infection.

(3) Inspection of tools

Needles should be inspected before the treatment. If the tip of the needle is found to have hook or defects or the tip of the needle is uneven, it must be replaced before proceeding. The connection between the needle handle and the needle must be firm to prevent slipping during tapping.

(4) Precautions

When tapping, attention should be given to the direction and sequence of tapping to avoid inversion or uneven density. After the treatment, the patient should be instructed to rest for a few minutes before leaving.

(5) Pay attention to observation

During treatment, pay attention to the patient's expression, ask about his feelings, and see if there are any abnormal reactions. Once the patient feels not all right, treatment should be stopped immediately and appropriate measures should be taken.

(6) Post-tapping treatment

After tapping, most patients will have rosy skin at the treated area and a few patients will have subcutaneous bleeding and other reactions. This does not require further treatment and can quickly turn back to normal. Subcutaneous bleeding will slowly disappear within 1 week.

(7) The practitioner must take extra care and possibly omit treatment with patients with the following conditions:
A. Acute disease and acute stages of disease,
B. Severe diseases,
C. Diseases that have a tendency to cause bleeding,
D. All kinds of fractures,
E. Pregnant women,
F. All kinds of skin diseases.

8.4 Clinical Research of Plum-Blossom Needling

Dai et al. [1] explained that combinations of plum-blossom needling provided moderate positive add-on effects in alopecia areata patients. Wu et al. [5] used a plum-blossom needle to relieve pain effectively for treating trigeminal neuralgia of wind and heat, and its therapeutic effect was superior to that of conventional acupuncture.

Fig. 17.3 Gua Sha scraper

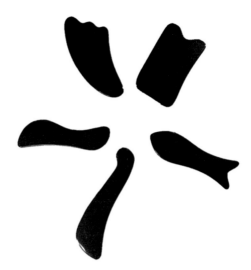

9 Gua Sha

9.1 Introduction to the Technique of Gua Sha

9.1.1 Definition

Gua Sha is a natural, alternative therapy that applies the Gua Sha scraper to scrape a certain skin area to increase the local blood circulation and correspondingly improve the function of local and remote areas or internal organs.(See Fig. 17.3).

9.1.2 General History and Development of Gua Sha

The Gua Sha treatment method has a long history and it is very difficult to track who and when it was created. The earliest time we can find is in the Yuan Dynasty, when the medical scientist Wei Yilin wrote *Shiyi Dexiao Fang* in 1337, and Sha (痧) comes from the sand (沙). Gua Sha can dispel the Sha toxin, the pathological product, out of the body to make the body recover from Sha syndrome. The skin will show corresponding red, dark red or dark blue dots after scraping the skin and this appearance is called 'Sha' after the treatment.

9.1.3 Features

In comparison with other acupuncture techniques, the Gua Sha scraper is especially designed to work on the skin area without any insertion into the skin. The local skin area can obtain more blood circulation after scraping and this treatment method is simple, safe and very convenient to practice and easy to learn after short-term training.

9.1.4 Detailed Techniques of Gua Sha

1 Posture of the Patient

- **Supine position**: This posture is good for the head, face, chest, abdomen, medial side of the upper limbs and lateral side of the lower limbs.
- **Prone position**: This posture is good for the nape, back and shoulders, lower back and back of the lower limbs.
- **Lateral position**: This posture is good for the sides of the head, neck, shoulder, back, lower back and lower limbs.

2 Choosing the Gua Sha Scraper

Bian Stone

Bian stone is a healing stone used in traditional Chinese medicine for thousands of years, the modality in which Gua Sha has its roots. It has healing properties which make Bian Stone an effective companion in self-care with a history of having powerful properties. Gua Sha scrapers are also made from rose quartz and jade stone which have their own properties.

Buffalo Horn

The Gua Sha scraper is made from the buffalo horn; it is one kind of traditional Chinese medicine Gua Sha scraper. The medicinal flavour is bitter, and its nature is cold. The function of Gua Sha includes heat clearing, detoxification, cooling blood and stoppingconvulsion. Gua Sha scrapers can also be made from plastic based products which emulate the buffalo horn but do not have the same properties as buffalo horn.

3 Direction and Sequence of Gua Sha

Generally, the sequence of Gua Sha is from upper to lower, for example, from the head, neck, back (thoracic vertebrae, lumbar vertebrae and sacral vertebrae), chest, abdomen, upper limbs and lower limbs.

4 Duration, Interval Time, and Course of Treatment

Duration: When using strong or medium force, apply a high or medium speed of Gua Sha, for no longer than one minute with approximately 10 times scraping for each part. For a mild force, use a low speed and up to 2–3 min for each part.

The scraping time and the body part for scraping will be determined according to the patient's age, constitution, problem or condition and course of the disease.

If Gua Sha is applied only for wellbeing, there will be no limitation regarding time and it will depend on the patient's preference, feelings and skin reactions.

Interval time: An interval of 3-6 days or when the scraping marks gradually disappear.

The course of the treatment can be 3–5 times as a course of treatment.

5 Detailed Scraping Methods

Direct Scraping Method

The practitioner cleans the local skin area with a warm towel, spreads the Gua Sha oil on the local area and then scrapes the local skin directly until the appearance of scraping marks. The characteristic of this treatment method lies in strong stimulation which will take effect quickly. This treatment method is suitable for people with a strong body constitution.

Indirect Scraping Method

The patient's body part that will be treated is covered with a layer of thin towel or material and then the practitioner scrapes over the towel until the local skin appears red, blood circulation is present along with scraping marks. It is called the indirect scraping method, which is a lighter method and suitable for children, the old, the weak and for some people with a high fever.

Gathering Scraping Method

The practitioner uses their own fingers instead of scraping tools to make the area of the body being treated acquire a purple colour. The colour indicates that the method will achieve an effective result for the patient. The gathering scraping method breaks down into the Che Sha (扯痧) method, Jia Sha (夹痧) method, Zhua Sha (抓痧) method and Ji Sha (挤痧) method.

Che Sha Method

The practitioner uses the thumb and index finger to pinch the patient's skin up; at the same time, the two fingers move up and down or circularly and release, and the process is repeated 3–5 times until the appearance of scraping Sha marks on the local area. This method is quite strong but should be bearable for the patient. The function is to disperse external pathogenic factors, activate Qi flow within meridians, stimulate the blood flow, and disperse stagnated Liver-Qi to relieve depression. The Che Sha method can be applied to the head, neck, back and Taiyang point on the face.

Jia Sha Method

It is also called the clamping Sha method or holding Sha method. The practitioner bends the five fingers and uses the second interphalangeal joints of the index and middle fingers to pull and twist the patient's skin, which means that the practitioner holds the skin tight with these two finger parts and lifts it to the highest.

The two fingers twist the skin combined with the manipulation of pinching up and release the skin to make the skin turn back to its original position. Do it repetitively approximately 6–7 times until the Sha marks appear on the skin.

Just because the Jia Sha method has a quite strong pulling force on the skin, it can cause the local or systematic reaction and make the local skin red and painful, but the patient will feel quite comfortable on the whole body after the local skin is pinched to a bruised condition. It is used on acupoints and its functions include inducing menstruation and promoting blood flow, stopping pain and guiding blood to go down. The Jia Sha method can be applied to the abdominal area, neck, shoulder, back and skin area where the tension is not too high.

Zhua Sha Method

The practitioner grabs the local skin evenly with the thumb, index and middle fingers; at the same time, the practitioner uses these three fingers to grab the skin firmly and move it to and fro and release the fingers until Sha marks appear. The function is to regulate the meridians, tonify the Spleen and Stomach, smooth Liver-Qi and activate blood to remove stasis.

Ji Sha Method

The practitioner squeezes the local places with the thumbs and index fingers 3–5 times until purple Sha marks appear. It is very commonly used on the forehead.

10 Clinical Applications of Gua Sha

Gua Sha is currently widely used for a variety of illnesses or diseases, including acute or chronic pain, stiffness and immobility, sunstroke, fever, common cold and flu, bronchitis, asthma and emphysema, headaches, migraines and hypertension.

Here is an example of a Sha clinical application:

10.1 Stiff Neck

Acupoints: Fengchi GB20, Dazhui DU14, Jianjing GB21 and Fengfu DU16.

Scraping from Fengfu DU16 to Dazhui DU14, applies Gua Sha oil to the local skin, and the practitioner uses the thin edge of the Gua Sha scraper at an angle of 45°–90° to the skin, scraping 6 to 7 times from top to bottom, with moderate force and speed, which is suitable for the treatment. Dazhui DU14 has no subcutaneous muscles, so the force should be gentle when scraping.

Apply Gua Sha oil to the local skin area from Fengchi GB-0 to Jianjing GB21. Use the thin edge of the Gua Sha scraper at an angle of 45°–90° to the skin. Scrape 6 to 7 times from top to bottom. The force and speed are moderate. The same technique can be used to scrape acupoints on the opposite side.

10.2 Precautions and Contraindications

a. Avoid treating the patients or take additional care to the patients with the serious mental health disorders, like phrenoplegia.
b. Deep Venous Thrombosis (DVT).
c. Thrombocytopenia.
d. Active haemorrhagic disease, haemophilia, leukaemia, any disorder of blood coagulation including taking blood thinning medication.

Precautions regarding location: Infectious skin disease, furuncle, ulcer, scar, abcess, any lump or problem on the skin with an unclear reason. The practitioner must avoid Gua Sha on these locations and furthermore the practitioners cannot scrape on the abdominal area of pregnant women.

10.3 Clinical Research

Saha et al. [3] stated that Gua Sha appears to be an acceptable, safe and effective treatment for patients with chronic low back pain. Ren et al. [2] concluded that Gua Sha therapy effectively improved the treatment efficacy in patients with perimenopausal syndrome.

Comprehension/Review Questions

1. How much blood does a three-edged needle need to release for each treatment?
2. Can a three-edged needle be used for deficiency syndrome?
3. What is the difference between a plum-blossom needle and a three-edged needle?
4. Which types of diseases are plum-blossom needles more effective for?
5. What is the biggest difference between Gua Sha and acupuncture?
6. How long is the suggested interval between Gua Sha treatments?

References

1. Dai T, Song N, Li B. Add-on effect of plum-blossom needling in alopecia areata: a qualitative evidence synthesis. Ann Palliat Med. 2021;10(3):3000–8. https://doi.org/10.21037/apm-20-1969. PMID: 33849090.
2. Ren Q, Yu X, Liao F, et al. Effects of Gua Sha therapy on perimenopausal syndrome: a systematic review and meta-analysis of randomized controlled trials. Complement Ther Clin Pract. 2018;31:268–77. https://doi.org/10.1016/j.ctcp.2018.03.012. Epub 2018 Mar 15 PMID: 29705467.
3. Saha FJ, Brummer G, Lauche R, et al. Gua Sha therapy for chronic low back pain: a randomized controlled trial. Complement Ther Clin Pract. 2019;34:64–9. https://doi.org/10.1016/j.ctcp.2018.11.002. Epub 2018;10. PMID: 30712747.

4. Wang M, Yin DS, Afulaha. Clinical observation on pricking blood therapy with three-edged-needle plus cupping on bisyndrome of wind-dampness type in yemenia. Zhongguo Zhen Jiu. 2006;26(1):48–50. Chinese. PMID: 16491760.
5. Wu MM, Liu XH, Wang LJ, et al. Clinical observation on deep needling at Xiaguan (ST 7) with round sharp needle combined with plum-blossom needle for trigeminal neuralgia of wind and heat. Zhongguo Zhen Jiu. 2021;12;41(10):1089–94. Chinese. doi: https://doi.org/10.13703/j.0255-2930.20210318-0003. PMID: 34628740.
6. Zhao JP, Piao YZ, Wang J. Effect of acupuncture combined with blood-letting by a three-edged needle on 50 cases of Bell's palsy at the acute stage. J Tradit Chin Med. 2010;30(2):118–21. https://doi.org/10.1016/s0254-6272(10)60026-x. PMID: 20653168.

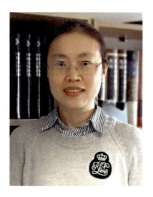

A/Professor and Dr. Bo Sheng (盛波) graduated from Heilongjiang University of Chinese Medicine. She received her BA degree for Acupuncture and Tuina in 2000, Master degree for Clinical Foundation in 2003, and PhD degree for Chinese Medicine Formula in 2008.

A/Professor Dr. Sheng worked as TCM lecturer in Confucius Institute for Traditional Chinese Medicine (CITCM), which is based at London South Bank University in 2008, and started her new role as Chinese Co-Director in 2020. She is also a registered practitioner at the Association of Traditional Chinese Medicine and Acupuncture (ACTM) UK. With over 20 year's experience, A/Professor Sheng devotes herself to TCM research and practice.

Electric Acupuncture and Laser Acupuncture

Electroacupuncture

Zunli Guo

Learning Objectives

- To help understand the principle of electroacupuncture.
- How to use electroacupuncture correctly.
- Learning about advantageous disease treatments using electroacupuncture.
- Precautions for using electroacupuncture.

1 Introduction

Electroacupuncture is a treatment method that connects acupuncture needles with a microcurrent close to the bioelectricity of the human body to treat diseases. Connecting currents of different frequencies, wavelengths, and intensities based on ordinary acupuncture and moxibustion can achieve the stimulation effect of traditional acupuncture and have the physiological effect of electrical stimulation. Choose the correct stimulation parameters to control different nerves and muscles. produce different physiological reactions and thus have a corresponding impact on the movement of qi and blood in the human body to achieve the purpose of treatment. This is a safe and effective treatment method. Because it is easy to use, it can replace manual needling for a long time to a certain extent and has relatively stable stimulation parameters, which can replace manual needling. As the electroacupuncture penetrates the skin and penetrates deep into the muscle tissue, the resistance of the muscle and nerve is less, so that the current passes through the needle and enters the muscle tissue to produce a greater stimulating effect, the affected area is wider, and the therapeutic effect is clear, but it also requires Acupuncturists to be familiar with the

Z. Guo (✉)
London Academy of Chinese Acupuncture, London, UK
e-mail: zguo176@hotmail.com

entire operation process in terms of disease types, selection of acupoints, compatibility, indications, and contraindications. It is recommended that acupuncturists receive relevant training before using electroacupuncture [1].

2 The Electroacupuncture Machine

There are many types of electroacupuncture devices. The electroacupuncture machine commonly used at present is a type of pulse generator, and it has a basic structure. It consists of 5 parts: a power supply circuit, a square wave generator circuit, a control circuit, a pulse main oscillator circuit and an output circuit. It uses an oscillating generator to output a low-frequency pulse current close to the bioelectricity of the human body. It can be used as electroacupuncture and can be directly placed on acupuncture points or affected parts with point electrodes or plate electrodes for treatment. Electroacupuncture devices are preferably those with a large stimulation volume, safety, battery use, no power supply limitation, low power consumption, small size, ease of transport, shock resistance and no noise.

Here is an introduction of an electric acupuncture treatment instrument, the AWQ-104 L digital electronic acupuncture instrument, commonly used in Europe (See Fig. 1).

The AWQ104E Digital Electronic Acupuncture machine with 4 outputs is a newly designed unit and features a digital display to show the frequency of stimulation during the operation and a numerical display to show the sensitivity of detection during the location of acupuncture points. This unit is fully equipped with distinguished features in appearance, circuitry and accessories. It is one of the most popular acupuncture stimulators with complete functions and stable performance in Europe.

The features include a digital display in Hz to show the frequency.

- Numerical digital display to show the sensitivity during point detection.
- Four [2] output channels.
- New IC circuitry, no crossover.
- Polarity reversal switch for each channel.
- Sensitive point location with numerical display, light and sound indication.
- Loc/Needle/Stim switch for selection of point location (Loc), needle treatment (Needle) and direct stimulation by probe (Stim).
- Hi/Lo voltage switch: Lo (low) for needles, Hi (high) for T.E.N S.
- Continuous, intermittent, and dense-disperse (modulated) wave forms.

Accessories Pointer probe and hand grip probe. Four connecting wires alligator type. 1 pc.9 V battery 1 artificial leather carrying case 1 instruction manual.

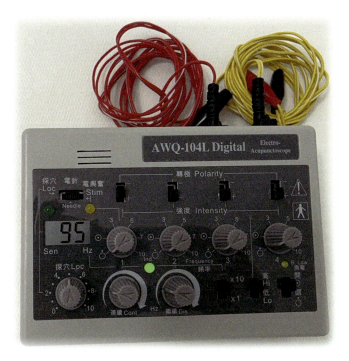

Fig. 1 An example of an electroacupuncture machine

3 Operation Method

3.1 Procedure to Use Electroacupuncture

Before using electroacupuncture, we checked whether the connection parts of the various electroacupuncture connectors were in close and firm contact and whether they were normal. You should also check whether the sockets and plugs are normal. The knob is consistent with the requirements.

Then, the output intensity adjustment knob was adjusted to zero, and the two electrodes of each pair of output terminals on the electroacupuncture instrument were connected to the two needles. After the treatment, all the output adjustment switches must be returned to the zero position; then, the power supply should be turned off, the wire plug should be removed, and the electrodes clamped on the needle should be removed. Usually, the same pair of output electrodes are connected on the same side of the body. Especially when performing electroacupuncture on the chest and back points, the two electrodes should not be straddled on both sides of the body. When turning on and off, special attention should be given to gradually increasing or decreasing the current intensity to avoid causing tension or injury to the patient due to electrical stimulation. If there is a stagnant needle, do not pull it out forcefully so as not to cause pain or even break the needle. At this time, we did not rush to withdraw the needle, lightly pressed the adjacent tissues to disperse the Qi and blood, and pulled out the needle after the air was not heavy when the needle was lowered.

3.2 Stimulation Parameters

Electroacupuncture parameters include waveform, frequency, intensity and duration. Among them, the amplitude, that is, the strength and frequency, are considered to be more important parameters. Different electroacupuncture stimulation parameters have different clinical effects on the body. Acupuncture manipulation is an important factor in determining the efficacy of acupuncture. When using electroacupuncture, different therapeutic purposes can be achieved by changing various parameters of electroacupuncture [3].

Repeated stimulation in a short period of time can accumulate stimulation volume, thereby improving the needle effect. Clinical practice has found that low frequency electroacupuncture with 2 Hz strong stimulation (wide wave width) has the best analgesic effect and is the most comfortable. Only by being familiar with and mastering the significance and characteristics of the stimulation parameters of the electroacupuncture device can we make the correct choice and improve the curative effect of electroacupuncture therapy [4].

3.3 Waveform

A pulse current is a sudden change in voltage or current that appears in an instant according to a certain rule and can produce a variety of different waveforms. The waveforms generally generated in electroacupuncture instruments are mostly pulse waves. Common pulse waves include square waves, spike waves, and sawtooth waves.

Square waves have the functions of anti-inflammatory and pain relief, calming and sleeping, relaxing tendons, relieving spasms, regulating muscle tension, promoting tissue absorption, relieving itching and lowering blood pressure.

Spike waves can excite muscles and motor nerves, improve muscle blood circulation, nourish muscle tissue, increase metabolism, and promote nerve regeneration.

Sawtooth wave: An undulating wave whose pulse amplitude changes automatically according to a zigzag shape, 16–20 times or 20–25 times per minute. Because its frequency is close to the breathing law of the human body, it can be used to stimulate the phrenic nerve, equivalent to the Tianding (LI-17) point, similar to artificial electric respiration, and rescue respiratory failure (the heart is still beating weakly), so it is also called a breath wave. It also improves neuromuscular excitability, adjusts meridian functions, and improves Qi and blood circulation [2].

3.4 Frequency

The frequency of electroacupuncture refers to the number of times the current changes per second, usually expressed in Hz. The electroacupuncture instrument stimulates the body by generating a regular bidirectional pulse wave. The output waveform has a continuous wave under different frequency settings, i.e. sparse waves, dense waves, sparse and dense waves, and intermittent waves. The effects produced by different waveforms are also different. In clinical use, the appropriate waveform should be selected according to the disease [5] (Table 1 for detail).

Low frequency (2–5 Hz) electroacupuncture can produce continuous analgesic effects and is suitable for the treatment of chronic pain and neuropathic pain. Medium-frequency (20–50 Hz) electroacupuncture can promote blood circulation and increase muscle tension and nerve excitability and is suitable for the treatment of muscle spasms and nerve dysfunction. High frequency (50–100 Hz) electroacupuncture can produce comfortable stimulation and is suitable for patients with mild pain, low tension and normal nerve function. Ultrahigh frequency (100 Hz) electroacupuncture needle stimulation can produce a strong stimulating effect and is used to treat patients with severe pain or muscle atrophy.

Table 1 Waves of electroacupuncture

Waves of electroacupuncture	Frequency	Functions	Indications	Wave patterns
Sparse wave (continuous wave)	< 30 Hz	Strong stimulation	Atrophy, pain, injuries of various muscles, joints, ligaments, tendons	
Dense wave (continuous wave)	> 30 Hz	Inhibit sensory and motor nerves	Relief pain and spasm, sedation	
Sparse and dense wave	Sparse waves and dense waves appear automatically alternately	Increase metabolism and eliminate inflammatory oedema	Sprains, arthritis, facial neuritis, etc.	
Intermittent wave	Automatically intermittently and continuously	Increase the excitability of muscle tissue	Atrophy, paralysis, etc.	

3.5 Electroacupuncture Intensity

The intensity of electroacupuncture is the intensity of the current, which is usually expressed in mA. Different intensities of electroacupuncture can produce different stimulation effects, so different intensities will be selected in different clinical situations. The intensity of stimulation should be determined according to the nature of the disease, the condition, and the patient's tolerance, and one should not stick to a certain amount of stimulation. Usually, clinical electroacupuncture stimulation intensity is divided into three types: strong, medium and weak.

Weak stimulation: usually using 0.1–0.2 mA electroacupuncture, the patient only has a slight comfortable feeling, no muscle contraction, no pain, suitable for spastic paralysis, neurasthenia, coronary heart disease and eye acupoints, mild symptoms, and sensitive patients.

Moderate stimulation: usually using 0.5–1 mA electroacupuncture to produce muscle contraction after electrification, no pain, but there is a needle feeling, suitable for the treatment of general diseases.

Intensity stimulation: 1–3 mA electroacupuncture is usually used, the amount of stimulation is large, the muscle contraction is obvious, the needle feeling is strong, accompanied by pain, and it is suitable for schizophrenia, muscle paralysis and certain chronic diseases.

Superstrength electroacupuncture: More than 3 mA superstrength electroacupuncture stimulation can produce a very strong sense of stimulation and is used to treat various severe chronic pain, neuropathic pain and other patients with serious conditions.

3.6 Sensory Threshold

When the current reaches a certain intensity, the patient will feel numbness and tingling, and the current intensity at this time is called the "sensory threshold". If the current intensity increases slightly, the patient will suddenly feel tingling pain, and the current intensity that can cause pain is called the "pain threshold" of the current. Due to individual differences in tolerance to electricity, the stimulation intensity should vary from person to person. Generally, it is appropriate to use a moderate intensity, which the patient can tolerate. At this time, the current intensity is between sensory and pain, which is the most suitable stimulation intensity for treatment. Too strong or too weak will affect the effect, and the intensity that the patient can tolerate should be used. Because the human body is adaptable to monotonous electric pulses, it is best to adjust the stimulation amount at any time when using monotonous pulses.

3.7 Electroacupuncture Time

Generally, the density wave is energized for 5–15 min each time; the intermittent wave is energized for approximately 15–20 min each time; and the continuous wave is energized for 30 min each time. Clinically, it is more common to retain the needle for 20–30 min. The course of treatment for various diseases is different. In Western countries, it is generally performed once a week, and for a few patients, it can be performed twice a week or once every two weeks [1].

4 The Mechanism of Electroacupuncture

Human tissue is a complex electrolyte electrical conductor composed of water, inorganic salts and charged biological colloids. When a pulse current with a constantly changing wave pattern and frequency acts on the human body, the ions in the tissue will move in a directional manner, eliminate the polarization state of the cell membrane, and cause significant changes in the concentration and distribution of ions, thereby affecting the function of human tissue. Changes in ion concentration and distribution are the most basic electrophysiological basis of pulse current therapy.

The commonly used setting frequency of electroacupuncture machines is 1–100 Hz. Different frequencies of electroacupuncture have different effects on the release of central neurotransmitters. Different frequencies of electroacupuncture stimulation can promote the release of different central neurotransmitters. A study on the analgesic effect of different electroacupuncture frequencies found that an electroacupuncture frequency of 2 Hz can cause the release of enkephalins and endorphins in the brain and spinal cord, and a frequency of 100 Hz can cause a large amount of release of dynorphins in the spinal cord. During the density wave, the above three substances can be released at the same time to achieve a synergistic analgesic effect. It also inhibits the production of endogenous pain-causing substances, intervenes in the intracellular signal transduction pathway of spinal dorsal horn neurons to exert analgesic effects, inhibits pain sensitization, and electroacupuncture may downregulate TRPV1 phosphorylation in injured dorsal root ganglia. Calcitonin gene-related peptide expression levels intervene in early peripheral sensitization of neuropathic pain and regulate ion channel function.

Danse waves can reduce nerve stress function. It first inhibits the sensory nerves and then also inhibits the motor nerves. It is often used for pain relief, sedation, muscle and vascular spasm relief, acupuncture anaesthesia, etc.

Sparse waves have a strong stimulating and emphasizing effect, which can cause muscle contraction and increase the tension of muscle ligaments. Inhibition of sensory and motor nerves occurs later. It is often used in the treatment of wilt and injuries of various muscles, joints, ligaments, and tendons.

The excitatory effect is dominant during the treatment of density waves, which can make the muscles contract and relax rhythmically, accelerate ion movement inside and outside the cells, stimulate the release of analgesic mediators, adjust the functions of the human body, strengthen the blood circulation of local tissues, promote metabolism, improve tissue nutrition, eliminate inflammatory edema, strengthen pain relief and sedation, and adjust muscle tension.

5 Clinical Applications

Electroacupuncture has the functions of relieving pain, sedation, promoting Qi and blood circulation, adjusting muscle tension, etc., to adjust human physiological functions. The scope of application of electroacupuncture is basically the same as that of filiform acupuncture, and electroacupuncture is widely used clinically. In almost all clinical subjects, it is often used for various pain syndromes, arthralgia syndromes, wilts and visceral functional diseases, as well as injury diseases of muscles, ligaments and joints. It can also be used for acupuncture anaesthesia.

5.1 Acupoint Selection

The correct selection of acupoints is closely related to the curative effect. Electroacupuncture points can not only be selected according to the meridian but can also be combined with the distribution of nerves to select the acupoints where the nerve trunk passes and the acupoints where the muscle nerves move. When needling the main and auxiliary points, it is best to switch on the electroacupuncture instrument after the acupuncture sensation reaches the diseased part.

5.2 Commonly Used Points

Head and face diseases: Tinggong SI-19, Yifeng SJ-17, Xiaguan ST-7, Yangbai GB-14, Sibai ST-2, etc.

Upper limb pain: Qingling HT-2, Xiaohai HT-3, Tianding LI-17, Jianliao SJ-14, Quze PC-3, Ximen PC-4. Shouwuli LI-13, Quchi LI-11, etc.

Lower limb pain: Huantiao GB-30, Zhibian BL-54, Yinmen BL-37, Weizhong BL-40, Yanglingquan GB-34, Chongmen SP-12, etc.;

Lumbosacral region: Qihaishu BL-24, Baliao points BL-31 to BL-34, etc.

5.3 Clinical Case

Similar to body acupuncture, electroacupuncture may help to treatment a great number of clinic conditions. Below are some sample commonly seen diseases in acupuncture clinic.

Facial paralysis: use Tinggong SI-19 or Yifeng SJ-17 as the main point, Yangbai GB-14 on the forehead, Sibai ST-2 Quanliao SI-18 on the cheekbone, ueing Dicang ST-4 if the disrobed of crooked tongue, using Tongziliao GB-1 if the insufficiency of eyelid closure. Electroacupuncture treatment: the dilatational wave frequency is 1–2 Hz, the intensity is based on the patient's tolerance or moderate stimulation, the time is about 30 min, the treatment cycle is once a day or twice a week, depending on the patient's condition.

Paralysis of the upper limbs: Tianding LI-17 or Quepen ST-12 as the main point, with Jianliao SJ-14 or Rushang LI-14, if the wrist flexor and finger extensor with Quchi (LI-11) and Shousanli LI-10 or Sidu SJ-9. Electroacupuncture treatment: the dilatational wave frequency is 1–2 Hz, the intensity is based on the patient's tolerance, or intensity stimulation the time is about 30 min, the treatment cycle is once a day or twice a week, depending on the patient's condition.

Spasm and Stiffness of the lower extremities: mainly ChongmenSP-12 and Weizhong BL-40, Biguan ST-31, Huantiao GB-30 Zhibian BL-54, Chengshan BL-57, Yanglingquan GB-34 etc.

Poststroke depression (PSD): Treated with acupuncture by soothing the liver and regulating the mind, with the principles of soothing the liver and regulating qi, regulating the mind, refreshing the brain and calming the nerves. Baihui, DU-20, Sishencong EX-HN 1, Yintang EX-HN 3, Shenting DU-24, Neiguan PC-6, Hegu LI-4, Taichong LR-3, etc., used scalp acupuncture of the Spiritual and emotional areas and Head area at the same time. Electroacupuncture treatment: the Intermittent wave wave frequency is 1–2 Hz, the intensity is based on the patient's tolerance or Moderate stimulation, the time is about 30 min, the treatment cycle is once a day or twice a week, depending on the patient's condition.

Gynecological Dysmenorrhea: Zusanli ST-36, Sanyinjiao SP-6 and Baliao points BL-31, BL-32, BL-33, BL-34 are the main points. Using Xuehai SP-10, GeshuBL-17 for period is Dark or purple colour, using Neiguan PC-6 for nausea, Zhongwan RN-13, Hegu LI-4 and Taichong LR-3for headache, etc. Electroacupuncture treatment: the Intermittent wave frequency is 2/100 Hz, the intensity is based on the patient's tolerance or intensity stimulation, the time is about 30 min, the treatment cycle is once a day or twice a week, depending on the patient's condition.

When needling the main and auxiliary points, it is best to switch on the electroacupuncture instrument after the acupuncture sensation reaches the diseased part.

6 Precautions

Before electroacupuncture, it is necessary to determine whether the patient meets the indications for electroacupuncture. Is electroacupuncture the best choice? Whether to choose the appropriate acupuncture point, body position? Whether to choose the appropriate electroacupuncture parameters? Acupuncturists should first be aware of individual differences in patients, different illnesses, psychological states and emotions of patients, all of which will affect the effect of electroacupuncture, so care should be taken during clinical application.

- The amount of current should be adjusted slowly from small to large and should not increase suddenly to avoid complete and broken needles due to strong muscle contraction.
- Try to avoid the current loop passing through the heart, close to the medulla oblongata, and the spinal cord. When using electroacupuncture, the point flow is easily small, so it does not stimulate too much. Attention was given to the depth of acupuncture on the chest and back.
- The distance between each pair of acupoints should not be too close. If the disease requires it, the current should be small.
- After a period of electrification, the patient may adapt, and the stimulation volume may become weaker. The current volume can be increased appropriately, depending on the tolerance.
- Pregnant women and uncooperative children should use electroacupuncture with caution. Old and weak, drunk, hungry, full, extremely tired, irritable, etc., are not easy to receive electroacupuncture.
- People with severe heart disease should be careful when applying electroacupuncture to prevent the current loop from passing through the heart to prevent accidents.

The stimulation volume of electroacupuncture treatment is greater than that of simple acupuncture treatment, so more attention should be given to prevent acupuncture fainting. When receiving electroacupuncture treatment, a comfortable posture is needed. Electroacupuncture treatment should not be accepted under the conditions of excessive fatigue, hunger, fear, etc. If treatment is necessary, it is best to choose the lying position. The patient's reaction was observed during the treatment to prevent needle fainting. The appropriate time for electrification is generally 20 min, which can be set by a fixed clock. If the amount of electroacupuncture stimulation is generally relatively large, you may feel a little tired after treatment, and you should pay more attention to rest.

7 Contraindications

- Patients with cardiac pacemakers and cardiovascular stents are prohibited from using it.
- For a very small number of patients who are particularly sensitive to electric current, if they feel uncomfortable after use, stop using this instrument for treatment.
- When you are tired, hungry or highly stressed.
- The acupoints on the top of the head when there are skin infections, scars or tumours, bleeding tendencies and high oedema, and children's fontanelles are not closed sed.
- It is not advisable to use electroacupuncture near important organs and large blood vessels in cases of stabbing internal organs and causing massive bleeding.
- Electroacupuncture should be used with caution or prohibited at the medulla oblongata, near the precordial area, and at the chest and back points to avoid the accidents of inducing epilepsy, heartbeat and respiratory arrest.
- People who are too afraid of electroacupuncture, those who have a history of fainting in the past, should not use electroacupuncture, and those who suffer from severe heart disease should pay strict attention to the application of electroacupuncture to avoid the current loop passing through the heart to prevent accidents.

8 Clinical Research

Li treated 120 patients with peripheral facial paralysis with sparse waves (frequency ≤ 30 Hz), dense waves (frequency > 30 Hz), dense waves and intermittent waves and found that the curative effect of intermittent waves was better than that of other waveforms [6].

Lv et al. [7] believed that electroacupuncture can improve lumbar spine dysfunction in patients with LDH and reduce multifidus muscle edema and fat infiltration. Sixty patients with LDH were randomly divided into an observation group and a control group, with 30 cases in each group. The control group was given symptomatic treatment; on the basis of the treatment in the control group, the observation group received acupuncture treatment at the L3–S1 Jiaji points and Dachangshu (BL25) and connected electroacupuncture at the L3 and L5 Jiaji points on the same side. If tolerance is appropriate, keep the needle for 20 min, once every other day, 10 times as a course of treatment, for a total of 2 courses of treatment.

Li's study showed electroacupuncture at the back-shu points of the five internal organs can improve the fatigue state of CFS patients and improve the quality of life of patients, which may be related to the increase in the excitability of the cerebral motor cortex [8].

The results from Wang's research show that electroacupuncture at four acupoints on the mastoid mainly treats nervous tinnitus, which can significantly reduce tinnitus loudness and tinnitus disability and relieve the pain and discomfort caused by tinnitus in patients. In clinical application, this method is effective for patients of any age within the study range. Those with a short course of disease can be basically cured, and those with a relatively long course of disease can also obtain a better curative effect [9].

Chen's study auricular point sticking combined with transcutaneous electrical acupoint stimulation can effectively reduce the degree of nicotine dependence in smoking cessation patients and improve tobacco withdrawal symptoms, and the curative effect is better than that of nicotine patch treatment [10].

Zhang et al. treated migraine with local acupuncture plus electroacupuncture with sparse and dense waves, and the total effective rate was 95.7%, which was better than that of simple acupuncture or electroacupuncture with continuous wave stimulation [11].

Han pointed out that low-frequency (2 Hz) and high-frequency (15 or 100 Hz) alternating density waves for 3 s each are the best analgesic [12].

Zhang's study divided into electroacupuncture frequency 2 Hz and electroacupuncture frequency 100 Hz, continuous wave, intensity 20–30 V. The results show that electroacupuncture can increase the content of serum complement C3, reduce the level of immunoglobulin IgM and IgG, and inhibit the hyperactivity of humoral immunity in patients with rheumatic arthralgia [13].

Chen indicated that EA is a great opportunity to remarkably alleviate pain and improve the physical function of KOA patients with a low risk of adverse reactions [14].

Comprehension/Review Questions
- What are the main functions of electroacupuncture?
- How to use electroacupuncture correctly?
- What are the advantageous disease treatments using electroacupuncture?
- What are the precautions for using electroacupuncture?

References and Key Reading Materials

1. Hou LQ, Xiong KR. Effect of electroacupuncture with different needle retention time on the expression of nitric oxide synthase in the septum. Chin Acupunct Moxibustion. 2006;12:879–82.
2. Ma GZ, Zhang Y, Chen L, et al. Comparison of therapeutic effects of electroacupuncture with different waveforms on lumbar disc herniation and its intervention on serum interleukin-6. Shanghai J Acupunct Moxibustion. 2014;33(02):153–6.
3. Zhou ZY. Research progress of acupuncture stimulation amount. Tradit Chin Med. 2021;10(4):534–9. https://doi.org/10.12677/tcm.2021.104072
4. Bian JL, Zhang CH. Academician Shi Xuemin's concept and core of acupuncture manipulation measurement. Chin Acupunct Moxibustion. 2003;23(5):287–9.

5. Han JS, Wang Q. Low-frequency and high-frequency electroacupuncture analgesia are, respectively transmitted by the arcuate nucleus of the hypothalamus and the parabrachial nucleus of the pons. Acupunct Res. 1991;16(3–4):181–3.
6. Li XY. Comparative study on the efficacy of different waveform electroacupuncture in the treatment of peripheral facial nerve paralysis. Shanghai J Acupunct. 2017;36(1):34–7.
7. Lv Y, Dai DC, Jiang HN, et al. The effect of electroacupuncture on the characteristics of the multifidus muscle in patients with lumbar disc herniation. Chin Acupunct Moxibustion. 2022;42(10):1103–7.
8. Li ZX, Zhang Y, Luda Y, et al. Effects of electroacupuncture at back-shu points of the five viscera on the fatigue state and cortical excitability of chronic fatigue syndrome. Chin Acupunct Moxibustion. 2022;42(11):1205–10.
9. Wang CY, Gao WB, Wang LJ, et al. Electroacupuncture at four acupoints on the mastoid mainly in the treatment of 30 cases of nervous tinnitus. Chin Acupunct Moxibustion. 2022;42(12):1377–8.
10. Chen SM, Liu ZY, Ji J, et al. Auricular point sticking combined with transcutaneous electrical acupoint stimulation for smoking cessation: a randomized controlled trial. Chin Acupunct Moxibustion. 2022;42(11):1235–9.
11. Zhang SQ, Yuan XS, Cheng YZ. 47 cases of migraine treated with local acupuncture plus electroacupuncture with sparse and dense waves. J Xinxiang Med College. 2002;19(02):134–5.
12. Han, JS, Chen XH, Sun SL, et al. Effect of low- and high-frequency TENS on Met-Enkephalin-Arg-Phe and Dynorphin an immunoreactivity in human Lumbar CSF. Pain. 1991;47:295–8. https://doi.org/10.1016/0304-3959(91)90218-M
13. Zhang HX, Huang GF, Zhang TF. Study on the analgesic effect of electroacupuncture at Jiaji point on lumbar disc herniation and its effect on plasma beta-endorphin. Chin J Orthop Traumatol. 2006;03:11–4.
14. Chen N, Wang J, Murelli A, et al. Electro-acupuncture is beneficial for knee osteoarthritis: the evidence from meta-analysis of randomized controlled trials. Am J Chin Med. 2017;45(05):965–85.

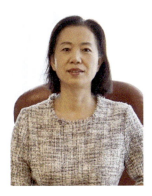

Dr. Zunli Guo (郭尊莉) has worked in a Chinese Medicine hospital for 10 years before moved to the UK. She has worked as practitioner of Chinese Medicine and acupuncture from 2002 till now. She established her Chinese Medicine centre since 2007.

Dr Guo has completed her master's degree of Traditional Chinese Medicine in the University of Middlesex UK in 2011. She completed her PhD study of acupuncture in Nanjing University of Chinese Medicine Nanjing China in 2021 and gained Doctor's degree of Medicine.

Dr Zunli Guo has talked as speakers in many seminars and conference in TCM and acupuncture. She is the executive director of the Academy of Scalp Acupuncture UK, and the senior member of the Chinese Acupuncture and Herbal Medicine Alliance UK.

Laser Acupuncture

Rongxian Zhang

Learning Objections

1. To learn the theoretical basis of laser acupuncture.
2. To understand the mechanism and therapeutic advantages of lasers.
3. To master the skills of laser operation on acupoints.
4. To evaluate which areas are suitable for common laser therapy.
5. To understand the current evidence of laser acupuncture from clinical research.

1 Overview of Laser Acupuncture

Laser acupuncture is applied under the model of traditional Chinese medicine and meridians theory and has a specific radiation power, energy density and wavelength of low-intensity laser beam directly irradiating the acupuncture points. The acupuncture points for effective photochemical or photothermal stimulation produce a series of biological regulation of reflex biological therapy, invigorating channels and collaterals, conditioning Zang Fu organs, qi and blood function. In 1960, Maiman in the United States developed the first ruby laser, and in 1961, Gavan developed the He–Ne laser and later developed the helium cadmium laser, nitrogen molecular laser Nd^{3+}-YAG laser, CO_2 laser and semiconductor laser. These lasers have been applied to laser acupuncture treatment. In 1966, Mester of Hungary proposed that a low-intensity laser had a biostimulating effect. In the early 1970s, YtemypaToBa reported that 118 patients with hypertension were treated by He–Ne laser irradiation of acupoints or reflex areas, 108 of whom recovered their blood pressure to normal. In 1972, Bopo-HuHa reported that 21 cases of bronchitis were treated with He–Ne laser irradiation,

---

R. Zhang (✉)
The Second Affiliated Hospital of Nanjing University of Chinese Medicine, 23 Nanhu Road, Jianye District, Nanjing City, Jiangsu Province, China
e-mail: 415322855@qq.com

21 cases had a good immediate effect, and the vital capacity was increased by 30%. In 1976, Plog first proposed the "light needle" instead of the traditional acupuncture needle and developed the Akuplas He–Ne laser acupuncture instrument, whose output power is 2 mW, wavelength is 632.8 nm, working mode can be continuous but also pulse with the pulse frequency at 0.2–50 Hz, and spot diameter at 1 mm. The action time can be precisely controlled in 10–30 s and the machine is also equipped with an instrument that can display skin resistance to accurately locate the acupoint, which can treat acute and chronic diseases previously treated by milliacupuncture. As early as the 1980s and 1990s, relevant scholars carried out comparative studies on the impact of metal needling acupuncture and laser acupuncture. They agreed that laser acupuncture is at least as effective as traditional (metal) acupuncture therapy and that painless laser acupuncture is the end point of the ongoing development of acupuncture medicine. In recent years, many scholars have studied the spectrum of diseases treated by laser acupuncture and found that it is effective in anti-inflammatory and analgesic treatments, promoting tissue recovery and regeneration, improving blood circulation, and regulating endocrine system functions [1].

2 The Function Characteristics of the Laser Acupuncture

The functional characteristics of laser acupuncture on acupuncture points include the following three aspects.

2.1 Accuracy of Stimulation

A low-level laser can be precisely placed at the stimulation position, similar to a metal needle. It affects an acupoint through the same biophysical primary and secondary effects as general biostimulation. One of the reasons for the stimulation is that the effect is triggered only within a narrow area of acupoint tissue. In other words, the more precise the stimulation, the more effective the stimulation, and only when the laser is aligned to a precision similar to that of traditional needle acupuncture can the desired effect on the acupuncture point be achieved.

2.2 Biological Regulation

Under normal circumstances, laser irradiation of the human body will produce a certain biological effect to stimulate the human tissue to start a series of feedback regulations to achieve the purpose of treating diseases. This is the biological regulation of lasers. The results show that when the laser irradiation dose is small, it will stimulate the biological regulation effect, but when the laser irradiation dose is large, it will inhibit the effect. In addition, with the increase in treatment courses and irradiation times, the biological effects produced by lasers will gradually accumulate, and after reaching the peak, the effects will gradually weaken, showing a typical parabolic phenomenon [2]. Therefore, when applying laser acupuncture to treat diseases, it is necessary to strictly control the course of treatment and treatment time to avoid negative effects.

2.3 *"Get Qi" Effect*

In the process of acupuncture, the emergence of effective qi sensation is the guarantee of successful treatment. When the metal is strongly stimulated against the acupoint to produce a sense of qi, if the stimulation is stopped, the sense of qi will be weakened in a short time. However, in the process of laser acupuncture treatment, energy accumulates slowly in the tissue, and the patient usually does not feel the laser device is turned on at the beginning. With the extension of the treatment time, the energy density in the tissue increases, and the stimulation effect on the acupuncture point also increases. After a few minutes of treatment, many patients report that they feel a tingling sensation on the acupuncture points where they are being treated, which is similar to the feeling of getting qi. Because the feeling of obtaining qi is delayed, it cannot be accurately placed on the acupoint as with traditional acupuncture. Some scholars have studied this and concluded that the core of qi sensation produced by laser acupuncture may be a phenomenon of conscious perception [3].

3 Principle of Action

3.1 *Anti-inflammatory Effects*

Low-level laser therapy has anti-inflammatory effects; for example, it promotes microcirculation by reducing the release of vasoactive amines, macrophages, leukocytes and fibroblasts migrate from tissues, and phagocytosis increases. The clearance rate of necrotic tissue, inflammatory mediators and pathogenic bacteria was accelerated.

3.2 *Analgesic Effect*

Low-level laser therapy relieves pain in different ways. It slows down the degranulation of mast cells, releasing vasoactive amines and inflammatory mediators. The concentration of prostaglandins that cause inflammation and pain and the pressure in the interstitial tissue are reduced, and the pain is alleviated (general pain is relieved). In addition, low-level laser therapy directly promotes the synthesis of ATP in pain receptors, which increases its hyperpolarization ability, as well as other effects. As a result, the threshold of pain receptors can be increased by 50% (local pain relief). In addition, a large number of opioid peptides (enkephalin, endorphin and dynorphin) inhibit, for example, the release of central neurotransmitters in the midbrain (central pain relief), which may gather in the small spinal nerve fibres responsible for the transmission of stimuli.

3.3 Tissue Regeneration Effect

In stage I of the wound (inflammation and necrosis), low-level laser therapy can promote anti-inflammation and anti-edema processes. In the wound II stage (proliferation stage) and III stage (epithelialization stage), low-energy laser therapy increases the oxygen supply of cells and the proliferation rate of fibroblasts to increase the formation of collagen and elastin. In addition, in stage III of the wound, it can promote the formation of a cellular lipid bilayer to improve the elasticity of the tissue. This stabilizes the refactoring process.

3.4 Effects of Improved Blood Circulation

In cases of trauma, inflammation, degenerative processes, vegetative state and other diseases, the regulation of the blood supply to organs and tissues may be interrupted. Low-level laser therapy affects this regulation in different ways. For example, it reduces adrenergic stimulation, thereby promoting peripheral microcirculation. It stimulates neuroreceptors. Induce them to release more neuropeptides to increase vasodilation. At the same time, it can activate lymphatic circulation, thereby reducing edema and reducing tissue pressure and blood circulation blockage. After injury, it can promote vascular reconstruction.

3.5 Elimination of Oedema Effect

Low-level laser therapy stimulated the absorption of edema. Due to the improvement of microcirculation, the pressure of liquid infiltration into blood vessels and tissue space is reduced. Therefore, the tissue can better supply oxygen and absorb the exudate back to the vascular system, thereby promoting its flushing. Due to the decrease in mast cell degranulation, the release of vasoactive amines and vascular permeability decreased. Low-level laser therapy further promoted the fibrinolysis and phagocytosis of macrophages and accelerated the dissolution of vascular exudates.

4 Laser Acupuncture Commonly Used Laser

(1) The He–Ne laser is a helium neon gas mixture, red light, wavelength of 632.8 nm, the first used for laser acupuncture. Due to its larger size, it is only suitable for hospital use. Its divergence angle is small, only 5 milliradians, the energy is highly concentrated, and the depth of its penetration into the tissue depends on the laser power. The penetration depth of the He–Ne laser with a power of 3.5 mW is 6–8 mm, and the maximum penetration depth can reach 8–10 mm when the power is 7 mW.

(2) The wavelength of the indium gallium aluminum laser is 632.8–635 nm, which has gradually replaced the He–Ne laser and red light. Because of its small size and similar power to the He–Ne laser, it has been used from hospitals to homes and individuals.

(3) Gallium indium, gallium indium aluminum laser wavelength 650 nm, is also used to replace He–Ne laser, red light, small, suitable for families and individuals, and cheap, the output power is higher than He–Ne laser.

(4) The wavelength of the gallium aluminum-arsenic laser is 780–890 nm, which is near-infrared light, and the penetration depth is deeper than visible light, which can reach 35 mm, and the periphery can reach 55 mm. The price is cheap, the analgesic effect is the best, and it can also be used to promote wound healing. Currently, it is more popular, can be irradiated at deeper points or acupoints, can perform hot moxibustion, and is suitable for deficiency cold stomach disease, abdominal pain, abdominal distension, diarrhea, wind cold cough and rheumatoid arthritis.

(5) The wavelength of the gallium-arsenic laser is 904 nm, the penetration depth is deeper, the laser can reach the deep tissue in the form of a pulse, and the continuous form can also be used.

(6) The N_2 laser wavelength is 337.1 nm, which is a pulse output, and the output laser is ultraviolet light. Good monochromaticity, narrow spectral line width, pulse width is also narrow, generally 6–10 ns, the shortest up to 0.4 ns, and the output peak is very high, up to tens of megawatts. Clinical point irradiation treatment of tonsillitis and pharyngitis and local irradiation treatment of vitiligo and psoriasis (psoriasis) are used, but because of their high prices, they are not widely used.

(7) The wavelengths of the Ar^+ laser are 514.5 and 488.0 nm, and its output power is up to 150 W. It has been clinically reported to be used for acupoint irradiation to treat paraplegic patients. Its cost is high, and it is not widely used.

(8) The He-Cd laser is a metal ion laser with a wavelength of 441.6 nm and an output power of tens of milliwatts to 100 milliwatts. It is clinically used for acupoint irradiation to treat hypertension, neurasthenia, etc., and its analgesic and sedative effects are better than those of red lasers.

(9) The Nd^{3+}-YAG laser wavelength of 1.06 nm is near infrared light, and its output power can reach hundreds of milliwatts, the deepest penetration of tissue, so it is often used for deep acupoint irradiation due to its expense, so clinical application is not common.
(10) A CO_2 laser wavelength of 10.6 nm belongs to the infrared output, with an output power up to hundreds of milliwatts. Due to the shallow effect on the tissue, the loss of normal tissue is small and more commonly used in the clinic. When used for laser acupuncture, because its thermal effect is more obvious, it is often used as moxibustion. However, due to its large size and inconvenient operation, it has recently been replaced by semiconductor lasers, which are more suitable for clinical use as laser scalpels.

The first 5 of the above 10 lasers are currently used in hospitals and families for laser acupuncture, and the last 5 are gradually replaced by other types of lasers due to their large size, slightly expensive price, inconvenient operation and other factors.

5 The Therapeutic Advantages of Laser Acupuncture

In the clinical application of laser acupuncture, in addition to the biological stimulation effect of laser acupuncture, compared with ordinary acupuncture, its advantages are also reflected in the following aspects:

(1) Painless: laser acupuncture is painless throughout the entire treatment process. This makes it possible for children and pain-sensitive patients to receive acupuncture treatment. At the same time, when acupuncture is performed on special acupoints, such as around the eyes, laser acupuncture can significantly relieve patients' fear and discomfort.
(2) No complications or side effects: laser acupuncture is not traumatic to the skin and can avoid the occurrence of acupuncture accidents such as syncope, infection and hematoma. It also allows beginners to treat potentially dangerous acupressure points.
(3) Produce additional effects: laser acupuncture has additional positive effects on the neurovascular bundles associated with acupuncture points. Due to the biological regulatory reflex of laser acupuncture, the imbalance of local tissues around acupuncture points can be corrected, and the uncoordinated patterns associated with acupuncture points can be reflexively adjusted.
(4) Inaccessible parts: Laser acupuncture can also reach parts inaccessible to ordinary acupuncture, such as inflamed and swollen tissues, directly promoting blood circulation in the tissues and improving edema.
(5) Shorter processing time: laser acupuncture determines the acupuncture treatment time by adjusting the laser power output and can continuously stimulate multiple acupuncture points at the same time, significantly shortening the treatment time and improving the treatment efficiency.

(6) Comprehensive treatment: laser acupuncture can be used in combination with other therapies, which can promote each other and enhance the comprehensive treatment effect to a certain extent.

6 The Operation Method

The operation method of each laser instrument is different. The following takes the German 3B laser acupuncture instrument as an example to introduce its treatment method: Before the treatment starts, the patient is fully exposed to the treatment site, the doctor will paste the disposable silicone gasket on the acupuncture point after local skin disinfection, and then insert the laser needle into the small hole of the silicone gasket. The insertion depth is 2–3 cm, the laser needle and the skin at the acupoint are fixed at 90°, and the power supply of the laser acupuncture treatment instrument is turned on. Set the corresponding parameters (power, wavelength, duration of treatment, energy, frequency (mode)), ask the patient to wear laser protective glasses, click the start button to activate the laser emission, and then the doctor leaves the treatment room, always paying attention to the occurrence of adverse reactions in the patient. The laser emission automatically stops after the end of the treatment, and the laser needle and silicone gasket are removed in turn after the end of the treatment. The specific treatment process is shown in Figs. 1, 2 and 3.

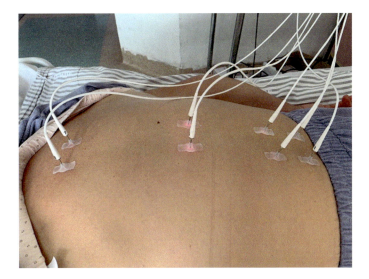

Fig. 1 Treatment process of laser acupuncture

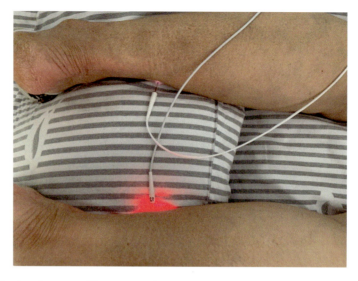

Fig. 2 Treatment process of laser acupuncture

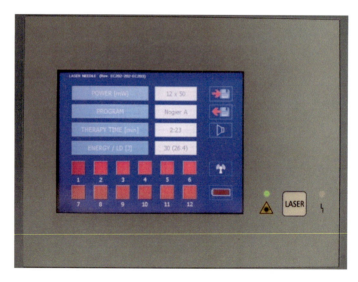

Fig. 3 Treatment process of laser acupuncture

7 Contraindications

Absolute contraindications: Irritation to the eyes, photosensitivity, tumor patients, fontanel insufficiency in children, epiphyseal plate, hyperthyroidism, high fever, decompensated cardiac insufficiency.

Relative contraindications: Patients with cardiac pacemaker (chest), epilepsy (head), pregnancy (stomach and back area), endocrine organs (thymus, testis, etc.), birthmark, acute posttraumatic hematoma, or acute skin streptococcal infection.

8   Side Effects

When low-level lasers are carried out correctly, the incidence of side effects is very small (approximately 2.5%) and rarely lasts longer. Usually, manifested as local redness of the skin, dizziness and fatigue, abnormal sensation and local pain, the reason is usually too long treatment time, too much stimulation, most of which can be relieved in a short time.

9   Precautions

(1) The skin was kept clean and free of oil before treatment, and treatment of the injured skin, wound or mucous membrane was avoided. Skin creams, lotions and serums should only be used after treatment.
(2) Do not look at the exit of the laser beam; even if the eyes are closed, do not shine the laser beam into anyone's eyes. It should be ensured that there are no mirrors or reflective surfaces (reflections of the laser) within a safe distance from the 3B laser needle. Laser goggles with corresponding wavelengths should be worn during treatment (by the patient and treatment operator). Laser goggles shall comply with the provisions of EU-standard EN207.
(3) Electric and magnetic fields affect the function of the laser system. Therefore, laser needles should not be used near devices that generate electromagnetic fields, such as electrotherapy unit devices or mobile phones.
(4) Adverse events such as photosensitization, local skin redness, swelling, pain and itching should be observed during treatment, or dizziness, nausea, palpitation, chest tightness and other similar reactions can be stopped at any time by pressing the laser button to stop treatment and related treatment.
(5) The principle of progressively increasing doses applies to all treatments. The duration of the initial treatment should not exceed 2 min.

10   Clinical Application

This section mainly introduces some laser acupuncture treatment schemes for some common clinical diseases [4]. For clinical treatment reference, they can be combined with other acupuncture therapies.

10.1 Cervical Spondylosis

(1) He–Ne or semiconductor laser acupoint irradiation: laser wavelength 632.8–650 nm, output power 5–20 mW, 5 min per acupoint, once a day, 10 times as a course of treatment. The Hua tuo Jia ji acupoint (EX-B2) at the neck of the acupoint is often selected, or He gu (LI4), Wai guan (SJ5) and other acupoints or the site of hyperosteogeny in the cervical intervertebral foramen can be added.
(2) CO_2 laser beam expansion local irradiation treatment: the output power was 15–20 W, irradiating the pain or acupoints, once a day, 10 min every time as a course of treatment.

10.2 Lumbar Disc Herniation

Semiconductor laser irradiation treatment: A semiconductor laser of 810 nm combined with CT and MRI and clinical signs was used to find the corresponding intervertebral space and then irradiated close to the left or right nerve root, such as Huan Tiao acupoint (GB30) irradiation, and the effect was better. The laser output power is 350–450 mW, which is the best when the patient has slight tingling or heat sensation. Eight minutes was irradiated at each point, and 2–3 sites were selected each time.

10.3 Scapulohumeral Periarthritis

(1) He–Ne or semiconductor laser acupoint irradiation: mainly at the pain point (A shi acupoint), irradiating 5 min per spot, 2–3 area, 10–15 min each time, once a day, 15 times as a course of treatment. The laser wavelength was 632.8–650 nm, and the output power was 25 mW.
(2) CO_2 laser beam expansion local treatment: The tenderness point around the shoulder joint was irradiated, and the power density was 300–500 mW/cm^2. Laser treatment of scapulohumeral periarthritis has an obvious analgesic effect.
(3) Semiconductor laser irradiation therapy: The semiconductor laser wavelength was 810 nm, the output power was 250–350 mW for acupoint irradiation, and each acupoint irradiation was 3–5 min, once a day, 10 times as a course of treatment. Commonly used acupoints are Jian zhen (SI9), Tian zong (SI11), Jian yu (LI15), Bi nao (LI14), and Tiao kou (ST38), and 2–7 acupoints can be selected for irradiation each time.

10.4 Chronic Gastritis

(1) He–Ne laser acupoint irradiation: The acupoints of Zhong wan (RN12), Nei guan (PC6) and Zu sanli (ST36) were often selected, the output power was 10–20 mW, the spot diameter was 1 mm, and each acupoint was irradiated for 5 min, 2–3 acupoints once a day, 10 times as a course of treatment.
(2) Local sensitive tenderness points were treated by He–Ne or semiconductor laser irradiation: these tenderness points were distributed 1.5 inches beside the 6th, 7th, 8th and 9th thoracic vertebrae, and there were generally 1–4 tenderness points. The irradiation method was the same as above.

10.5 Migraine

He–Ne or semiconductor laser acupoint irradiation: output wavelength 632.8–650 nm, output power 5–30 mW, 3–20 min per acupoint, once a day, 6–10 times as a course of treatment. Tai yang (EX-HN5), Yin tang (DU29), Cuan zhu (BL2), Bai hui (DU20), Feng chi (GB20), Wai guan (SJ5) and Shuai gu (GB8) were often selected.

10.6 Ischemic Heart Disease

(1) He–Ne laser or semiconductor laser local and acupoint irradiation therapy: laser wavelength 632.8–650 nm, output power 20–30 mW, diffused beam, light diameter 5 cm, irradiation on precordial area, 10–15 min 10–20 times each time as a course of treatment. At the same time, the curative effect is better if the acupoints Nei Guan (PC6), Xin Shu (BL15), Shen Men (HT7) and Dan Zhong (RN17) are selected, and each acupoint is irradiated for 5 min.
(2) CO_2 laser focused irradiation: laser irradiation in the precardiac area, power 15–20 mW, with temperature sensation as the degree, once a day, 15 min each time, 10 times for a course of treatment.

10.7 Dysmenorrhea

(1) He–Ne or semiconductor laser auricular point irradiation treatment: laser wavelength 632.8–650 nm, output power 2.5 mW, each acupoint irradiation 5 min, once a day, acupoints: Zi gong (TF2), Jiao gan (AH6a), Pi zhixia (AT4), Shen men (TF4).
(2) Laser acupoint irradiation therapy: The laser treatment method was the same as above, selecting acupoints San yinjiao (SP6), Guan yuan (RN4), Zhong shu

(DU7), Zu sanli (ST36), Xue hai (SP10), Yang lingquan (GB34), etc., generally using the left side, and treatment 2–3 times was effective.

10.8 Chronic Cholecystitis

He–Ne or semiconductor laser acupoint irradiation: Yang lingquan (GB34), Qi men (LR14), Ri yue (GB24), Zhong wan (RN12), Dan nang (EX-LE6), Zu sanli (ST36), Gan shu (BL18), Dan shu (BL19), Nei guan (PC6), tenderness point irradiation and local irradiation of gallbladder area. Laser wavelength 632.8–650 nm, power 20–25 mW, 5–10 min per acupoint. Two to three acupoints were selected as a group, once a day, 7 days as a course of treatment.

10.9 Occipital Neuralgia

Semiconductor laser (810–830 nm) local and acupoint irradiation: the tenderness point of the great occipital nerve was on the Feng Chi (GB20) acupoint, the output power was 200–250 mW, and local irradiation was 3–5 min, once a day, 10 times as a course of treatment.

11 Research on Laser Acupuncture

11.1 Clinical Research

Laser acupuncture has a wide range of clinical applications, such as orthopedics, neurology, psychosomatic disorders, otorhinolaryngology, internal medicine, dermatology, pediatrics, gynecology, dentistry, ophthalmology and more than 200 kinds of diseases. The following is a brief introduction to the research progress of laser treatment of type 2 diabetes.

Zhang [5], through low-intensity laser irradiation on Cun Kou (radial artery) and Nei Guan (PC6) in patients with type 2 diabetes mellitus, found that laser acupuncture had obvious advantages in reducing blood sugar compared with conventional intervention treatment, with a total effective rate of 91.67%. Liu [6] used a 10 mW semiconductor laser to irradiate He gu (LI4), Qu chi (LI11), Zu sanli (ST36) and other acupoints in patients with type 2 diabetes. The results showed that the blood glucose and physical fitness indexes of the patients were improved to some extent, which was significantly different from that of the Western medicine alone group. This conclusion was also confirmed by a clinical trial by Xiong [7]. Dong [8] was treated with laser acupuncture combined with traditional Chinese medicine. The results showed that not only did the blood sugar and urine sugar of the patients return to normal levels, but the corresponding clinical symptoms were also significantly alleviated, and there was no obvious aggravation during the late follow-up. Qian [9] conducted a cross-control trial to study the clinical effect of compound laser acupuncture on type 2 diabetes. The results show that this method can not only reduce the fasting blood glucose of the patients but also improve the mental state and physical quality of the patients and help to prevent the occurrence of complications.

In addition, laser acupuncture has also made some progress in the study of related complications of type 2 diabetes. Meyer-Hamme [10] designed a prospective, partially double-blind, placebo-controlled randomized trial to explore the possible effect of laser acupuncture on diabetic peripheral neuropathy with the amplitude of sural sensory nerve action potential as the main outcome index. The results suggest that laser acupuncture has significant advantages in improving nerve conduction and repairing nerve injury. Zhang [11] compared Western medicine with Western medicine plus laser acupuncture to explore the clinical effect of both on diabetic peripheral neuropathy. Laser acupuncture selected the corresponding main acupoints and reinforcing and reducing modes according to TCM syndrome differentiation. After the course of treatment, the results showed that laser acupuncture combined with Western medicine not only significantly improved nerve conduction function and symptom scores but also significantly improved blood sugar levels. Lu [12] used laser acupuncture to treat early diabetic retinopathy. Tai yang (EX-HN5), Yang bai (GB14), Yu yao (EX-HN4) and Cuan zhu (BL2) acupoints were selected and irradiated by a 10 mW semiconductor laser once a day, 5 times as a course of treatment. The results showed that the blood glucose, visual acuity and the range of visual field defects in the laser acupuncture group were improved compared with those before treatment, and the curative effect was significantly better than that in the control group. Liu [13] collected 58 patients with gastric dysfunction of type 2 diabetes, irradiated Nei guan (PC6), Zhong wan (RN12), Zu sanli (ST36) and other main acupoints with a semiconductor laser therapeutic apparatus and selected the other acupoints according to the corresponding TCM syndrome differentiation. The treatment results showed that 38 cases were markedly effective, and the total effective rate was 96.55%.

11.2 Mechanism Research

The mechanism of laser acupuncture in the treatment of type 2 diabetes may be related to the following factors: because human acupoints are rich in nerve endings and receptors, they are highly sensitive and easily excited by external stimuli [14]. Under the irradiation of a low-intensity laser, it will produce a series of biological effects similar to electromagnetic waves, acupuncture, moxibustion and so on. Under the action of physical factors such as heat energy, light energy and electromagnetic energy, it is easy to stimulate acupoint activity. The therapeutic effect of acupoints is initiated by sensory transmission along meridians to regulate the qi and blood of

Zang-fu organs and improve endocrine metabolism. In addition, through the stimulation of acupoints, laser acupuncture can significantly improve the biological activity of enzymes related to glucose metabolism and the mitochondrial respiratory chain, improve mitochondrial function, restore the balance of islet cell membrane potential, and enhance islet cell sensitivity. promote the utilization of glucose [15]. Some studies have also shown that laser acupuncture can contribute to the normal output of the insulin PI3-K/Akt2 signaling pathway and activate the activities of glucose transporters and glycogen synthase, thus improving insulin resistance [16].

The mechanism of inflammation runs through the occurrence and development of diabetes. Some scholars have found that low-level laser irradiation can reduce the release of inflammatory biomarkers such as IL6, TNF-α and adiponectin, control the inflammatory state, reduce insulin resistance, and promote an increase in fibroblast growth factor-21 (FGF-21) concentration [17]. Because FGF-21 affects the glucose and lipid metabolism of hepatocytes and adipocytes, it may be helpful to treat hyperglycemia and hyperlipidemia [18]. Some scholars have confirmed through animal experiments that laser acupuncture can effectively inhibit islet β-cell apoptosis and enhance islet function in diabetic rats, thus reducing blood sugar [19].

12 Summary

An increasing number of patients like to use laser acupuncture to alleviate their pain, but different diseases need treatment via different acupoints and laser frequencies, as well as different treatment cycles and research on the mechanism of laser acupuncture is not very established. Further exploration is needed. In addition, the therapeutic dose, irradiation time, 'tonifying' and 'diarrhea' of laser irradiation, acupoint selection of laser irradiation, depth adjustment acupuncture mode and so on need to be further standardized and scientific to realize the individual demand in treatment.

Laser acupuncture requires lasers and related accessories, such as laser trocars, the price is higher, the operation is not as convenient as acupuncture, and the acupoints are easy to move, so it is often not accepted by acupuncturists. In particular, for some deeper acupoints, such as the Huan Tiao (GB30) acupoint, the depth of laser transmission cannot be reached, so it can only be used as a supplementary treatment and cannot replace traditional acupuncture therapy.

Comprehension/Review Questions

1. What is the main principle of laser acupuncture treatment?
2. What are the therapeutic advantages of laser acupuncture compared with traditional acupuncture?

References

1. Zhu P, Feng YH. Manual of clinical application of low intensity laser. Beijing: People's Military Medical Press; 2011. p. 22–32.
2. Yan HJ, Wang ZG. Laser acupoint irradiation dose and mechanism of a preliminary study. J Laser Biol. 2006;15(5):550–51+444.
3. Salih N, Bäumler PI, Simang M, et al. Deqi sensations without cutaneous sensory input: results of an RCT. BMC Complement Altern Med. 2010;54(2):27–8.
4. Zhu P, Ma N. Practical handbook of laser acupuncture. Beijing: China Science and Technology Press; 2019.
5. Zhang KK. Effect of weak laser irradiation on Cunkou and Nei guan(PC6) points on glycosylated hemoglobin in type 2 diabetes mellitus. Henan Tradit Chin Med. 2010;30(1):47–8.
6. Liu HH, Xiong GX, Zhang LP. Effects of laser acupoint irradiation on blood glucose and glycosylated hemoglobin in type 2 diabetes mellitus. Laser Phys. 2016;26(6):065604.
7. Xiong GF, Jia JY. Effect of laser acupoint irradiation on blood glucose and glycosylated hemoglobin in patients with type 2 diabetes mellitus. Clin J Tradit Chin Med. 2015;27(11):1577–9.
8. Dong G, He AM, Tian LQ, et al. Discussion on different treatment of the same disease in the treatment of diabetes mellitus with traditional Chinese medicine combined with internal moxibustion laser acupuncture needle. Hebei Tradit Chin Med. 2013;35(5):701–2.
9. Qian ZY. Effect of compound laser acupoint irradiation on blood glucose in patients with type 2 diabetes mellitus. Shanghai University of Traditional Chinese Medicine; 2016.
10. Meyer-Hamme G, Friedemann T, Greten HJ, et al. ACUDIN—acupuncture and laser acupuncture for treatment of diabetic peripheral neuropathy: a randomized, placebo-controlled, partially double-blinded trial. BMC Neurol. 2018;18(1):40.
11. Zhang L, Chen GZ, Xu YX. Clinical study of photon traditional Chinese medicine information therapy in the treatment of diabetic peripheral neuropathy. J Laser Biol. 2017;26(3):232–6.
12. Lu XJ, Jiao SX, Liang KS, et al. Observation on the efficacy of compound Danshen dropping pills combined with laser acupoint irradiation on early diabetic retinopathy. J Binzhou Med College. 2017;40(6):464–6.
13. Liu FY, Song WX. 58 cases of diabetic gastric dysfunction treated with semiconductor laser. Laser Mag. 2004;25(4):6.
14. Li XZ, Liang FR. Progress and present situation of research on tissue morphology specificity of human acupoints. Tissue Eng Res Clin Rehabilit China. 2008;12(33):6535–8.
15. Zhu P, Feng YH. Clinical application manual of low intensity laser. Beijing: People's Military Medical Publishing House; 2011. pp. 117–119.
16. Gong LL, Jiang XX, Huang L, et al. Low power laser irradiation activates P13-K/Akt2/GLUT4 signal to promote glucose absorption and glycogen synthesis to alleviate insulin resistance in skeletal muscle. In: Proceedings of the 2013 symposium of guangdong biophysics society; 2013. p. 1.
17. Da Silveira Campos RM, Dâmaso AR, Masquio DCL, et al. The effects of exercise training associated with low-level laser therapy on biomarkers of adipose tissue transdifferentiation in obese women. Lasers Med Sci. 2018;33(6):1245–54.
18. El-Kadre LJ, Tinoco ACA. Interleukin-6 and obesity: the crosstalk between intestine, pancreas and liver. Curr Opin Clin Nutr Metab Care. 2013;16(5):564–8.
19. Xiong GX, Xiong LL, Li XZ. Effects of low intensity laser acupoint irradiation on inhibiting islet beta-cell apoptosis in rats with type 2 diabetes. Laser Phys. 2016;26(9):095605.

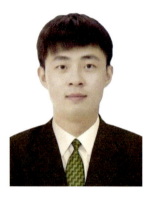

Dr. Rongxian Zhang (张荣贤) a Chinese medicine doctor in the acupuncture and moxibustion Department of the Second Hospital of Traditional Chinese Medicine in Jiangsu Province, has a master's degree, is a member of the acupuncture and moxibustion Massage Health Care Branch of the Jiangsu Health Preservation Society of Traditional Chinese Medicine, a member of the acupuncture and moxibustion Society in Nanjing. He graduated from acupuncture and moxibustion Massage in Nanjing University of Traditional Chinese Medicine in 2020, and has published several papers in core journals, Participated in a number of research projects and the compilation of monographs such as Zhaojun Gu's acupuncture and moxibustion Clinical Medical Records, participated in the drafting of a group standard of the Chinese Society of Traditional Chinese Medicine, was good at using various characteristic acupuncture and moxibustion techniques to treat nervous and motor system diseases.

Summary

Summary and Combination

Weixiang Wang and Tianjun Wang

Learning Objectives

1. Understand the historical evolution of acupuncture from ancient China to its adoption in Western healthcare.
2. Explore the foundational principles of classical needling techniques and their enduring significance.
3. Familiarize with diverse acupuncture techniques and their clinical combination with other needling techniques.
4. Recognize the potential benefits and applications of integrating various acupuncture techniques in Western healthcare.

Acupuncture, once a traditional healing practice confined to China and other Asian countries, has now become an integral part of healthcare in the Western world. In the last two decades, there has been a growing interest as more individuals seek natural and holistic ways of living and healing. Nowadays, acupuncture is widely accepted, with cities and countries recognizing its therapeutic advantages. However, in the midst of this widespread adoption, a group of Chinese Medicine and Acupuncture practitioners, joined by some colleagues from the West, have identified gaps in the understanding and application of acupuncture techniques in Western practices. This realization has prompted the creation of this comprehensive guide.

The roots of acupuncture run deep in the ancient traditions of China, where it originated over 2500 years ago. Rooted in the belief that the body possesses a vital energy known as Qi, acupuncture involves the precise insertion of thin needles into

---

W. Wang (✉)
Dutch Acupuncture Academy, Amsterdam, The Netherlands
e-mail: tcmdao@gmail.com

T. Wang
London Academy of Chinese Acupuncture, 70 Springfield Dive, London IG2 6QD, UK
e-mail: info@tjacupuncture.co.uk

specific points along meridians to harmonize the flow of Qi, aiming to restore health by balancing the Yin Yang and harmonizing the body and mind. The journey of acupuncture from its ancient roots in China to its widespread adoption in Western countries has been marked by a fascinating evolution.

In ancient China, acupuncture was deeply integrated into the culture and medical practice. Passed down through generations, the practice was traditionally learned through an apprenticeship model, fostering a profound connection between practitioners and their craft. This model emphasized a holistic approach to healthcare, considering the interconnectedness of the body, mind, and spirit.

The spread of acupuncture to Western countries gained momentum in the early 1970s. American journalist James Reston played a pivotal role in raising awareness about acupuncture's potential benefits. After undergoing an appendectomy in China, Reston shared his positive experience with acupuncture as part of postsurgical pain management. This sparked curiosity and interest in the West, leading to increased exploration and adoption of acupuncture practices [1].

As acupuncture found its way into Western countries, its techniques evolved. While retaining its traditional roots, acupuncture practitioners in the West began integrating other additional traditional therapies such as cupping, moxibustion, and ear acupuncture. This blend of traditional and modern approaches has contributed to the diverse landscape of acupuncture practice we see today.

In China, for the past 70 years, acupuncture has been a part of the official medical system. Almost every hospital in China has a department dedicated to acupuncture, thanks to the acupuncture education provided at the university level. The education covers bachelor's, master's, and Ph.D. levels and combines traditional Chinese medicine with modern medicine. In China, acupuncturists working in hospitals are also medical doctors, providing them with a broader vision, deeper knowledge, and more experience when practicing acupuncture.

In contrast, in Western countries, acupuncture is not commonly considered a part of medical practice. Practitioners receive brief education in modern medicine, focusing on basic subjects like anatomy, physiology, and pathology. Acupuncture education in the West mainly concentrates on filiform needles, without incorporating a full range of diverse acupuncture techniques. This limited focus may restrict their approach to treatment and their understanding of diagnosis and therapy.

The difference in educational approaches has significant implications. In China, the integration of acupuncture into the medical system, along with comprehensive education, enables practitioners to view patients holistically. Acupuncturists in China consider a broad range of techniques and applications in their clinical practice, drawing from both traditional and modern medical perspectives. On the other hand, the Western model often separates acupuncture from mainstream medical practice. This may limit practitioners in terms of diagnostic capabilities and the range of therapeutic interventions they can offer, and it may not capture the full potential of acupuncture's therapeutic modalities.

The comprehensive manual presented here aims to bridge the gap in understanding and application of acupuncture techniques in the West. By providing a more inclusive acupuncture techniques and perspective similar to the approach seen in China, this guide aspires to enhance the practice of acupuncture in Western healthcare settings. Through shared knowledge and collaborative efforts, the goal is to contribute to a more holistic and effective application of acupuncture techniques, benefiting acupuncturists and patients in the West.

The significance of introducing diverse acupuncture techniques to the West extends beyond merely enriching the diversity of acupuncture practices. It addresses a broader goal—that of bridging the gap between Eastern and Western acupuncture traditions. By embracing a variety of needling techniques, Western practitioners not only expand the scope of acupuncture practice but also offer patients a more extensive spectrum of treatment options. In addition to the fundamental and traditional acupuncture needling techniques, as well as complementary therapies like moxibustion and cupping which can be combined with any other needling techniques, this comprehensive guide delves into an array of advanced acupuncture techniques. These include Burn-Penetrating needling, Dao-qi technique, Ear acupuncture, scalp acupuncture, wrist-ankle acupuncture, cheek acupuncture, fire needling, Yuan Li needling, Plum blossom needling, three-edged needling, electric acupuncture, and laser acupuncture.

One of the key advantages of introducing this diverse range of acupuncture techniques to the Western acupuncture landscape is the enhancement of treatment options for patients. Traditional acupuncture, which is often called Body Acupuncture, Ti Zhen, with its focus on filiform needle insertion, is combined by more specialized approaches.

Classical needling techniques from ancient Chinese texts such as Huang Di Nei Jin, Nan Jing, and Jin Zhen Fu form the foundational basis of acupuncture practices. These techniques have withstood the test of time and have been integral to the development of acupuncture over centuries. While there have been numerous evolutions in needling approaches across different dynasties in China, the core principles have remained remarkably consistent.

Over the past five decades, acupuncture has gained widespread acceptance and usage globally. During this period, various needling techniques have emerged, reflecting the dynamic evolution of this ancient practice. Notable among these techniques are Dao-qi manipulations, simple Burn-Penetrate needling, sinew needling, and many others. However, even with the introduction of these innovative methods, practitioners often find themselves tracing back to the classical needling techniques. This phenomenon is succinctly expressed in a Chinese saying: "万变不离其宗"—translated as "thousands of changes, but you cannot escape from the root."

The development of classical needling techniques has not only broadened the treatment range of acupuncture but has also enhanced its overall effectiveness. By adhering to the fundamental principles outlined in ancient texts, practitioners can achieve optimal outcomes in their treatments. The emphasis on balancing Yin and Yang, harmonizing the body's energy flow, and addressing imbalances within the meridian system remains central to classical acupuncture, contributing to its enduring success.

The "**Burning-Penetrate Needling**" technique, which serves as a simplified version of the "burning mountain fire to cool the sky" needle technique. This technique has the functions of warming, supplementing, cooling, and purging, and it aims to balance Yin and Yang. It is a versatile method applicable in the treatment of various conditions such as pain syndromes, rheumatic disorders, and a range of diseases affecting women and children. In acupuncture practice, it can be used independently based on the specific condition of the illness or combined with other acupuncture treatments as a routine method for tonification and reduction [2].

Scalp acupuncture (SA) is a highly advantageous technique for the treatment of neurological and psychological disorders, as a primary acupuncture modality in clinical practice for these conditions. It is especially effective on the nervous system and psychological health. Scalp acupuncture is often integrated into comprehensive treatment plans, combining with the filiform acupuncture and other specialized techniques like auricular acupuncture, and electro-acupuncture.

In clinical scenarios involving paediatric patients, scalp acupuncture frequently takes precedence as a standalone treatment, due to the fact that children tend to be scared of needles when they see the needles. Scalp acupuncture insert the needles without being visible to the child, providing a discreet and less intimidating experience. It is crucial that the paediatric patients have a more positive and cooperative attitude which contributing to the overall success of the treatment [3].

Auricular acupuncture is a microneedling system for diagnosis and treatment that normalises the body's function by stimulating certain points of the ear. It plays a much bigger role in western acupuncture practice than in China. Some western acupuncturists only practice auricular acupuncture while in China, auricular acupuncture is mostly used as a complementary for body acupuncture. It is rather common for auricular acupuncture to be combined with cupping, moxibustion, scalp acupuncture, electric acupuncture etc.

The wrist-ankle needling boasts several advantages, including simplicity, convenience, painlessness, wide applicability, and rapid efficacy. It can be used independently in clinical practice or combined with other needling techniques for a synergistic effect. Particularly in the treatment of painful conditions or diseases associated with pain, it demonstrates a prompt and significant impact.

Cheek needling can be independently applied in clinical practice and is typically not combined with other needling techniques. However, it is not precluded that, with proficient mastery, cheek needling can be concurrently utilized with other needling methods. For acupuncture professionals, it can be coordinated with traditional acupuncture techniques. Those who have acquired proficiency in additional needling methods may incorporate cheek needling to enhance therapeutic efficacy, alongside techniques such as scalp acupuncture. If the therapeutic outcome is satisfactory through cheek needling alone, concurrent use with other methods is unnecessary [4].

Fire needling is an ancient yet innovative acupuncture method where the needle is first heated until it becomes red-hot, and then rapidly inserted into acupuncture points to treat various diseases. This technique introduces a powerful combination of heat and kinetic energy into the patient's body instantly, playing a leading role in promoting meridian circulation and facilitating the movement of Qi and blood. From this, more than ten subsidiary effects have been derived. Fire needling is suitable for both cold and heat-related conditions, as well as deficiency and excess patterns. It can be applied as a standalone technique or in conjunction with other needling methods, especially when combined with warm needling.

The Yuan Li Needling is the sixth needle among the ancient Nine Needles. Its therapeutic methods are divided into ancient Yuan Li Needling and modern Yuan Li Needling based on its historical evolution. In ancient times, Yuan Li needles had a large needle tip, making it difficult to penetrate during insertion, and it was challenging to operate, causing discomfort for patients. Modern Yuan Li Needling has a needle shape that has been changed to a fine needle shape, similar to a filiform needle but slightly thicker. It is a new type of acupuncture tool with a needle body slightly thicker than that of a filiform needle. This modification eliminates the pain during needle insertion experienced with the ancient Yuan Li Needling while retaining the large characteristics and therapeutic principles of the ancient Yuan Li Needling. As a result, it is more easily accepted by clinical patients. When the method and techniques of needle insertion are mastered, it can achieve a nearly painless experience similar to filiform needles. Yuan Li Needling is mainly used in clinical pain conditions such as neck, shoulder, lower back, and leg pain, which are common in orthopaedics. It is also widely applied to sinew-related visceral diseases and is often used in conjunction with filiform needles.

The plum blossom needle belongs to the category of superficial needling techniques within traditional acupuncture therapy. It is proficient in promoting local blood circulation, facilitating the flow of meridians qi, and alleviating obstruction. Operating through the cutaneous meridian—minor meridians—connecting vessels—meridian system, this technique regulates the Yin and Yang, as well as the Qi and blood of internal organs, thereby serving a preventive and therapeutic role. In clinical practice, it is commonly combined with body acupuncture, especially in cases of facial paralysis, hemiplegia resulting from stroke, where it is often complemented with electroacupuncture. Additionally, for certain chronic and persistent skin conditions, it is frequently used in conjunction with cupping therapy.

The three-edged needling plays a crucial role as an integral component of acupuncture, contributing significantly to the advancement of acupuncture in clinical settings. This technique involves puncturing specific points on the body's surface to release a small amount of blood or extrude fluids, or even to puncture subcutaneous tissues, serving as a method for treating various diseases. The therapeutic application of three-edged needling primarily targets conditions associated with heat toxicity and blood-heat. Possessing the effect of clearing heat and expelling toxins, three-edged needling aids in the elimination of pathogenic factors through blood release. By regulating the circulation of qi and blood, this technique facilitates the restoration of normal physiological functions. In clinical practice, three-edged needling can be applied independently or in conjunction with body acupuncture, cupping, and other needling techniques, thereby expanding the scope of treatment and enhancing therapeutic outcomes.

Electric acupuncture is a therapeutic technique that builds upon the foundation of filiform acupuncture, utilizing a microcurrent output from an electric acupuncture device that closely mimics the body's bioelectricity. This method involves applying filiform needles to specific areas of the body, integrating electrical stimulation for the prevention and treatment of various diseases. It is introduced and popularized in China in the 1950s, electric acupuncture combines filiform acupuncture with electric stimulation. This approach not only reduces the workload of needle insertion but also enhances the therapeutic effects of filiform acupuncture, broadening the scope of its application while allowing precise control over the stimulation intensity.

Electroacupuncture has multifaceted effects, including pain relief, sedation, improvement of blood circulation, and adjustment of muscle tension. Its application range is essentially similar to that of traditional filiform acupuncture. Clinically, electric acupuncture is commonly employed for treating various pain syndromes, rheumatic disorders, functional dysfunctions of organs such as the heart, stomach, intestines, gallbladder, bladder, uterus, as well as disorders like mania. It is also used for injuries to muscles, ligaments, and joints, and can even be utilized in acupuncture anaesthesia.

Laser acupuncture is a natural treatment method that combines traditional Chinese medicine principles with modern medical knowledge. It features characteristics such as painlessness, sterility, and safety. Widely applied in clinical settings, laser acupuncture can be used independently. Additionally, after the primary treatment, it can be combined with other acupuncture methods, such as body acupuncture and wrist-ankle needling, to enhance therapeutic efficacy. It's important to note that laser acupuncture cannot replace traditional needle acupuncture.

This book goes beyond being a compendium of acupuncture techniques; it serves as a guide to their practical application in clinical settings. The inclusion of detailed explanations and insights into each technique equips practitioners with the knowledge needed to integrate these methods into their practice effectively.

By expanding the toolkit available to Western practitioners, this guide facilitates a more personalized and adaptable approach to patient treatment. The integration of diverse acupuncture techniques has the potential to significantly enhance patient care in Western healthcare settings. As acupuncture becomes more standardized globally, the exchange of knowledge and techniques fosters mutual communication and cooperation in clinical treatment, research, and education. This collaborative approach contributes to the evolution of acupuncture as a science and ensures that patients worldwide benefit from a standardized and enriched acupuncture practice.

The development of the book is not an endpoint but a starting point for ongoing education. It recognizes that acupuncture originated from practice and emphasizes the need for practitioners to engage in continuous learning. This includes participation in seminars, workshops, and practical training to deepen their understanding and refine their techniques.

In the spirit of collaboration, exploration, and continuous growth, we invite practitioners, educators, and enthusiasts to join us on this journey of advancing acupuncture practice and education worldwide. May the fusion of Eastern wisdom and Western innovation in the acupuncture field create a harmonious and thriving landscape for the benefit of patients across the globe.

Review Questions

1. What are the key principles of classical needling techniques, and how have they contributed to the effectiveness of acupuncture over time?
2. How has the adoption of acupuncture in Western countries led to the evolution and integration of diverse needling techniques?
3. In what ways do advanced acupuncture techniques, such as Burning-Penetrate and Yuan Li Needling, enhance the scope of treatment options for practitioners?
4. How can the integration of diverse acupuncture techniques contribute to a more personalized and adaptable approach to patient care in Western healthcare settings?

References

1. Xia LJ. Clinical observation on essential hypertension with "Green Dragon Wagging Tail and White Tiger Shaking Head" acupuncture technique in Europe". J Changchun Univer Chin Med Changchun. 2012;04:659–61.
2. Li CQ. The improvement and clinic applications of burning mountain fire and penetrating sky cool, 2nd ed. National Medical Forum; 1994. pp. 32–3.
3. Wang TJ. Acupuncture for brain-treatment for neurological and psychological disorders. Chan, Switzerland: Springer; 2021.
4. Wang YZ. Cheeks acupuncture therapy, vol. 287. People's Health Publishing House Co. Ltd.; 2017.

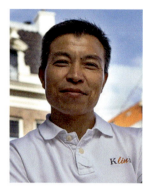

Prof. Dr. Weixiang Wang (王维祥) A Ph.D. graduate of Nanjing University of Chinese Medicine (NUCMNUJCM), has played a pivotal role in advancing TCM in the Netherlands. Formerly serving at the Second Clinical College of NUCM until 2003, he co-founded the European Academy of Traditional Medical Science and currently act as the academic dean of the Dutch Acupuncture Academy (DAA). With a rich background, Dr. Wang has led the Dutch Association of TCM (NVTCG Zhong) as chairman for six years, contributing an additional three years as a board member. Additionally, he serves as an executive member of the European Association of TCM (ETCMA). Driven by a commitment to elevate educational standards and integrate TCM into healthcare systems, his lectures on the integrative practice of TCM are highly sought-after in academic institutions and TCM congresses. An accomplished author, Dr. Wang has written and co-authored 11 TCM books in China since the commencement of his TCM career in 1989. Currently practicing at Klinic in Amsterdam, he holds the prestigious position of president for one of the most influential TCM events, the International Dutch TCM Congress (DTCMC).

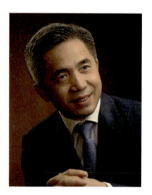

Prof. Dr. Tianjun Wang (王天俊) graduated from Nanjing University of Chinese Medicine (NUCM) in 1989. He completed his PhD of Acupuncture at NUCM. Tianjun moved to the UK and joined the University of East London UK as a Senior Lecturer and the Director of Acupuncture Clinic 2007–2014. He is a Guest Professor of NUCM.

Current Prof. Wang is the Principal of the London Academy of Chinese Acupuncture (LACA). He is also the Vice President of the Scalp Acupuncture Committee of World Federation of Chinese Medicine Societies (WFCMS) and the president of the Academy of Scalp Acupuncture UK (ASA). He owns TJ Acupuncture Clinic and Brain Care Centre in London.

Prof. Wang has authored and co-authored more than 50 academic papers as well as peer reviewers to many international journals. His authored book "Acupuncture for Brain: Treatment for Neurological and Psychologic Disorders" published by Springer 2021.